SEATTLE BABY RESOURCE GUIDE

2ND EDITION

Including Bellevue, Bothell, Kirkland, Issaquah, Renton, Auburn, Everett, Lynnwood, Edmonds, Burien and more!

Completely revised and updated

i'm expecting · the baby resource company

Publisher: Kari E. Hazen
Local Editor: Shelley Arenas
Copy Editor & Layout Production: Troy Maslow Smith
Resource Verifier: Janine Jijina
Cover and Illustrations: Karen Olson
Baby Pages Representatives: Kari Hazen and Julie Varon
Photography: Craig Larsen and Mary Anne Maberry

Disclaimer

The authors have made every reasonable effort to provide the most accurate and updated information at the time Seattle Baby Resource Guide went to print. The authors have not solicited or accepted payments or consideration of any kind from any person as an inducement to exclude or include material in this book, or to influence its content. However, the reader should bear in mind that the very nature of this book required that the authors receive their information from sources who may have had a bias or who may have been mistaken and that much of the material in this book is based entirely on the personal opinions of the authors and their sources and thus may be inaccurate. Therefore, the readers would make their independent evaluations of any product, service, or course of conduct mentioned herein prior to buying, using or engaging in the same and should not rely on this book as being authoritative in any respect. The authors strongly recommend that the reader discuss all health related issues, services and products with their medical professional and not rely on any health related "advice," suggestions, or information contained in this book. This book is simply intended to provide its readers with a starting point in their quest for information and, hopefully, a certain degree of entertainment.

Published by I'm Expecting, Auburn, CA (916) 823-3659
For information regarding custom editions or for information on reproducing the Baby Resource Guide in another city or for the Seattle Baby Pages contact Kari Hazen at (916) 823-3659. To be listed in the next Seattle Baby Resource Guide contact Shelley Arenas at 367-4305. The Seattle Baby Resource Guide and the Seattle Baby Pages are copyrighted. Other brands and names are the property of their respective owners.

Also, look for the Sacramento, Central Valley, Portland and Phoenix Baby Resource Guides for friends and family expecting!

Manufactured in the United States of America.

TABLE OF CONTENTS

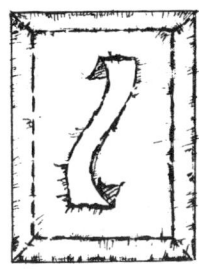

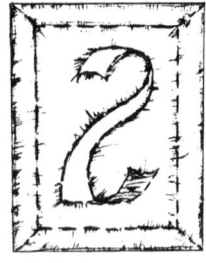

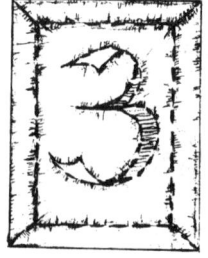

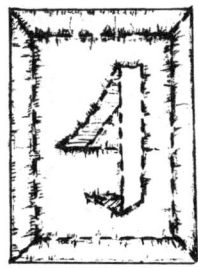

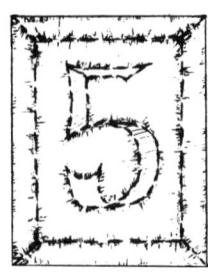

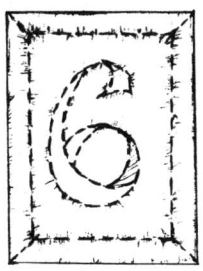

INTRODUCTION

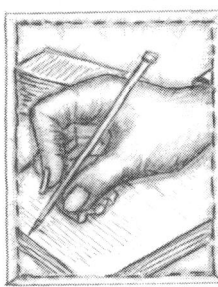

Every day is a miracle. Nothing is more true than when you think about the birth of a child.

Think about it. It all starts with two people coming together, creating two cells that offer the blueprint to a human being. These cells multiply to create a heart, a mind and a soul. Every day a fetus is in its mother's womb it gains strength to face this miracle... life.

As a parent, there are times when you will sit back and look with amazement at your child, overcome with awe that you created this special human being. It is frightening to think of the new responsibilities given to you, all with no instructions and no exam by which to validate your proficiency as a parent.

There are so many questions that come with the birth of a new baby. In today's complex society it may be difficult to find the answers you need. We may find ourselves living thousands of miles away from our families, with no support network and possibly working through pregnancy and beyond, while at the same time wanting to be an involved and educated parent.

Because of this, a company named *I'm Expecting* was born. Its mission was to compile a resource guide for area parents. It started as a simple idea, yet grew as many area parents and experts contributed their thoughts and experiences to our endeavor, all with the hope of helping you in your new parenting role. And now, through the support of the baby business community and parents, the Seattle Baby Resource Guide is in print.

The Seattle Baby Resource Guide is meant to be many things, none of which is to replace medical advice or treatment, or to take the place of Consumer Reports. Please take care of yourself and your baby. Cherish these special days. As a soon-to-be parent, you are experiencing our greatest miracle... life!

❧

In today's complex society it may be difficult to find the answers you need.

❧

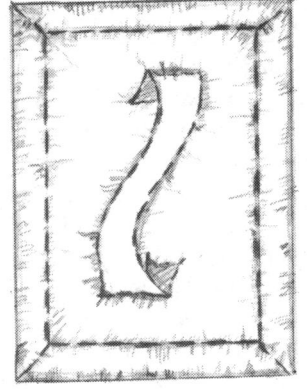

SO,
YOU'RE
HAVING
A
BABY!

CHOOSING YOUR PRACTITIONER

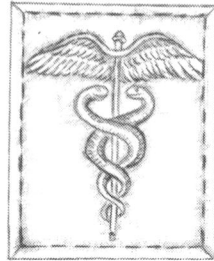

If you're thinking about becoming pregnant, or are pregnant, your very first step should be to get prenatal care; it is important for you and the unborn life that depends on you. It is also equally crucial for you to not wait for your initial prenatal visit to begin preparing your body for the birth of your child.

The first trimester is when your baby is forming every single vital organ—not to mention its fingers and toes. So, until your practitioner confirms your pregnancy, take care of the basics: eat healthy, don't drink alcohol, stay out of hot tubs, and if you smoke, try to quit as soon as possible. Also, if you are taking a prescription drug or need to take an over-the-counter drug, call your practitioner first, as many drugs may cause problems during pregnancy. Your practitioner is the expert on prenatal care; listen to his or her instructions and establish an open and honest relationship. Your practitioner's goal, as is yours, is to bring a new, healthy life into this world.

Before you meet with a practitioner, you may have questions on where to find one. Many expectant mothers may already have an obstetrician or a general practitioner that they are completely satisfied with. Others may choose to "shop around" or simply do not have a provider at all.

There are a variety of providers and referral agencies who can help you with prenatal care. A good place to start is with your insurance or DSHS program to find out if you can select a provider of your choice, or if you must use a plan's specific provider. You may also have friends or relatives that have children; ask for their recommendations. Remember the personality of the person referring you. Every individual has different needs and a communication style—keep that in mind when considering a referral.

What you will probably find is the types of practitioners will vary considerably in their philosophy, training, experience and expertise. The following information on providers' qualifications can help you make your choice.

❧

Your practitioner's goal, as is yours, is to bring a new, healthy life into this world.

❧

PERINATOLOGIST

Perinatologists are physicians who have spent two to three additional years of schooling after having completed a residency in obstetrics and gynecology. They have had four years of medical school, four years of specialty training in obstetrics and gynecology, plus the addition of the two to three years sub-specialty training. Usually you will only see a perinatologist if you have a very special problem and are referred by another practitioner.

OBSTETRICIAN

An obstetrician has completed college, four years of medical school and four years of specialty training in obstetrics and gynecology. Obstetricians are trained specifically in pregnancy and are acknowledged "experts" in their field. Obstetricians are able to identify pregnancy risks and perform surgical procedures as needed. Obstetricians who have successfully passed an oral and written examination given by the American Board of Obstetrics are known as "Board Certified." The initials FACOG verify that they have completed this training and joined the organization called the American College of Obstetrics and Gynecology.

FAMILY PHYSICIAN

A family physician has been trained to care for a broad variety of patients—from obstetrics to pediatrics to geriatrics. This allows a patient to have one physician overseeing not only her medical and obstetrical treatment, but also that of her family members. Check with your family physician to see if he or she delivers babies. Family physicians have completed four years of medical training followed by three years of specialty training in family medicine that includes obstetrics and pediatrics. Those family physicians who have successfully passed a written examination given by the American Board of Family Practice are known as "Board Certified."

NURSE PRACTITIONER

Some physicians' offices have either a nurse practitioner or physician's assistant. Depending on your physician, they may do some or the majority of your prenatal office visits. A nurse practitioner has a bachelor's degree in nursing and then attends graduate school and completes an internship before practicing. A physician's assistant attends a specialized medical program, although it may not necessarily be in obstetrics.

CERTIFIED NURSE MIDWIFE

A certified nurse midwife has a degree in nursing and then receives one to two years of further education in nurse midwifery. A certified nurse midwife generally works in several different settings. She may be in practice with a physician or she may work through a hospital or a county health department. Many midwives also practice independently. In Seattle, a certified nurse midwife offers everything from prenatal care to delivery of your baby. The hospital chart in this book indicates which hospitals have midwives on staff. In case of a medical emergency, a midwife will have a physician backup.

LICENSED MIDWIFE

In Washington, a midwife may also be licensed. A licensed midwife must go through three years of training and pass a state licensing exam. She also must attend 100 births and manage or deliver 50 births during this period. Most licensed midwives deliver babies either at home or at a birth center.

INTERVIEWING

The referral numbers in this section may help you find a qualified practitioner during your pregnancy. Once you have a number of possibilities, call these offices to see if they are accepting new patients, whether they accept your insurance carrier, and if an interview is available. While some providers are willing to provide a free, short consultation in person or by telephone, others charge for an interview and many are too busy with patients. In the latter case, the only way to know if the provider is right for you is during or after your first prenatal visit. If you do decide to "interview" a provider, here are some questions to consider asking:

- What is your educational background and experience?
- How often will I see you?
- Will I be seen by other staff members, and who are they?
- What is your policy when you are not on call (including during labor and delivery) and who covers for you during such a time?
- At which hospitals do you have admitting privileges?
- Under what conditions do you recommend that an ultrasound be performed?
- At what maternal age do you recommend an amniocentesis?
- How do you feel about VBAC (Vaginal Birth After Cesarean) birth?
- What is your policy regarding induction of labor if I go beyond my due date? What is your induction rate?
- What is your Cesarean birth rate?
- Will insurance or DSHS pay for treatments and delivery with this provider?
- Are there any legal considerations in choosing this provider?
- Are you licensed?
- What medications are routinely used during labor?

After the interview or first visit, ask yourself if you and/or your partner will feel comfortable with the qualifications and communication style of the practitioner. Also, consider how comfortable you feel with your provider's office staff. You probably will have more encounters with the office staff during your pregnancy than with the actual provider. Therefore, a friendly, open and available office staff may make a difference about how you feel about your provider.

Only your own special circumstances and criteria can determine your provider-patient relationship. Use your judgment and trust your intuition when making your decision. Finding a provider that you can work with and trust completely will make for a happier and less stressful pregnancy.

❧ RESOURCES ❧

A simple phone call puts you in contact with these free doctor referral services.

■ **AMERICAN COLLEGE OF NURSE MIDWIVES**
(202) 728-9860
818 Connecticut Ave. N.W., Ste. 900
Washington, DC 20006
The American College of Nurse Midwives offers information about nurse-midwifery services in the Seattle area and also a listing of accredited university-affiliated nurse-midwifery education programs.

■ **COMMUNITY HEALTH REFERRAL SERVICES**
800-756-5437
This is a free referral service for expectant moms that specializes in locating health care and community resources for low income, DSHS, and uninsured families. It serves King and Snohomish counties.

■ **COMMUNITY OBSTETRIC REFERRAL PROGRAM**
284-5291
This is a community based and supported non-profit agency that can refer you to an OB/GYN or pediatrician in King and Snohomish counties. They can also help you find certain health care providers who accept your specific insurance. This was one of the friendliest groups we spoke to!

■ **MIDWIVES ASSOCIATION OF WASHINGTON STATE**
860-4120
You'll most likely receive a recorded message at this number that will ask you to leave your name and number. A volunteer will call you back with information to help you find a local midwife.

■ **NORTHWEST HOSPITAL/ MED-INFO**
633-4636
Sponsored by Northwest Hospital, this informative service provides free health information and will help match you with a health care provider who delivers at Northwest. Provider names are given out on a rotating basis. The staff personnel asks for your name and address to send out a confirmation of your referral request.

■ **OVERLAKE MEDICAL CENTER**
688-5211
This is a 24-hour service for individuals looking for a physician referral from Overlake Hospital.

■ **PACIFIC ASSOCIATION FOR LABOR SUPPORT (PALS)**
325-1419
PALS provides expectant parents a list of local labor support persons (doulas). Members of the association have completed a training program offered by either the Seattle Midwifery School or by Informed Birth and Parenting. Many of the support people are childbirth educators; many have given birth; many also work in health-related fields. Support is available before, during, and after labor. Fees for this service vary with most charging on a sliding scale.

■ **PROVIDENCE MEDICAL CENTER**
554-7768
This is a 24-hour referral number for individuals looking for a Providence physician, including an OB/GYN or pediatrician.

■ **SEATTLE MIDWIFERY SCHOOL**
322-8834
2524 16th Ave. S., Ste. 300
Seattle, WA 98144
By calling this accredited midwifery school, you can receive the names and phone numbers of all licensed and certified nurse midwives in the greater Seattle area. This school also trains midwives and doulas.

■ **STEVENS HEALTH SOURCE**
640-4066
This service links you with a health care provider employed by Stevens Memorial Hospital.

■ **SWEDISH MEDLINK**
386-6066 or 800-443-2762
Registered nurses are available to answer general medical information. They can also help you find a health care provider who practices through the Swedish system.

■ **VALLEY MEDICAL CENTER**
251-5129
If you want a health care provider who delivers at Valley Medical Center, this number will connect you.

HOSPITAL CHOICES

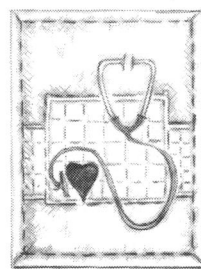

During your pregnancy you are faced with many choices. Deciding where to have your baby is probably one of your biggest decisions. Hospitals today offer expectant parents a wide array of services that make your stay comfortable and more "homelike" than ever before. Because mothers may spend such a short time in the hospital, the education and postpartum programs may be more of a consideration factor. Here are some things you may want to consider in choosing your hospital:

- Where your health care provider delivers
- Hospital location
- The nursery facilities
- The number and type of labor and delivery rooms
- The hospital and nursing staff
- The quality of care
- Whether your insurance covers care at that hospital
- The types of education programs offered
- Postpartum care provided, if any
- Your overall feelings about the hospital

❧

Remember,

you are a

consumer

here, and

you do have

a choice

about where

your baby is

born.

❧

Before making your choice, try to obtain as much objective information as possible. Tour the local hospitals; ask friends, relatives, and coworkers for referrals; and ask questions to ensure the hospital meets your needs. Remember, you are a consumer here and you do have a choice in where your baby is born.

When talking to others about their birth experiences, you'll find patients who have received exceptional care at one hospital and others who were not completely satisfied at the same facility. The nurses and hospital staff make the personal difference and depending who cares for you, experiences may vary.

To assist you in making your choice, this section provides data and a hospital chart to compare the different facilities. Information was obtained from responses to a mail survey of all area hospitals. The number of babies born may not indicate the quality of care provided in any hospital.

ANNUAL BIRTHS

In the greater Seattle area, the number of babies delivered in hospitals was fairly comparable. As indicated in the hospital chart, most hospitals delivered between 1,000 and 2,000 babies per year during the time period surveyed (August 1994-July

1995). Swedish Medical Center's staff delivered 3,885 babies at their Seattle and Ballard hospitals—the most babies of all the area hospitals. An annual total of 28,974 babies were born at the hospitals we surveyed in King and south Snohomish counties.

CESAREAN DELIVERY RATES

Cesarean deliveries take place on average just less than one out of five births (or approximately 20 percent of the time) at the hospitals we surveyed. The Cesarean delivery rate may vary from hospital to hospital for many reasons, including the number of high-risk maternity patients and the patients' individual or medical needs. Expectant parents may want to discuss the possibility of a Cesarean delivery with their health care provider and find out under what circumstances the procedure would be done. Know that Cesarean delivery rates at hospitals are a sensitive issue. Also, realize the hospital does not perform the Cesarean, the physician does. So, open communication with your provider will make you more aware of how a Cesarean delivery may affect you. The statistic listed is a combination of the primary and secondary Cesarean delivery percentage rate. A primary Cesarean delivery statistic is the number of first-time Cesarean deliveries and the secondary statistic gives you the number of repeat Cesarean deliveries. If you have specific questions regarding Cesarean delivery rates, ask a hospital representative for a breakdown of this statistic.

NURSERY LEVELS

All hospitals surveyed offer at least a Level I nursery, also called a primary care nursery. The majority of babies only need Level I care. If your baby was delivered at a Level I nursery and had complications that needed more specialty treatment, chances are the infant would be transferred to a Level II or Level III hospital.

A Level II nursery means it is equipped for handling most newborn emergencies. Most of the hospitals in Seattle offer a Level II nursery. If your baby had a medical condition that was serious, but not necessarily life-threatening, then a Level II nursery could care for the child. Most local Level II nurseries do care for premature infants who are at least 30-32 weeks gestation.

The most sophisticated type of nurseries are Level III. They are equipped with the high-technology equipment and specialists who are capable of handling the most serious types of newborn emergencies. Local hospitals with Level III nurseries include Swedish Medical Center (Seattle), University of Washington Medical Center, and Children's Medical Center. Each Level III nursery is equipped to care for premature infants.

FETAL MONITORING

All hospitals surveyed require patients to receive an initial fetal monitoring reading in accordance with the American College of Obstetrics and Gynecology (ACOG) guidelines. ACOG advises women to be monitored for an initial 20 minutes upon admission to the hospital. How long you will be monitored depends on your medical condition and the hospital or your doctor's policy.

MIDWIVES

Nearly half of the hospitals we surveyed have midwives on staff, available for prenatal/postnatal care and for labor and delivery assistance. Midwives carefully monitor your progress and have the support and facilities of the hospital and physicians and staff as a necessary backup, should complications arise.

ROOMS

A variety of rooms, from a traditional shared hospital cubicle to a specially furnished private "homestyle" suite, are what you'll find at local hospitals. The latter style of room has become the most common in area hospitals. Called Labor/Delivery/Recovery/Postpartum (LDRP) rooms, this concept was first introduced in 1984 by Northwest Hospital with their "Birth Suites." The single-room suite offers the comfort and convenience of not being moved from room to room, as well as allowing more privacy and involvement by partners and other family members. Several area hospitals' birthing centers—including Evergreen, Northwest, Providence (Pacific campus), Stevens, and Swedish (Ballard)—provide all of their rooms in this style. Others are planning on adding LDRPs as part of remodeling plans at their birthing centers in 1996 and 1997, including Swedish (Seattle), which will have 17 LDRPs with individual whirlpool baths in late 1996.

Besides LDRPs, the next most common rooms are Labor/Delivery/Recovery (LDR) rooms. These rooms offer patients the advantage of remaining in one room during labor, delivery, and recovery. Following delivery and recovery, mothers are then moved to a "postpartum" room. Most LDR and LDRP rooms offer the comforts of home with the sophistication of advanced medical technology. These rooms are equipped with all the necessary medical equipment, often stored out of sight in custom cabinetry until needed. They also may offer such amenities as custom decor, whirlpool baths, televisions, VCRs and a hide-a-bed for your partner or guest.

Hospitals usually offer many of these same amenities in their regular postpartum rooms as well, recognizing the need to treat the birthing experience as a life event, rather than simply a medical procedure.

ROOMING-IN

All hospitals we surveyed accommodate patients who want to keep their babies in their room day and night. At several hospitals, the policy is for all well newborns to stay in the same room as their mother for their entire stay.

ANESTHESIOLOGISTS

All hospitals have anesthesiologists on-call (or in-house) on a 24-hour basis.

OVERNIGHT GUESTS

All the hospitals allow your support person to stay with you during labor, delivery, and recovery. Support persons are also allowed to stay overnight in postpartum rooms, except when you're sharing the room with another patient. But even hospitals that don't guarantee private rooms usually assign you to one unless all the rooms are full. Most hospitals offer a sleeping chair or daybed for your support person's convenience; this is generally a standard feature of LDRPs.

	HOSPITAL COMPARISONS	Annual Births	Nursery Level	% C-Sections
1	Auburn General Hospital	723	I	23
2	Evergreen Hospital Medical Center	2647	II	17.9
3	Group Health Hospital Central	1366	II	11
4	Group Health Hospital Eastside	1200	I	15
5	Highline Community Hospital	893	I	21
6	Northwest Hospital	1740	II	20.4
7	Overlake Hospital Medical Center	2727	II	21.2
8	Providence General Medical Center - Colby	2396	II	17
9	Providence General Medical Center - Pacific	703	I	18
10	Providence Medical Center	1920	II	18
11	St. Francis Community Hospital	1721	I	18
12	Stevens Memorial Hospital	1483	II	18.7

Midwifery Services	Beds in OB Unit	LDRs	LDRPs	Postpartum Program
Yes	9	4	0	Yes
No	36	0	36	Yes
Yes	22	0	12	Yes
Yes	20	5	15	Yes
Yes	11	4	0	No
Yes	26	0	20	Yes
No	28	10	0	Yes
Yes	42	13	5	No
No	12	0	12	No
No	22	5	0	Yes
Yes	22	8	0	No
Yes	14	0	11	Yes

HOSPITAL COMPARISONS		Annual Births	Nursery Level	% C-Sections
13	Swedish Medical Center Ballard	564	I	18
14	Swedish Medical Center Seattle	3321	III	20
15	University of Washington Medical Center	1481	III	21.4
16	Valley Medical Center	2937	II	15
17	Virginia Mason Hospital	1152	II	10

VISITORS AND VISITING HOURS

Most hospitals surveyed allow visitors, including non-immediate family members, during labor and delivery. Most also allow siblings to be present during a vaginal delivery with the supervision of an adult (other than the primary support person), but recommend that siblings attend a sibling class beforehand. You should consider the child's age in determining whether their attendance is appropriate. Most hospitals have open visiting hours and even those with structured hours do not restrict the support person or significant other. Given the relatively short postpartum stay for many mothers, several hospitals advise that you limit your number of hospital visitors (other than support people and immediate family), so that you can focus on rest and recovery.

SAFETY PRECAUTIONS

Extreme care and safety precautions are taken to secure your baby in area hospitals. Security personnel, video camera surveillance of all entries, staff identification, alarm systems, and patient education are the most common security measures. All hospitals use the Identaband systems in which babies and parents/partners are banded at birth using the same numbers and names. Most hospitals will not reveal details of their security programs until you are admitted into the hospital to protect you and your infant. The more informed you are about the hospital's security program, the more knowledgeable you will be in the rare case a security issue arises.

Midwifery Services	Beds in OB Unit	LDRs	LDRPs	Postpartum Program
Yes	12	8	8	Yes
No	27	12	0	Yes
Yes	15	4	0	Yes
No	11	11	0	Yes
Yes	18	6	0	Yes

CLASSES

Childbirth and parenting classes are available through area hospitals. Many also offer additional resources, such as exercise classes, support groups, and lending and resource libraries. In most cases, classes are available to the general public, whether or not you plan to deliver at that hospital. Nominal class fees are charged to participants. For a complete listing of childbirth preparation and postpartum (including parenting) classes, see the Childbirth Education section of this book.

POSTPARTUM CARE

Often hospital stays for normal vaginal births are very short, most likely only one day. This happens for several reasons: mother's choice, insurance limitations, a desire to reduce costs. But sometimes the time between the discharge from the hospital to the first visit with the pediatrician can be filled with questions and concerns, especially for first-time parents. Most of the area hospitals have addressed this need by providing different options for postpartum follow-up soon after discharge.

Evergreen Hospital has a Postpartum Care Center, where you can bring your baby for a visit soon after birth. They also offer a free support group for parents of infants up to three months old, which meets weekly. Northwest Hospital provides a postpartum follow-up program, which includes a phone call within 24-48 hours from a postpartum follow-up nurse, who will check to see how you're getting along and answer your immediate baby care questions or concerns. You can also schedule a home visit by a nurse, if needed. Overlake Hospital offers one hour postpartum follow-up appointments with either a mother-baby nurse or a public health nurse. Other hospitals offer home visits and/or follow-up phone calls. Most of the hospitals have lactation consultants and consulting nurses available by phone, and can also refer you to a public health nurse for continued support if needed.

Hospital Phone List	
Auburn General	833-7711
Evergreen	899-3500
Group Health Central	326-3000
Group Health Eastside	883-5151
Highline	244-9970
Northwest	364-0500
Overlake	688-5326
Providence General (Colby)	261-2000
Providence General (Pacific)	258-7123
Providence Medical Center (Seattle)	320-2190
St. Francis	927-9700
Stevens Memorial	640-4000
Swedish (Ballard)	781-6344
Swedish (Seattle)	386-3606
University of Washington	548-3300
Valley Medical Center	228-3450
Virginia Mason	624-1144

BIRTH CENTERS

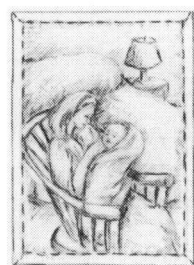

By Chris Thain, Licensed Midwife

There are eight licensed free-standing birth centers in the State of Washington as of 1996. Birth centers offer a viable option for low-risk, healthy maternity clients, and their families, who are interested in an out-of-hospital birth experience.

Birth centers are owned and operated by licensed midwives, certified nurse midwives, or naturopathic/licensed midwives. There are consulting and referral physicians available to each birth center. Washington law outlines a program and set of guidelines for birth centers, which require clients to be low-risk and healthy, and to fulfill certain other criteria.

Midwives are specialists in out-of-hospital birth, and offer families the opportunity to engage in a more intimate, personal, participatory experience. Moms and babies are seen by the midwives for their entire maternity care, including prenatal care, labor and delivery, postpartum, and early newborn care. Emergency medications and equipment are available at each birth center, including oxygen, resuscitative equipment, IV material, and certain medicines. Moms plan an unmedicated birth without anesthesia or instruments, such as forceps.

State law mandates that a physician be consulted if there is a deviation from normal during pregnancy, labor or delivery. In 90 percent of cases, there are no such complications. If mother or child should need special medical attention, immediate access to specialists in high-risk obstetrics, obstetrical anesthesia and newborn care is provided.

The setting for birth centers is similar to a bed and breakfast (without the breakfast), though families may bring foods of their choice to the birth, and design the atmosphere to include choice of music, lighting, friends and loved ones present. The length of stay for a normal delivery is a minimum of two to four hours, with a maximum stay of 24 hours after delivery.

Most major insurance companies cover midwife/birth center deliveries, recognizing the safety and cost effectiveness of this setting for birth. Midwives will help clients determine eligibility. In Washington, medical assistance (DSHS) is available for many maternity clients, and complete maternity care is covered when birth takes place in a licensed birth center.

❧

Birth centers offer a viable option for low-risk, healthy maternity clients, and their families, who are interested in an out-of-hospital birth experience.

❧

ها RESOURCES *ها*

■ **ARLINGTON BIRTH CENTER**
Chris Campbell, C.N.M.
(360) 435-5323
P.O. Box 8
Arlington, WA 98223

■ **GREENBANK WOMEN'S
CLINIC AND BIRTH CENTER**
Cynthia Jaffee, L.M.
(360) 678-3594
P.O. Box 67
Greenbank, WA 98352

■ **LAKESIDE BIRTH CENTER**
Nancy Spencer, L.M.
862-6533
800-862-6533
2722 214th Ave. E.
Sumner, WA 98390

■ **PUGET SOUND BIRTH
CENTER**
Lee Anne Shelley, L.M.
Chris Thain, L.M.
823-1919
13128 Totem Lake Blvd. N.E., Ste. 101
Kirkland, WA 98034

■ **SEATTLE HOME MATERNITY
SERVICE & CHILDBIRTH
CENTER**
Suzy Myers, L.M.
Marge Mansfield, L.M.
722-3426
3830 S. Ferdinand
Seattle, WA 98118

■ **SEATTLE NATUROPATHY,
ACUPUNCTURE & BIRTH
CENTER**
Rich Postmantur, N.D., L.M., C.A.
Felice Barnow, N.D., L.M., R.N.
328-7929
2705 E. Madison
Seattle, WA 98112

■ **THE BIRTH CENTER**
Les Griffith, N.D., L.M.
771-9000
19514 64th Ave. W.
Lynnwood, WA 98036

■ **WENATCHEE MIDWIFE
SERVICE AND CHILDBIRTH
CENTER**
Laurie Braunstein, L.M.
(509) 663-2770
310 S. Mission
Wenatchee, WA 98801

THE 24-HOUR HOSPITAL STAY

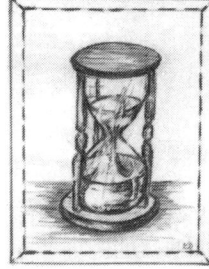

By Nanci J. Newell, R.N.C., M.S. Candidate

As health care policies unfold in our nation, state and city, how will expectant and new parents be affected? What changes are occurring now? What changes might occur in the future? And, most importantly, how can you prepare now for your own needs and those of your baby?

One major trend seen in nearly all area hospitals (and in most geographic areas of the state and country as well) is a shorter length of stay in the hospital following birth. Other major changes are being seen by expectant and new parents in the coverage they may have by their insurance companies. For most families having a normal vaginal delivery, a one-night stay follows birth and discharge takes place sometime the next day. And, unless there are medical complications, insurance coverage usually does not include more. For mothers having a Cesarean birth, a two-night stay following birth is now normal procedure unless there are medical complications. Also, some aspects of care may not be covered by insurance companies, such as immunizations for the baby. Other complications of pregnancy such as pre-term labor may sometimes be managed at home instead of in the hospital. Some insurance companies provide coverage for home care and others do not. These trends are likely to continue. And, in some hospitals and birth centers, a woman may go home just a few hours following birth.

There is actually a great deal to do in advance to make the transition to parenthood far more enjoyable.

WHAT YOU CAN EXPECT

A typical hospital experience for women having a normal, uncomplicated vaginal delivery might go like this one:

Lisa and Mark spend the first hours of early labor at home, and are admitted to the hospital childbirth center in active labor at 2 p.m. on Tuesday. Lisa gives birth at 9 p.m. to 8 lb., 2 oz. Michael. Between 9 p.m. and midnight, Lisa receives her immediate postpartum care and breastfeeds Michael. Michael also receives a newborn assessment, eye care, and vitamin K. The pediatrician will come to the hospital the following morning to examine him. Lisa is taught postpartum care for herself. She and

Mark eat a late dinner and they both continue to hold Michael as they call their parents and other family members.

At 1 a.m., Lisa, Mark and Michael are encouraged to try to get some rest. Mark and Lisa are too excited to sleep more than about three hours all night. In the morning, Lisa's doctor arrives to check her, finds everything normal and says she can go home after lunch. Michael's doctor arrives also, checks Michael and gives Mark and Lisa instructions for Michael's care at home, and says Michael can go home, too. Two friends and four relatives call. Flowers arrive. The lab tech comes to draw blood from Lisa for a complete blood count (CBC) and from Michael for a phenylketonuria (PKU) test. The birth certificate worksheet is completed with the help of the unit secretary. Information on how to get Michael a social security number is explained. Michael seems too sleepy to nurse, even though he cries. The lactation specialist is called and visits, reviews the basics of breastfeeding, and shows Lisa how to hold and encourage Michael to latch on properly. After Lisa takes a quick shower, lunch and 30-minute nap, Mark brings in the car seat, belongings are gathered and they are all *discharged home* at 2 p.m. Lisa is a normal mother with a normal baby and has no medical complications. Her total length of stay is 24 hours.

As the famous vocalist Peggy Lee sings, "Is that all there is?" Unless Lisa and Mark are well prepared and have good support, the normal physical and emotional changes they are about to experience as they become parents may be difficult, if not overwhelming, exhausting, and extremely stressful.

BE PREPARED

What can be done now to plan for and be prepared for a short length of stay in the hospital so that new parents can assume the care of themselves and their infants without feeling totally overwhelmed and exhausted? There is actually a great deal to do in advance to make the transition to parenthood far more enjoyable. Take a look:

THE PRENATAL PLAN

- Contact your insurance company to determine what coverage is available for pregnancy, birth and for the care of the newborn.
- Ask about home care coverage.
- See if lactation services are covered.
- What are the length of stay limitations? Do they differ with complications?
- Ask your health care provider what the usual length of stay is for patients.
- Tour your hospital.
- Talk to a financial counselor (usually located in admissions).
- If you have any unusual circumstances or additional needs, talk to the case manager or social worker at the hospital.
- Attend early discharge and breastfeeding classes.
- Read as much material on prenatal and baby care as you can.

It is nearly impossible to absorb all of the new information about yourself and the care of a newborn during a short hospital stay where you are laboring, giving birth, and getting to know your new baby. It helps a lot to have attended some classes in advance, even if you don't have a baby with which to practice.

THE POSTPARTUM PLAN

In addition to your birth plan, you will find it helpful to develop a postpartum plan. Here are some suggestions:

- Make a list of who might be of real help to you when the baby is born.
- Cross off the list anyone who needs to be entertained or those you're not comfortable asking for help.
- If you don't have a partner or have inadequate help available to you, contact the social worker or care manager at your hospital.
- Make a list of your home responsibilities and add infant tasks to that list.
- Keep a calendar to book helpers.
- Implement a visitor-control and telephone screening plan.
- Find out what postpartum programs are available.

New parents need to be in charge of *the plan* and of their baby. Helpers need to support new parents in ways which are perceived as helpful by the new parents. Rocking the baby may be grandmother's favorite helping activity but it may not be what the new mom needs most.

Ask your provider and hospital what (if any) postpartum services are available and are included along with your hospital stay. Some hospitals offer a follow-up program that extends professional nursing care into the postpartum period. Families may receive a telephone assessment by a registered nurse and a home visit, if needed.

With careful advance planning, expectant parents can learn much to reduce the normal stress associated with the early weeks at home with a new baby and enjoy being new parents!

Life Experiences ...

ROCHELLE , BILL AND ISABELLA

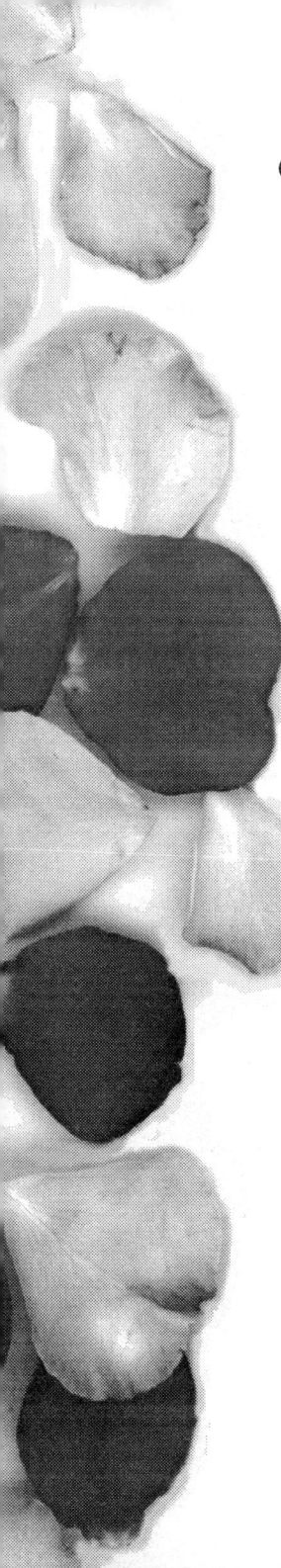

"WITH A LITTLE HELP"

By Rochelle Barcellona

I always assumed that I would sail through pregnancy like Doris Day in some 1950s movie. After all, none of the women in my family had ever had any problems during pregnancy or been sick. Little did I know that my pregnancy was more likely to resemble "The Nightmare on Elm Street" than a Doris Day movie. The first five-and-one-half months of my pregnancy were spent horizontally, on my office floor, in bed, anywhere. When I needed to be flat, I was. I learned that morning sickness was a misnomer, as mine lasted 24 hours a day.

With my immediate family about 800 miles away, my husband Bill became my lifeline. He was more involved in my pregnancy than any other husband I've met. He would get up at 5 a.m. and bring me food in bed so I could nibble. He took care of the house, the yard, the pets, basically everything in our lives, for that time period. As I lay on the bathroom floor one morning, telling him that I couldn't go on anymore, he held me and listened to my hormone-induced ranting.

When I became pregnant with our second child, everyone told me that pregnancies are different and I should expect this one to be quite different from the first. I hoped for it, and, unfortunately, got my wish. I was sicker than with our first. Bill again stepped into his usual role, but this time it was more difficult. We had an extremely active toddler in the house. And I was self-employed. If there was work to be done, I had to do it. The extra responsibilities at home and no support at work made things worse.

That's where some very good friends of ours stepped in. John and Cassy, the parents of Isabella's best friend, Ben, took over when Bill couldn't be there for me. They would have me over to lie on the couch while the kids played. They fed me more lunches and dinners than I can remember. They would take

Isabella for a play date with Ben so I could get some much-needed sleep. This time around, I couldn't have gotten through my first five-and-a-half months without them.

It was through this experience that I realized how important friends have become. It used to be that grandmothers, mothers, sisters and aunts helped during the pregnancy, birth and raising of children because extended families lived in the same town. Now, friends have really taken over that role. I am so grateful that I have friends who are willing to help out and that I've gotten over the initial embarrassment of admitting that I need help. They've been in my situation before and are offering their help out of love and empathy. And, they know that I'm here for them the next time they need help. I'll watch the kids, go grocery shopping or help clean up the house.

These two pregnancies have made me realize two things. One, how much I appreciate my loved ones and the extra mile they'll go for me. And, two, whoever came up with the term "Supermom" had it all wrong. You are a Supermom if you love and care for your children. There is no rule that says you have to do it all on your own. Life is more joyous when you share the good times with loved ones and more precious when you share the difficult times. ❧

QUESTIONS AND ANSWERS
Your Insurance Provider

Medical insurance coverage during pregnancy is a financial necessity today. Recent studies show the average cost of a vaginal delivery to be $6,200. The average price of a Cesarean birth is a lofty $11,200. And, these figures only include routine prenatal care and delivery of your child; they do not include laboratory fees or costs for ultrasound or anesthesia.

Although the cost of prenatal care may seem high, don't be tempted to cut corners by skipping this important care for you and your baby. The benefits far outweigh any savings to your budget. Studies have linked good prenatal care with a decrease in low birth-weight babies and infants born with other serious medical problems. Because of the importance of prenatal care, it is essential that you have a plan for covering the costs.

The following interview on the many different aspects of insurance coverage and pregnancy includes information provided by an independent insurance brokerage, R.L. Evans Company Inc., as well as the Washington State Insurance Commissioner's office.

Q. *If I do not have insurance and am pregnant, what options are available to me?*

A. Until recently, most insurance policies either didn't cover "pre-existing conditions" or had such a long waiting period (typically 12 months)

before they would, that you basically wouldn't be able to get maternity coverage if you were already pregnant. Thanks to Washington State's Health Care Reform legislation, that practice has changed. Since July 1995 pregnant women have had at least some options to purchase maternity coverage. The variety of options and their costs are difficult to predict and even the time frame of their availability may change, so we suggest contacting the Office of the Insurance Commissioner, listed at the end of this section, for the most up-to-date information on health care reform and how it affects you.

Besides purchasing insurance, there are two other options to pay for your health care. For women who qualify based on income, state assistance is available through DSHS's First Steps program (described in the next section in this chapter). The other option is cash payment. A decision to pay cash can be a more expensive route, since you won't have the advantages of the pricing structure afforded to insurance companies that channel patients to the doctors and hospitals. If cash payment makes the most sense for your situation, take the time to call around to some of the local hospitals and compare prices, as they can vary considerably.

Q. If I do not have insurance now and am planning to become pregnant soon, what are my options?

A. Two options to consider are private insurance and the state-sponsored First Steps program if you meet the income guidelines.

A private insurance program insures you individually. In the past, it was very expensive to receive personal insurance. Today there are some affordable options for individuals. Finding the best plan for you, in this time of ever-changing health care laws, can be a complicated job to do yourself. It's best to contact a private insurance broker (look in the Yellow Pages under Insurance, and note the ones that specialize in health insurance). Your broker can help you through the confusing maze of terms like HMO, PPO, and POS, so you can better understand your options. As your representative, they'll look at your individual needs and resources and help you make an educated choice. Your insurance policy will cost the same if you buy it from the broker as it would from the insurance company itself, but by working with a broker you get both an advocate and an expert source of information on the latest developments in the health care industry.

Q. If your spouse has separate insurance coverage from you, is it worthwhile to join his/her health plan to get double coverage to reduce your final medical bill for maternity care and delivery?

A. This is basically a question of economics. You should sit down and calculate your savings when making this choice. For example, if your current insurance company will only cover $1,000 of your maternity care and the final bill should equal approximately $5,000, then you would need $4,000 in cash to pay for your child's delivery. Let's say you could sign up for health insurance on your spouse's plan for $100 a month during one year. In this example, you would pay $1,200. For this couple, using double coverage would save approximately $2,800 and would definitely be a smart cost-saving move.

However, each couple's situation is different. You must look at the coverage each health insurance company provides and examine the financial implications before deciding whether double coverage is a feasible option. You'll need to investigate exactly when you can join your spouse's plan; some insurance plans only allow changes during annual open enrollment periods, and this timing could also affect the total cost. You should also carefully review each plan's section on "coordination of benefits" to find out exactly how the plans coordinate with each other.

Q. **What questions should I ask my insurance company about maternity coverage?**

A. Here are a few to consider:
- What is the cost per provider visit?
- Does the insurance offer a co-payment plan or pay a percentage of each visit?
- What is the calendar year deductible that you must fulfill before coverage begins?
- Is there a separate maternity deductible from a general services deductible?
- What hospitals accept your insurance plan?
- Does the insurance company have a list of doctors from which to choose?
- How are laboratory charges handled and which laboratories may you go to and still receive coverage?
- Is there a difference in coverage for a Cesarean or vaginal birth?
- Are twins or other multiple births handled any differently?
- What coverage is provided if complications arise?
- Are Cesarean births considered a complication?
- How many days of hospital stay are covered?
- How is emergency care covered?
- Is insurance provided for pediatric or neonatal care?
- Is the newborn child covered under your policy for the first 72 hours automatically or do you need to immediately enroll the child as a dependent?
- What is the procedure for payment of bills?

- Do you have to pay provider and hospital bills up front and then be reimbursed by your insurance company? Are claim forms necessary?
- Who should you contact if you have questions about your insurance policy?

Q. **What questions should I ask my insurance provider regarding well-baby care for my new baby?**

A. Well-baby care is defined as general checkups, immunizations, and other preventive care office visits when your infant is not ill. The checklist below provides questions for your insurance provider.
- Does your insurance plan cover well-baby care?
- What specifically is included with well-baby care?
- What does each office visit cost?
- When the baby is born, does well-baby care cover hospital visits?
- Are immunizations a part of well-baby care?

Q. **How soon should I add my new child to my insurance plan?**

A. The standard time is 30 days. This ensures that your new baby will be covered under the plan without any gap in coverage.

RESOURCE

- **OFFICE OF INSURANCE COMMISSIONER**
800-562-6900 (Seattle)
(360) 753-7300 (Olympia),
P.O. Box 40255
Olympia, WA 98504

FIRST STEPS PROGRAM

Through the First Steps Program, Washington State's Department of Social and Health Services (DSHS) offers expanded Medicaid eligibility and other support services for pregnant women and their babies. First Steps helps pay for medical expenses and helps to locate health care. It also assists with personal problems, child care, and transportation.

CALL FIRST

Finding out about First Steps begins with a phone call to the Healthy Mothers, Healthy Babies toll-free bilingual number, 800-322-2588. When you call, you'll receive at no charge:

- Resources and referrals to link you with maternity care providers in your community
- A packet of written information about pregnancy and maternity care
- An incentive—a baby book—to make an appointment for your first prenatal checkup. Books are now available in English, Spanish, Korean, Vietnamese and Chinese.

≈

If you have any doubts about your ability to pay your prenatal and delivery costs, it's to your benefit to consider the First Steps program.

≈

They'll also give you current guidelines regarding the state medical financing options and the eligibility requirements. If you have any doubts about your ability to pay your prenatal and delivery costs, it's to your benefit to consider the First Steps program. The income guidelines may surprise you. Even if you have insurance, the program can pick up costs of deductibles and other non-covered expenses if you qualify. A major difference between this and other public assistance programs is that your assets (home, car, etc.) are not considered when qualifying for aid, only your monthly income. And, once you've qualified, your medical benefits can't be terminated during your pregnancy, even if your income changes. While the eligibility levels change from time to time, here's a general idea of the cutoff point for First Steps medical assistance (based on 1995 figures):

Family Size	Yearly Income	Monthly Income
2*	$18,564	$1,547
3	$23,292	$1,941
4	$28,032	$2,336

*Note that a pregnant woman counts as two people for this program.

VISIT A FACILITY

To apply for medical financing, you'll need to visit a DSHS Community Service Office (CSO). The office you visit is determined by your zip code; offices are listed in the blue pages of the phone book, under Washington State, and in this chapter. You can call first and have an application mailed to you (this may add about a week to the process), or go to the office to complete the application. Along with the application you'll need to provide the following: written proof of pregnancy, verification of income, social security or alien registration card, and picture ID.

Once you've submitted the application, you'll be given an appointment to return within five days to meet with a financial counselor. The counselor will review your application and explain the programs you qualify for. You'll be informed of your rights and responsibilities and, if eligible for First Steps assistance, you can then receive your DSHS medical identification card (formerly called medical coupons). The counselor will also ensure that you make contact with the First Steps social worker, if you haven't already.

MEET WITH A SOCIAL WORKER

Each CSO has a social worker who will explain the specific First Steps program services available. If the social worker is available on your first visit, you can meet then, even before your application has been reviewed. Otherwise you'll make an appointment to meet with the social worker either in the office or in your home.

WIC AND OTHER SERVICES

Besides medical financing, you may qualify for the Women, Infants & Children (WIC) Supplemental Food Program. This program provides nutritious foods, education and assessments, breastfeeding promotion, and referrals to health and social services. Income guidelines are similar to those listed, although pregnant women are counted as one person for WIC eligibility. In addition, you must have a nutrition health risk to be eligible. Some of these risk factors are anemia, underweight, obesity, and smoking during pregnancy. Call Healthy Mothers, Healthy Babies for the WIC clinic nearest you at 800-322-3498.

First Steps also offers:

- Transportation to medical appointments
- Child care
- Maternity support services
- Childbirth classes
- Drug/alcohol counseling and treatment
- Assistance in obtaining public assistance and food stamps
- Dental coverage
- Case management with home visits by a public health nurse
- Family planning services (includes medical costs, and prescription and non-prescription supplies) for one year after pregnancy ends
- Automatic medical coverage for your newborn for one year

HEALTHY OPTIONS PLAN

DSHS/First Steps provides prenatal care and delivery coverage by paying a premium to a health maintenance organization (HMO) called a Healthy Options Plan. Plans available vary depending on where you live. You must select a plan and a primary provider (physician or nurse practitioner) within the plan. All of your medical care must be provided by your primary provider, or specialists that your primary provider refers you to, otherwise the care will not be covered. There are no deductibles or co-payments. Prescriptions, medical supplies, dental care, and maternity support services are provided outside of the Healthy Options Plan and paid directly by DSHS to the provider.

Your local CSO will give you enrollment forms and a list of medical plans available for your selection. If you don't select a plan or primary provider, one will be selected for you. You can change plans monthly and providers within the plan on a daily basis. If you have other insurance, your Healthy Options plan will act as your secondary insurance plan. If you have already been receiving medical care for your pregnancy from a provider outside a plan, you can ask to be exempt from having to use an HMO if you wish to continue with the same provider. Instructions on how to do this are available from the CSO.

You'll receive a medical ID card from DSHS monthly. This is used for billing purposes so you will have to show it to your providers. It's very important to keep DSHS informed of any address changes to ensure you receive your ID card monthly. Coverage continues under First Steps for two months after delivery.

❧ RESOURCES ❧

■ HEALTHY MOTHERS, HEALTHY BABIES

800-322-2588

Statewide referral number which will link you to resources and referrals for maternity care providers in your area that participate in the First Steps program. You can find out current guidelines regarding state medical financing options and eligibility requirements.

DSHS COMMUNITY SERVICE OFFICES (CSO)

■ BELLTOWN CSO

464-7060
2106 2nd Ave.
Seattle, WA 98104
Hours: M-F   8:00 a.m.-5:00 p.m.
Serves zip codes 98101, 98104, 98121

■ BURIEN CSO

433-1336
15811 Ambaum Blvd. S.W.
Burien, WA 98146
Hours: M-F   8:00 a.m.-5:00 p.m.
Serves zip codes 98062, 98146, 98148, 98158, 98166, 98168, 98188, 98198

■ **CAPITOL HILL CSO**
720-3170
1700 E. Cherry
Seattle, WA 98122
Hours: M, T 8:00 a.m.-11:00 a.m.
M-F 1:00 p.m.-3:00 p.m.
Serves zip codes 98102, 98112, 98122

■ **FEDERAL WAY CSO**
872-2145
1617 S. 324th
Federal Way, WA 98023
Hours: M-F 8:00 a.m.-5:00 p.m.
Serves zip codes 98003, 98023, 98054, 98063, 98093

■ **KING EASTSIDE CSO**
649-4000
15821 N.E. 8th
Bellevue, WA 98008
Hours: M-F 8:00 a.m.-5:00 p.m.
Serves zip codes 98004-98009, 98011, 98014, 98019, 98024, 98027, 98033, 98034, 98039, 98040, 98041, 98045, 98050, 98052, 98053, 98056, 98065, 98073, 98083

■ **KING NORTH/BALLARD CSO**
545-7607
907 N.W. Ballard Way
Seattle, WA 98107
Hours: M-F 8:00 a.m.-5:00 p.m.
Serves zip codes 98103, 98105, 98107, 98109, 98117, 98119, 98133, 98177, 98199

■ **KING NORTH/LAKE CITY CSO**
368-7200
11536 Lake City Way N.E.
Seattle, WA 98125
Hours: M-F 8:00 a.m.-5:00 p.m.
Serves zip codes 98115, 98125, 98155

■ **KING SOUTH CSO**
872-2145
25316 74th Ave. S.
Kent, WA 98035
Hours: M-F 8:00 a.m.-5:00 p.m.
Serves zip codes 98001, 98002, 98010, 98015, 98022, 98025, 98031, 98032, 98035, 98038, 98042, 98047, 98048, 98051, 98055, 98057, 98058, 98064, 98071, 98092

■ **RAINIER CSO**
721-2775
3600 S. Graham
Seattle, WA 98118
Hours: M-F 8:00 a.m.-5:00 p.m.
Serves zip codes 98108, 98118, 98124, 98134, 98144, 98178

■ **WEST SEATTLE CSO**
933-3300
4045 Delridge Way S.W.
Seattle, WA 98106
Hours: M-F 8:00 a.m.-5:00 p.m.
Serves zip codes 98013, 98018, 98070, 98106, 98108, 98116, 98126, 98136

STAYING IN SHAPE

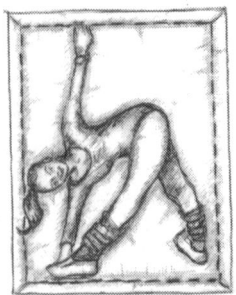

❧

The goals of

prenatal

exercise

should

include

preventing

discomfort,

backache,

and fatigue.

❧

By Lisa Yount, Physical Therapist

Many different approaches and educational opportunities have been available to assist a woman in preparing for the exciting event of birth and newborn care. Unfortunately the importance and opportunities of prenatal and postnatal exercise have been essentially neglected. Today not only is exercise during pregnancy accepted by most physicians, it is highly recommended. Even someone who does not exercise routinely can safely perform exercises that will make her pregnancy more comfortable. Just as every pregnancy is different, the exercise program should be designed for the individual woman with special attention to the pregnancy and postpartum periods.

Pregnancy creates several changes in a woman's body. Her balance, coordination, endurance, and strength can be altered. The obvious structural and hormonal changes cause the stretching of muscles, shortening of ligaments, and the loosening of joints. The curve in the lower back becomes more pronounced as the baby grows and the woman's center of gravity moves forward. If adequate muscular support is lacking, the stress to the pelvis and back is increased, resulting in poor posture, fatigue, and backache. It is important to exercise and maintain control of the voluntary muscles to help support the backbone and pelvis, which are put under significant stress. If she is to be at her best during the pregnancy and is to prevent future problems, it is essential that she improve her physical condition. The important key muscle groups are the abdominal muscles, the pelvic floor, and the postural muscles.

The goals of prenatal exercise should include preventing discomfort, backache, and fatigue. This is done by toning the essential muscle groups by stretching, relaxation, and proper body mechanics.

GUIDELINES FOR PRENATAL EXERCISE

- Exercise regularly (three times a week).
- Avoid increasing the body core temperature; strenuous exercise should be limited to 15 minutes and exercise should not be performed in hot, humid weather.
- Exercise heart rate should not exceed 140 beats per minute.
- Begin the exercise program with warm-ups and end gradually.
- Repeat each exercise only a few times; change your body position to work the same muscle groups in different positions.
- Do not hold your breath during exercises and avoid any exercise that causes you to do a Valsalva maneuver (bearing down).
- Exercises should be performed slowly; bouncing motions should be avoided.
- Avoid heavy resisted exercises overhead or with long leverage.
- Avoid positions that increase the curve in your lower back.
- Drink plenty of fluids.
- Limit time spent exercising on your back, and stop exercising in this position if you feel any tingling or dizziness.

WARNING SIGNS

Although exercise during pregnancy is recommended, it is important to be aware of the signs indicating that exercise should cease or a physician be contacted:

- Bleeding
- Frequent uterine contractions during or after exercise
- Sciatic nerve numbness
- Pain, numbness, or tingling in the wrist/hand
- Lower back or pubic pain
- Pain in the pelvic area
- A breathless, dizzy, light-headed feeling or fatigue
- Palpitations or rapid heart beat

Difficulties with present or previous pregnancies or general health problems may be contraindications to exercise during pregnancy. These areas should be discussed with the physician.

Prenatal exercises strengthen the body and decrease the discomforts of pregnancy (there is limited evidence that they shorten labor). You will have greater endurance for a long labor, and recovery is thought to be quicker. Feeling good physically also helps you to feel good mentally. Participants in exercise programs report decreased fatigue, decreased "moodiness," wonderful peer support, and shorter recovery periods.

There are inherent benefits to exercise that can be appreciated during pregnancy and the postpartum period. The program should be individualized to provide the highest level of fitness without compromising the health or safety of the fetus or the pregnant mother.

EXERCISE PROGRAMS

There are several on-going exercise programs offered by Seattle area hospitals that directly address physical fitness during pregnancy. Other programs are offered by individuals, health clubs, and park and recreation districts. Since programs are constantly changing, you should verify time and locations. Before beginning any exercise program, be sure to talk to your health care provider and follow his or her instructions.

■ SEATTLE BIRTH FITNESS AND EDUCATION (BIRTHWORKS)
932-1687
411 Fairview Ave. N.
Seattle, WA 98109
Seattle Birth Fitness and Education is owned by a mother, fitness instructor, and certified childbirth educator. Through this unique training, members receive much more than just a prenatal/postnatal exercise program. Besides the usual non-impact aerobics and stretching, Seattle Birth Fitness and Education also offers practical information to participants concerning the labor and parenting process. Classes run $6 for drop-ins or $40 per month. Some partial scholarships are available.

■ EVERGREEN HOSPITAL MEDICAL CENTER
899-3480
12040 N.E. 128th St.
Kirkland, WA 98034
Maternity Fitness and Education is an exercise and fitness program for pregnant women and new mothers. This pre/post pregnancy low-impact aerobics and exercise program is a fun and easy way to shape up before and after delivery. You'll improve muscle tone, relieve discomforts of pregnancy, ease tension, and make new friends. The cost is $35 per month for as many sessions as you want to attend.

■ HOLISTIC CHILDBIRTH EDUCATION AND YOGA CENTER
547-9882
4649 Sunnyside Ave. N., Rm. 300
Seattle, WA 98103
As the name implies, this center offers an assortment of classes for expectant and new parents, all with a focus on promoting personal growth and body/mind awareness through yoga, massage, and holistic health education. For pregnant women, there's Prenatal Yoga, offered in an ongoing eight week series. A once-a-week series costs $80, twice a week is $128, and drop-in classes are $12. And after your baby is born, you can continue with Postpartum Yoga With Infant, a bring-your-baby class that includes not only yoga, but also support with other mothers. The cost ranges from $38 for four classes to $72 for eight classes, and $12 for drop-in.

■ NORTH SEATTLE YMCA
524-1400
5003 12th Ave. N.E.
Seattle, WA 98105
The "Y" offers a Prenatal/Postpartum Aerobics class, which is geared towards preparation for and recovery from childbirth. The workout includes low impact aerobics for cardiovascular fitness, muscle conditioning with emphasis on abdominals and upper body, and stretching to relax and relieve tension. Babies are welcome and this is a great support group for new moms, too. Classes cost $1 for members, $3.50 for nonmembers and meet twice a week for one hour.

■ OLYMPIC ATHLETIC CLUB
789-5010
5301 Leary Ave.
Seattle, WA 98107
OAC offers a safe, low-impact workout program that is modifiable for all levels of fitness. Floor and Step Aerobics are combined with upper and lower body strengthening to provide a well-rounded workout for women in all stages of their childbearing year, from pregnancy to postpartum. The class is designed to improve the strength of those muscles most challenged by the condition of pregnancy and the event of childbirth: the abdominal, back, and perineal muscles. OAC also offers monthly seminars on topics related to pregnancy and child care. Infants are welcome to attend class with their moms; child care for babies over four months is also available. The class cost is $24 per month for members or non-members.

■ SWEDISH HOSPITAL
386-2035
747 Summit Ave.
Seattle, WA 98104
Swedish Hospital offers both a prenatal and postnatal exercise class. When calling the number listed, a staff person may connect you with a recorded message line regarding the programs. Here is what we found:

The Prenatal Fitness class meets in the aerobic room downtown and costs $40 for eight weeks or is free to Swedish Hospital Baby Club members. This fee includes a free copy of the book *Exercise in the Childbearing Years,* by Elizabeth Nobel. This class also offers a lecture series and informal discussions on fitness, exercise, and general childbearing related topics. If you do not use all your sessions during your pregnancy, you may receive a credit for their Moms and Babies postpartum exercise class.

The Moms and Babies class costs $20 or is free to Swedish Hospital Baby Club members for four classes of your choice. Classes are offered twice per week on a drop-in basis and focus on aerobics, floor exercises, and posture awareness work with an emphasis on safe resumption of activity following pregnancy. Babies are incorporated into exercises to keep them happy and interactive. Both classes are taught by physical therapists.

CHILDBIRTH EDUCATION

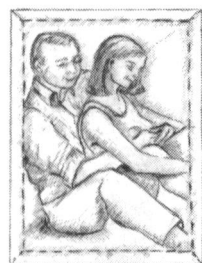

By *Laura Kremer, ICCE*

As with anything else, the more prepared for childbirth you are, the better off you will be. A parent's goal, no matter what, is to deliver a healthy child into the world. Childbirth education gives parents the opportunity to learn of the risks, benefits, and alternatives available for their labor and birthing experience. It teaches them skills and strategies to meet the demands of labor and delivery. Once this knowledge is gained, parents are better prepared to take an active part in the birth of their child.

To provide you with a better understanding of different childbirth educators and methods, here is some information to help you in making a choice.

BRADLEY

This was the first approach to establish the husband-coached delivery. Its focus is on understanding the process of labor and conditioning yourself to work with your body. The Bradley method also stresses a need for healthy diet and exercises that will help prepare the muscles of the body for the birth. This method teaches deep abdominal breathing and recommends that the woman concentrate within herself and work with her body. Many Bradley classes begin during the fourth or fifth month of pregnancy, believing that it takes that much time to prepare both physically and emotionally for labor and delivery.

LAMAZE

This style of childbirth preparation uses a combination of distraction and focus to help the laboring woman deal with pain. Lamaze is famous for teaching the pregnant woman and her partner how to "breathe" in labor. This is usually referred to as the "hee hee hee hoo" breathing pattern. Lamaze also made popular the use of fingertip massage during pregnancy and labor. An accredited Lamaze instructor is certified through ASPO, the American Society of Psychoprophylaxis in Obstetrics. She may then list ACCE after her name as an ASPO Certified Childbirth Educator.

≈
A parent's goal, no matter what, is to deliver a healthy child into the world.
≈

HYPNOBIRTHING

One of the newest concepts in childbirth preparation is HypnoBirthing™. Taught by certified HypnoBirthing practitioners, the technique emphasizes maintaining a relaxed state of mind and body, while remaining fully awake, alert, in control and aware through childbirth. Proponents say mothers trained in hypnobirthing typically experience a shorter, easier delivery with about ten minutes of pushing, and are refreshed and very much present for postnatal bonding and breastfeeding.

ICCE CERTIFICATION

A childbirth educator with the designation ICCE is certified through the International Childbirth Education Association. ICEA does not promote a specific style of childbirth education, but rather promotes the concepts of "family centered maternity care" and "freedom of choice based on the knowledge of alternatives." ICCEs may, or may not, be certified by another affiliation (Bradley or Lamaze). They may combine different aspects of several childbirth education styles in their curriculum. Most "hospital" childbirth educators are certified through ICEA.

HOSPITAL CLASSES

Most expectant parents attend a childbirth course through the hospital where they will be giving birth. Classes usually have 10 to 15 couples, but they may vary with the size of the hospital. Hospitals recommend scheduling your childbirth classes between your fourth and sixth month in order to complete all of your classes by your delivery date. Many hospitals now offer a wide variety of classes that include baby basics, first aid and CPR, breastfeeding and much more. Prices range from $30 to $90.

LABOR DOULAS

Many childbirth assistants (labor doulas) have started independent companies not affiliated with any medical establishments. Although the basic information you will receive in any childbirth class will be similar, the interpretations and emphasis may be different. Independent labor doulas can teach their independent philosophies through their classes without having to follow hospital or medical establishments guidelines. They can also assist you during childbirth as a coach. Classes are usually taught out of a home or in a small community setting. Pricing is usually competitive with hospital classes.

USING A LABOR DOULA

The labor doula is a person specially trained and paid to give additional support throughout the labor and delivery process. Since most physicians are unable to remain by your side during the entire labor, and a hospital's nursing staff has a multitude of other responsibilities, a labor doula is a great option for parents who want a person to remain with them to assist and support. The average cost for a doula is $250. Many charge fees on a sliding scale—some labor doulas work for free and others charge as much as $500.

❧ RESOURCES ❧

■ **AMERICAN SOCIETY OF PSYCHOPROPHYLAXIS IN OBSTETRICS (ASPO)**
800-368-4404
1101 Connecticut Ave. N.W., Ste. 700
Washington, DC 20036
Lamaze instructors are certified through this organization. By calling the toll-free number you may obtain a list of instructors in your zip code area.

■ **BIRTH AND BEYOND**
324-4831
2610 E. Madison St.
Seattle, WA 98112
Birth and Beyond offers customized personal classes on childbirth, breastfeeding, newborn care, and parenting. Call for current schedules and information. This organization also rents tubs for those interested in a water birth.

■ **BRADLEY METHOD OF**
NATURAL CHILDBIRTH
800-422-4784 or 800-423-2397
329-1799
P.O. Box 5224
Sherman Oaks, CA 91413-5224
This referral line provides a free pamphlet describing the Bradley method, classes available, teachers in your area, and professional labor support. All inquiries are responded to by mail. These are the only numbers through which you can reach a certified Bradley instructor.

■ **CHILDBIRTH EDUCATION & TRAINING**
565-0393
3406 Olympic Blvd. W.
University Place
Tacoma, WA 98466
Suzanne Grandon teaches classes for expectant parents in HypnoBirthing and trains HypnoBirthing practitioners for certification through the HypnoBirthing Foundation. Call for class information.

■ **CHILDBIRTH EDUCATION ASSOCIATION OF SEATTLE (CEAS)**
789-0883
10021 Holman Rd. N.W.
Seattle, WA 98177-4920
The Childbirth Education Association of Seattle, a nonprofit organization, provides classes to families on a variety of subjects including Labor and Birth, Childbirth Preparation, Newborn Care, Fathering, Infant Safety and CPR, Breastfeeding, and much more. Teachers are health professionals who have additional training in their specialty areas.

■ **CHILDBIRTH AND PARENTING RESOURCES**
781-0858
This is an advocacy association of consumers and professionals which campaigns for improvement in all aspects of maternity care by promoting birth and parenting options, offering resources and referrals and providing support and encouragement to parents and the community.

■ **PACIFIC ASSOCIATION FOR LABOR SUPPORT (PALS)**
325-1419
PALS provides expectant parents a list of local labor support persons (doulas). Members of the association have completed a training program offered by either the Seattle Midwifery School or by Informed Birth and Parenting. Support is available before, during, and after labor. Fees for this service vary with most charging on a sliding scale.

■ **PENNY SIMKIN INC.**
325-1419
1100 23rd E.
Seattle, WA 98112
Instructors Penny Simkin, PT, and Sandra Szalay, ARNP, offer classes on home birth preparation and also contract with local hospitals to provide childbirth education.

■ **PREPARATION FOR EXPECTANT PARENTS (PEP)**
282-1729
This nonprofit organization offers support and education for childbearing families through a variety of classes and workshops, including Birth Preparation Workshop, Breastfeeding Support Program, Homebirth/Clinic Birth Classes, Early Pregnancy Class, New Parenting Course, Sibling Preparation Class, Previous Cesarean Class, and private instruction. Their instructors are certified by the International Childbirth Education Association (ICEA) and most are also available to help with labor support.

■ **PUBLIC HEALTH CENTERS**
Many of the local public health centers offer a basic childbirth series, with payment by donation or DSHS medical card. Call the center nearest you for schedules.

Auburn:	296-8400
Columbia (S. Seattle):	296-4650
Downtown:	296-4755
Eastgate (Bellevue):	296-4920
Federal Way:	838-4557
North District (N. Seattle):	296-4765
Northshore (Bothell):	296-9787
Renton:	296-4700
Southwest (Burien):	296-4646

■ **AUBURN REGIONAL MEDICAL CENTER**
833-7711
20 2nd St. N.E.
Auburn, WA 98002
● Prepared Childbirth
● Refresher
● Big Brothers & Sisters

■ **EVERGREEN HOSPITAL MEDICAL CENTER**
899-3000
12040 N.E. 128th St.
Kirkland, WA 98034
● Labor & Birth
● Labor & Birth (Christian)
● Labor & Birth for Teens
● Labor & Birth Refresher
● Prenatal & Infant Nutrition
● Preterm Birth Prevention
● Cesarean Birth
● Vaginal Birth After Cesarean (VBAC)
● Planning for the Newborn
● Breastfeeding & the Working Mom
● Breastfeeding Basics
● For Dads Only
● Sibling Class
● Grandparents Class
● Infant and Child CPR

- Infant Massage
- Baby-Parent Time
- Feeding Fundamentals: Starting Solid Food
- Breastfeeding the Older Baby

■ GROUP HEALTH CENTRAL & EASTSIDE

287-2527 (800-462-5327)
Courses are held at Group Health centers throughout the community and are open to non-enrollees.

- First, Second & Third Trimester
- Birth Preparation
- Birth Preparation for Teens
- Refresher Workshop
- Vaginal Birth After Cesarean Refresher
- Our New Baby: Sibling Preparation
- Newborn Care
- Lactation
- Breastfeeding Support

■ HIGHLINE COMMUNITY HOSPITAL

244-9970
16251 Sylvester Rd. S.W.
Seattle, WA 98166

- Prepared Childbirth (Lamaze)
- Refresher Course
- Breastfeeding Preparation
- Kangaroo Kapers (sibling program)

■ NORTHWEST HOSPITAL

368-1784
1550 N. 115th St.
Seattle, WA 98133

- Baby??? Maybe
- Expecting Changes
- Breastfeeding
- Mother and Baby Care
- Preparation for Labor
- Survival Skills for New Dads
- Infant CPR and Safety
- Grandparents Class

- VBAC: Vaginal Birth After Cesarean Refresher Course
- Siblings Class
- Parenthood: The First Two Months
- Parenthood: The Developing Infant
- Parenthood: Eating and Sleeping the First Year
- Parenthood: Guiding the Older Infant
- Blended (Step) Families
- Trying Temperaments, Terrific Kids
- Tea for Two (for expectant working moms)
- Positive Parenting
- Parenting Your Teen

■ OVERLAKE HOSPITAL MEDICAL CENTER

688-5259
1035 116th Ave. N.E.
Bellevue, WA 98004

- Early Pregnancy
- Preparation for Childbirth
- Refresher
- Siblings Are Special
- Vaginal Birth After C-Section (VBAC)
- Fitness & Health Options for the Childbearing Years
- You and Your New Baby
- Breastfeeding
- Just for Dads: Post Partum
- Infant CPR & Safety Proofing

■ PROVIDENCE GENERAL MEDICAL CENTER (COLBY CAMPUS)

261-2000
1321 Colby
Everett, WA 98206

- Healthy Beginnings: Planning for Pregnancy
- Childbirth Preparation
- Preterm Birth Prevention

- Once Again With Style (Childbirth Refresher)
- Breastfeeding Basics
- Teens 'n Birthing Childbirth Preparation
- A New Baby is Coming to Our House (for siblings ages 3¹/₂ to 9 years)
- Kangaroo Kapers (for siblings ages 2¹/₂ to 6 years)
- Living With Baby Weekly Support Class
- Infant Safety and CPR
- Systematic Training for Effective Parenting (STEP)

■ PROVIDENCE GENERAL MEDICAL CENTER (PACIFIC CAMPUS)
258-7711
Pacific and Nassau
P.O. Box 1067
Everett, WA 98206
Classes offered at Providence General's Colby Campus listed above are also available at the Pacific Campus.

■ PROVIDENCE MEDICAL CENTER
320-2190
500 17th Ave.
Seattle, WA 98124
- Childbirth Preparation & Refresher
Many other classes through Childbirth Education Association

■ ST. FRANCIS COMMUNITY HOSPITAL
838-9700
34515 9th Ave. S.
Federal Way, WA 98003
- Preparing for Childbirth
- Preparing for Childbirth: Lamaze Refresher
- You and Me, Babe (for pregnant teens)

- Cesarean Birth
- Breastfeeding
- Infant Preparation
- Kangaroo Kapers (sibling)

■ STEVENS MEMORIAL HOSPITAL
640-4066
21601 76th Ave. W.
Edmonds, WA 98026
- Childbirth Preparation
- VBAC (Vaginal Birth After C-Section)
- Childbirth Refresher
- Preterm Birth Prevention
- Breastfeeding
- Sibling Class
- Newborn Care
- Pediatric CPR
- Kid Safety Plus

■ SWEDISH MEDICAL CENTER—BALLARD
386-3606
N.W. Market & Barnes
Seattle, WA 98107
- Preparation for Parenthood
- Childbirth Refresher
- Big Kids and Babies
- Infant CPR
- Everything You Always Wanted to Know About Babies

■ SWEDISH MEDICAL CENTER—SEATTLE
386-3606
747 Broadway
Seattle, WA 98114
- Childbirth Preparation Series
- Childbirth Preparation Seminar
- Refresher Series
- Sibling Preparation
- Dads Only Class
- Grandparents Class

- Breastfeeding
- Newborn Care
- Infant CPR & Safety
- Newborn Preparation Seminar
- New Mother Seminar/Support Group
- Babies & You (series of free seminars)

Swedish also offers "Baby Club" memberships which include admission to the classes above, as well as exercise classes and other benefits.

■ UNIVERSITY OF WASHINGTON MEDICAL CENTER
548-4003
1959 N.E. Pacific St.
Seattle, WA 98195
- Prepared Childbirth Series
- Refresher Childbirth Series
- Breastfeeding and Newborn Parenting
- Early Pregnancy
- Preventing Preterm Birth
- Pregnancy Planning for Women With Diabetes
- Southeast Asian Prepared Childbirth Series
- Sibling Preparation
- Baby Safety & CPR
- Childbirth Classes in Spanish

■ VALLEY MEDICAL CENTER
575-BABY
400 S. 43rd
Renton, WA 98055
- Planning for Pregnancy
- Care During Pregnancy
- Labor & Birth
- Planning, Packing, Parking, Pushing
- Refresher Course
- Teens: Pregnant & Prepared
- Expecting a Grandbaby
- Breastfeeding and the Working Mother
- Infant Feeding
- Infant Child CPR and Early Childhood Safety
- Postpartum Care/Infant Interaction

■ VIRGINIA MASON MEDICAL CENTER
623-8655
1100 Ninth Ave.
P.O. Box 900
Seattle, WA 98111
A variety of childbirth education classes are offered through PEP & CEAS.

Life Experiences ...

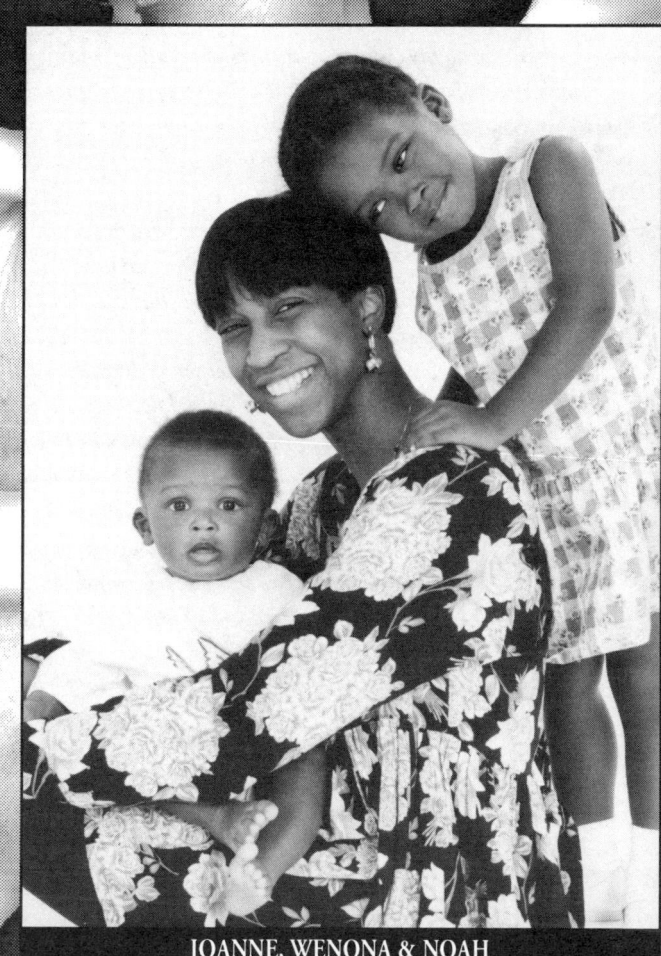

JOANNE, WENONA & NOAH

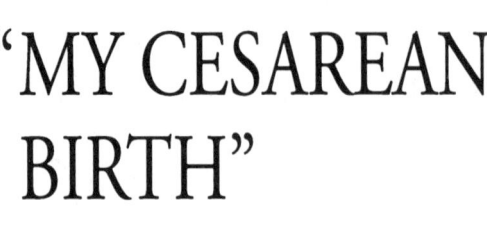

"MY CESAREAN BIRTH"

By Joanne Brice

I remember during my pregnancies how I worried about my children's futures. I recall agonizing over the birth process and about what long-term consequences it might have for them. Both my children, who are now two years old and five months old, were born by Cesarean section after pregnancies so uneventful, thank God, that I could spend countless hours worrying about nebulous future events.

The first time around we did what most prospective parents do: take childbirth classes, buy a video camera, and make the inevitable mental preparation for an event that would be painful, but ultimately wonderfully fulfilling, bordering on the spiritual. I read every book (several times), explored every option, met with an anesthesiologist (I am a realist), and even picked out which birthing suite I wanted at the hospital. I was intellectually prepared.

So when my water broke two weeks early, one would think that I would take this in stride and proceed to the hospital as instructed. Instead, I washed, and rewashed, everything in sight, in complete denial about what was obviously about to happen. Five hours later I went to the hospital. My tardiness was encouraged by the fact that I had not begun to have any signs of labor. Another five hours was spent on pitocin drip to induce labor, with no success. External fetal monitors, internal fetal monitors, two relatively mild contractions, one centimeter dilation and absolutely no response from the baby from the pitocin. That was when the doctor on call became... concerned. When he broke this news to me, I began having concerns of my own.

My obstetrician was out of town, my husband had just left to pick up the video camera (we somehow managed to forget

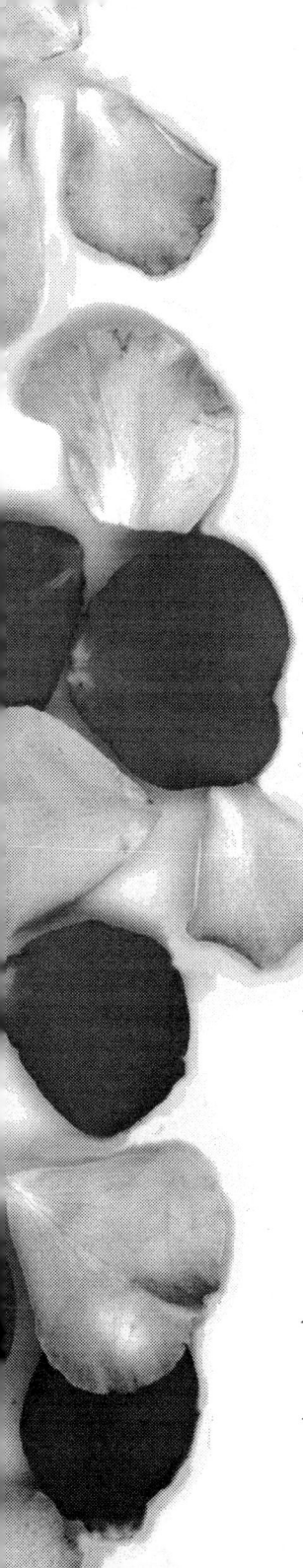

it) and I had my first anxiety attack. There is nothing quite like making a decision about an operation you had no reason to anticipate, with a doctor you've never seen before who is worried about your baby's lack of responsiveness, when at the same time, you're hooked up to several machines and you're temporarily all alone. What was I going to say when he suggested a Cesarean? Of course I would go ahead!

After I made the decision, however, things improved dramatically. Once my husband returned (barely in time) I no longer felt as vulnerable to forces I could not control. The procedure went smoothly, from the spinal anesthesia to the delivery of my healthy, screaming daughter. Even my recovery seemed idyllic. There was pain, yes, for two or three days, and walking or climbing stairs was a challenge. But I have no recollection of the prolonged, painful recovery associated with Cesarean births that you read about in so many books. Breast-feeding was going well, I felt strong and was back at work, with my daughter in tow, in a month.

It was a small wonder that when I was pregnant with my son I was so willing to go this route again. This pregnancy, though similarly medically uneventful, was significantly more stressful. My husband and I were now both in medical school and we had a bright and busy two-year-old. The pace of our lives had definitely quickened. When presented with the predictability of another Cesarean, I grabbed it. No one I talked to, including my obstetrician, could understand my willingness to undergo this procedure again. Many talked about the joy of giving birth the "natural way," as I, in polite silence, wondered what was so natural about enduring ten or more hours of medicated yet excruciating pain while I tried to squeeze my child through an orifice obviously several times smaller than he was?

Anyway, it was clear almost from the beginning of the procedure that my son had no intention of being a clone of his sister. When the epidural somehow managed to numb only one side of my body, I knew things would be different this time. Another epidural did the trick, but a little too well, so that as my newborn was being brought to me, I started feeling light-

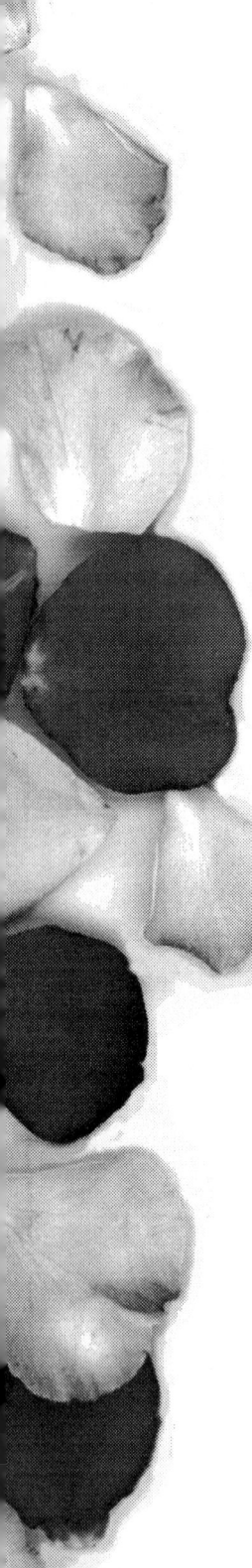

headed and unable to control my breathing. Knowing that this happened from two doses of anesthetic only partially controlled the tendency to panic, but I think I managed not to become too obnoxious (the nurses were still nice to me afterward) until the drug wore off somewhat. Still, it was several hours before I could feel my toes again.

In short, this experience did not gel with my rosy recollection of the previous Cesarean. After the anesthetic wore off, I was left with an uncontrollable itch over my whole body that lasted for several days. Though the pain from my incision was manageable, a small urethral tear which occurred during catheterization caused my urethra to go into spasm at the mere thought of passing any fluid. The three-day hospital stay, which had been such a welcome respite the last time, this time seemed fraught with an ever-changing stream of people wanting to prod, poke, question, feed, measure or record every bodily fluid that I or the baby passed. I got no rest and our son, whom we had the audacity not to name yet, was also cranky.

I only felt like I was starting to recover when I was among familiar people and surroundings at home. Even then, it was not a straightforward process: I had an inquisitive and demanding two-year-old around, our new home had more stairs to climb and curiously, the skin around my incision (not the incision itself) felt stretched, and hurt for many weeks afterward. I will not even describe how long it takes for a urethral tear to heal completely.

Through both of my Cesareans, I have learned a few lessons. Birth experiences are as individual as the children they produce. In recovery, age and stress must definitely be factors. In the end, the decision about what type of birth experience you have should be made by you and your partner. Also, realize sometimes you may not have a choice. Try to stay flexible, remembering that birth is a process. The important part is the outcome: having a healthy child. Almost everything else either heals or passes with time. We feel as blessed with our two healthy children as we would had they been delivered to us in any other way. 🌿

QUESTIONS AND ANSWERS
The Emergency Cesarean Birth

In this section of the resource guide, we address many birth experiences. The majority of women will not experience our final topic—an emergency Cesarean birth. This interview with Dr. Ralph Neighbor, a North Seattle obstetrician and gynecologist, will offer a glimpse of an emergency Cesarean birth.

Q. What is an emergency Cesarean birth and why would it be medically necessary?

A. An emergency Cesarean birth is a response to a rapidly deteriorating situation. The fetus may be acutely deprived of oxygen and is in distress. The mother may start to hemorrhage. When these events occur, immediate intervention is life-saving. The American College of Obstetricians and Gynecologists (ACOG) recommends that once the decision for an emergency Cesarean birth is made, the operation should begin within 30 minutes. Often the time is shorter.

Q. How does the emergency Cesarean birth differ from a non-emergency Cesarean birth?

A. With non-emergency and scheduled Cesarean births, there is plenty of time to discuss and answer questions so parents understand the procedures and the order of events. With the emergency Cesarean birth, the rapid safe delivery of the child and the physical safety of the mother are paramount. Things are moving very quickly and there is often little time for explanations or discussion. Additional hospital staff may appear "out of the woodwork," so there may be an appearance of confusion. Rest assured that each of the professionals is preparing for the baby's immediate birth and attending to the comfort of the mother.

Q. What happens to the father or support person during an emergency Cesarean birth?

A. In an emergency, the father or support person may be sent to a waiting area or be asked to stay in the mother's room. The team handling the emergency can respond with the greatest speed and efficiency without extra people in the way. If feasible, the father might be able to be included, and if not, someone should be available to explain to him what is happening.

Q. Is a woman awake during an emergency Cesarean birth?

A. That depends. If the mother has an epidural anesthetic in place when the emergency is declared, then that may be used as anesthesia for the Cesarean birth. If there is no anesthesia in place, a general anesthetic (where mother is put to sleep) renders her pain-free in a few minutes. The general anesthetic is preferred because of this rapid onset of action. Spinal anesthesia takes around 15 minutes to result in adequate "numbness" for surgery to proceed comfortably, and the epidural block takes more than 30 minutes. On rare occasions, an emergency Cesarean is done under local anesthesia, but that alternative is not a favorite.

Q. *What should a woman expect during recovery from an emergency Cesarean birth?*

A. Usually the recovery from an emergency Cesarean birth is little different than the recovery from other Cesarean births. The general anesthetic may leave the mother drowsy for several hours and delay holding the baby, delay the initiation of the bonding process, and postpone the first nursing. The newer drugs used for general anesthesia wear off more rapidly than the old pentothal, and mothers are alert much quicker than they used to be.

It is important that the physician sit down with the new parents and give a thorough debriefing concerning the emergency and the team's response to it. This should be done at a time after the couple has had a chance to rest and the mother is feeling better. The new mother and father should be encouraged to voice their feelings and have all their questions answered.

The average hospital stay after Cesarean birth is two to five days. After the operation, the mother is "recovered" by a specially trained nurse for an hour or so until all effects of the anesthesia have reversed. Monitoring of vital signs continues. Deep breathing is encouraged to avoid the complication of pneumonia. It may be a day before the mother's stomach is ready to tolerate food. The incision can be quite sore for about a week and the mother will have to take medication to help with the pain. Full recovery from the Cesarean birth takes four to six weeks, but the mother is usually able to take care of her new baby and attend to most of her own personal needs three to four days after the operation.

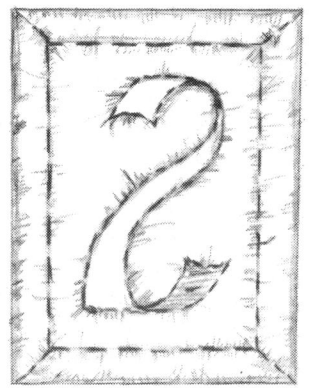

PREPARATION
FOR
BABY

THE LIGHTER SIDE OF PREGNANCY

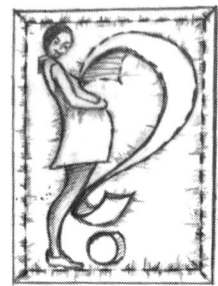

A dear friend, Claire Voyant, who has had experience dealing with over six pregnant couples, has graciously agreed to answer the most often asked questions about pregnancy, childbirth and babies, no matter how ridiculous they may be (the questions, not the babies).

By Joyce Armor

Q: I'm two months pregnant now. When will my baby move?

A: With any luck, it will be right after he finishes college, but some kids hang on a few years longer.

Q: What is the most common method of determining a baby's sex?

A: Childbirth.

Q: Will my baby be born with strawberry birthmarks if I eat too many strawberries while I'm pregnant?

A: No, and the baby won't be born with shingles if you re-roof the house while you're pregnant either.

Q: My brother says that, since my husband has a big nose and big noses are dominant, the baby I'm expecting will have a big nose as well. Is this true?

A: The odds are greater that your brother will have a fat lip.

Q: What's the easiest way to figure out exactly when I got pregnant?

A: Have sex once a year.

Q: *Why don't more women carry twins?*

A: They don't have enough womb.

Q: *All the expectant women I know seem so sure of themselves. Am I the only pregnant woman who has ever had second thoughts about becoming a mother?*

A: Yes.

Q: *My wife is six months pregnant and so moody that she overreacts to the simplest problem. Sometimes she's borderline irrational.*

A: So? What's the question?

Q: *Should I stay away from funerals while I'm pregnant?*

A: Yes, unless you know the deceased.

Q: *What is this pregnancy "glow" I've heard so much about?*

A: When someone tells you you have the pregnancy glow, it can be roughly translated into: "No, really, you don't look fat."

Q: *Will my wife's breasts stay this big after our baby is born?*

A: If she's nursing, her breasts will get even bigger, but you probably won't be allowed near them.

Q: *When is it safe to have sex during pregnancy?*

A: When your wife agrees to it.

Q: *How will I know if my baby has dropped?*

A: He'll start crying. Be more careful.

Q: *Where should my husband stand during our baby's delivery?*

A: By your head, infringing on your view in the mirror.

Q: *My childbirth instructor says that it's not pain you feel during labor, but pressure. Is she right?*

A: Yes, in the same way that a tornado might be called an air current.

Q: *Is there any reason I have to be in the delivery room when my wife gives birth?*

A: Not unless the word "alimony" holds any meaning for you.

Q: *Under what circumstances should a baby not be circumcised?*

A: When it's a girl, for starters.

Q: *Do newborns have a sense of taste?*

A: Apparently not, or why would so many of them wear those shapeless sacques and washed-out colors?

Q: *Please settle an argument I'm having with my sister. Can a mother get pregnant while nursing her baby?*

A: Yes, but it's much easier if she removes the baby from her breast and puts him down for a nap first.

Q: *Does nursing make breasts sag?*

A: Not any more than doctoring or lawyering.

Q: *What is the biggest difference between cloth diapers and disposable diapers?*

A: Disposable diapers make lousy dust rags.

Q: *Does pregnancy affect perms?*

A: Yes, and it also affects temps.

Q: *Will I love my dog less when my baby is born?*

A: No, but your husband will probably get on your nerves.

Q: *When does a woman's biological clock start ticking?*

A: Right after the stroke of "Oh, my God, crow's feet!"

Q: *Does pregnancy age a woman?*

A: Of course not. That's ridiculous. It's raising children that makes women old before their time.

Q: *Does pregnancy cause dandruff?*

A: Pregnancy causes anything you want to blame it for. That's the least it can do.

Q: *Should I be flushed while pregnant?*

A: Not unless you're a toilet.

Q: *What happens to disposable diapers after they're thrown away?*

A: They are being stored in a silo in the Midwest in the event of global chemical warfare.

Q: *I'm pregnant for the first time, and I'm already worried about how far apart I should space my children. What do the experts say?*

A: Most experienced parents space their children at least 6 feet apart.

WHERE TO SHOP

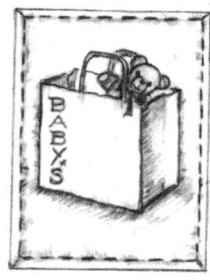

The list below should give you an idea of local stores, pricing, quality of merchandise and service. Keep in mind that although we tried to be as objective as possible, the shopping team may have had personal biases. Most stores were shopped only once and at only one location. We tried to highlight the unique things each store offers. We do not endorse any particular store nor were we paid for these reviews.

There are many places to shop in the greater Seattle area for maternity and baby items. You have the choice of shopping at department stores, discount chains, boutiques or consignment shops. Depending upon what you are looking for, each type of store has its advantages.

First-time parents who have little or no experience shopping for maternity or baby products may want to visit a variety of stores before making their purchasing decisions.

BABY PRODUCT STORES

■ BABY DEPOT—BURLINGTON COAT FACTORY

776-2221
24111 Hwy. 99
Edmonds, WA 98020
Hours: M-Sat. 10:00 a.m.-9:30 p.m.
          Sun.   11:00 a.m.-6:00 p.m.

575-3995
17900 Southcenter Pkwy.
Tukwila, WA 98188
Hours: M-Sat. 9:30 a.m.-9:00 p.m.
          Sun.   11:00 a.m.-6:00 p.m.
As the name implies, Burlington sells coats (lots and lots of them!), but they also

have a complete baby department, with everything from clothing to furniture. Their furniture department is one of the largest in the area, with many cribs and toddler beds on display, all featuring co-ordinated bedding and accessories in attractive themes. There are also plenty of strollers, car seats, playpens, swings, rocking chairs, lamps, and other furniture items. The Baby Depot carries major brands like Childcraft, Century, Simmons, Graco, Aprica, and Perego, and prices are discounted about 20-30% from other retail outlets.

Besides furniture, a well-stocked accessories section includes nursing supplies, safety items, baby bottles, bibs, toys, books, car seat covers, diaper bags, bedding, and more. You can also sign up for the mother-to-be registry.

The store has a large baby clothes section where they carry popular brands in both casual and dressy styles, again at discounted prices. They have preemie sizes available, as well as some christening gowns. There's also a small maternity section with casual and career wear, nursing lingerie, and maternity hose.

The Baby Depot offers a 10% discount when you buy an identical item for a twin (or triplets!). The staff were very helpful and considerate, and quite knowledgeable about the wide range of products they carry. One store policy to be aware of at Burlington is that they don't do cash (or credit card) returns, only exchanges or in-store credits.

■ BELLINI JUVENILE DESIGNER FURNITURE [Baby Pages]
451-0126
201 Bellevue Way N.E.
Bellevue, WA 98004
Hours: M-Sat.   10:00 a.m.-6:00 p.m.
        Th   until 8:00 p.m.

Just a few blocks from Bellevue Square, in the Park Row Shopping Center, is Bellini Juvenile Designer Furniture. Bellini presents a beautiful display of cribs, bedroom sets, and accessories. The products are high quality with a definite designer feel. You can think of Bellini as the kind of store that sells only the best. The store also carries Perego strollers as well as beautiful quilts and linens both affordable and heirloom quality. Bellini is best known for their cribs. Every Bellini crib converts into a youth bed, saving parents the extra expense of purchasing a toddler bed later. The furniture you purchase at Bellini will last for years and retain its quality. Prices are more affordable than you may think, with cribs in the $400 range.

Bellini carries birth announcements that can be custom ordered and offers numerous wallpaper and nursery decoration catalogs to help you design that very special room. They also offer free gift wrapping and a baby registry.

■ CHILDREN'S WORLD
451-0833
10843 N.E. 8th St.
Bellevue, WA 98004
Hours: M, T, W 10:00 a.m. - 6:00 p.m.
        Th, F   until 8:00 p.m.
        Sat.   10:00 a.m.-6:00 p.m.
        Sun.   12:00-5:00 p.m.

South of Bellevue Square is a great baby products store that offers expectant parents a wide array of merchandise from the usual to the unusual. Children's World carries everything from cribs to strollers to bedding to mobiles. I found an excellent buy manufactured by Baby's Dream for parents who want furniture to grow with their child—a crib that eventually converts to a double bed. Parents buy a conversion kit and the crib grows to a youth bed and then a double bed. This product ran about $289.

Bassinets, youth beds, dressers, and rocking chairs are also available at this unique store. Ask about their free gift wrapping, baby registry, and layaway plan.

■ A CHILD'S ROOM

643-7050
15123 N.E. 24th St.
Redmond, WA 98052
Hours: M-Sat.   10:00 a.m.-6:00 p.m.
       Sun.   Noon-5:00 p.m.

Located off the 148th N.E. exit from the 520 freeway, A Child's Room is just east of the Overlake Sears store. There's a dreamy feel to this place as you walk in and notice the bedroom sets, attractively outfitted in themes from Winnie the Pooh to the Wild West. Although the store specializes in furniture for bigger kids, they do have a baby section that includes a selection of lamps, mobiles, wall hangings, night lights, and picture frames.

A Child's Room also carries a nice assortment of books, rattles, stuffed animals and toys for baby, as well as baby books and family memory books. They have some clothing in infant and toddler sizes too, by such makers as Little Me and Gear Kids.

■ GO TO YOUR ROOM

453-2990
13000 Bel-Red Rd.
Bellevue, WA 98007
Hours: M-Sat.   10:00 a.m.-6:00 p.m.
       Sun.   Noon-5:00 p.m.

528-0711
6411 12th N.E. (Roosevelt Square)
Seattle, WA 98115
Hours: M-Sat.   10:00 a.m.-6:00 p.m.
       Sun.   Noon-5:00 p.m.

Go To Your Room offers an extensive selection of furniture, bedding, and accessories for both infants and older children. Their vast array of cribs, lamps, rockers, mobiles, strollers, wall hangings, posters, and other room decor enables you to put an entire nursery together in a relaxed, friendly atmosphere. Started by two mothers, their stores reflect what they feel meets the needs of other parents. A good selection of more than a dozen popular cribs that include Simmons, Childcraft, and Ragazzi, are fully outfitted with coordinated bedding from Nojo, California Kids, and Pine Creek Bedding, to name a few. There are also quite a few strollers from such makers as Emmaljunga, Combi, and Racing Strollers (of Yakima). They feature two sleek yet practical high chairs from Baby Trend and Chicco. Both are easy-to-clean with multiple position seats (one lifts off for attaching to the table), and have a wide base with swivel wheels that lock. They have the biggest selection of glider rockers from Dutailier in the area. You may choose from chairs in stock, or custom order one from the catalog in a different finish or fabric. Go To Your Room also has their own on-site warehouse which makes furniture pick-up easy. Delivery and assembly are also available. As parents, the owners believe in making the stores as kid (and parent)-friendly as possible. They encourage your children see, touch and sit on the furniture. Duplo tables and puzzles are also available for your children to play with, so they won't get bored during shopping.

Go to Your Room offers in-store financing and a baby gift registry too.

■ GRANDMOTHER'S HOUSE

771-4640
7331 196th S.W.
Lynnwood, WA 98036
Hours: M-Sat.   9:30 a.m.-5:30 p.m.
Sun.   Noon-5:00 p.m.

Located west of Hwy. 99 on 196th S.W., the store occupies both the upstairs and downstairs of a house-turned-store. Outdoor items (trikes, bikes, strollers, play equipment) fill the front yard, and it seems that every available space inside is used to display something. Part of the reason for the (over)abundance of merchandise is that this store has been in business for over 20 years. The majority of items are used, and since the store buys items outright (no consignment), that makes for an ongoing and growing accumulation of merchandise.

There's definitely lots to choose from here, with rooms full of baby swings (at least 20, priced from $25-$30), high chairs (at least 15, from $16-$45), and play pens (more than 6, from $40-$60). They've got plenty of toys, books, bedding, and clothes (including a whole rack of Osh-Kosh) too. I found shopping here a bit overwhelming, something like shopping in a too-crowded thrift store, but other parents were delighting in their discoveries. The prices on many items seemed a bit high for used, especially compared to local consignment store prices for similar items, and even compared to new items at discount stores. There were also several signs posted that warned that not all items met federal safety standards; presumably store staff could advise on that further before you make a purchase.

■ IKEA

656-2980 or 800-570-4532
600 S.W. 53rd St.
Renton, WA 98055
Hours: M-F   10:00 a.m.-9:00 p.m.
Sat.   10:00 a.m.-7:00 p.m.
Sun.   10:00 a.m.-6:00 p.m.

IKEA is more than just the largest home furnishing store in the Northwest, it's also a shopping adventure. It's a great place to spend a few hours on a rainy afternoon: covered parking, free strollers, a restaurant with Swedish meatballs, kids' menu, and other treats, and even a play area for kids (toddlers and older) to stay while you shop. If the possibilities seem overwhelming on the first visit, just pick up a catalog to take home and browse at your leisure.

In the Kids Corner, they carry several cribs, changing tables, wardrobes, and high chairs, as well as room accessories, bedding, wooden and stuffed toys, and more. Brands include Mandrill, Bra, Narvik, Bandiller, and Marmosa. A crib by Gulliver is priced at just $89; a high chair and tray set by Kameleont costs $89 too, and features an adjustable seat and footrest to grow with baby. For toddlers and older, the Mammut line of furniture features whimsical designs with funny shapes and patterns and cartoon colors. Items include a flip-out sofa bed for $199, a bed and mattress set for $229, and oversized striped armchair for $98, and a wooden chair for $19. The emphasis at IKEA is on quality products that are affordably priced. Since they have many of their large stores around the world, they're able to buy in volume. Getting items home is easy too; most are packed in flat boxes for home assembly. In-store assembly is also available, as well as home delivery for large furniture items and rooftop carrier rentals.

■ **KIDS CLUB** [Baby Pages]
643-5437
15600 N.E. 8th
Bellevue, WA 98008
Hours: M-Sat. 10:00 a.m.-9:00 p.m.
            Sun.   11:00 a.m.-6:00 p.m.

524-2553
2676 N.E. University Village Mall
Seattle, WA 98105
Hours: M-F   10:00 a.m.-8:00 p.m.
            Sat.   10:00 a.m.-6:00 p.m.
            Sun.   Noon-6:00 p.m.

Located in the south end of Crossroads Mall, the Bellevue Kids Club store is a complete department store for kids. It's bright, clean, colorful, and very welcoming—the kind of store that you'll want to walk through slowly, so you don't miss anything. There's a well-stocked shoe department, with Keds Prewalkers, Weeboks, and more, all affordably priced. There's lots and lots of cute clothing for infants and children, and plenty of hats, bows, and other items for accessorizing.

The toy section is quite complete too, with items for all ages from infants to school-age—toys, puzzles, Brio kits, stuffed animals, books, cassettes, and more. Near the toy section, the store offers a complete Medela nursing display, with nursing supplies and pillows. They also sell feeding products of the Avent line, including bottles and bottle sterilizers, a manual breast pump, and breastfeeding accessories. Other baby products include a full line of safety items.

Kids Club's furniture and equipment section takes up about half the store. There's a full selection of cribs (more than 20 on display when I visited) by such makers as Simmons, Ragazzi, and Childcraft. Prices were reasonable and some items were on sale. A rocking bassinet by Simmons caught my eye, as did the rows of strollers and high chairs. Cribs were adorned with attractive bedding options and accessories by Nojo, Cotton Tale Designs, and other manufacturers. Special orders are welcome too, and the sales associates here go out of their way to help you and to make you feel welcome. Kids Club has several play areas to keep your children occupied while you shop; they also offer a baby registry and from time to time they have free parenting classes and story hours.

The Kids Club at University Village is a smaller store, featuring the high-quality clothing and accessories that the Bellevue Kids Club is well-known for. They also offer toys, breastfeeding supplies, and other baby items. Furniture is carried from time to time and can be ordered from the Bellevue store for delivery directly to your home. An added plus when shopping at this store are the new features of the upgraded University Village shopping center. There's an outdoor play area for kids ages 2-6 and some fun cow sculptures, as well as an assortment of new and remodeled restaurants and the Barnes and Noble superstore.

■ KYM'S KIDDY CORNER
361-5974
11721 15th Ave. N.E.
Seattle, WA 98125
Hours: M-Sat.   10:00 a.m.-5:30 p.m.
       Sun.   Noon-5:00 p.m.

In business for more than ten years, Kym's Kiddy Corner is a popular destination for north Seattle parents looking for one-stop shopping. Here you'll find a great mix of both new and used items—clothing, equipment, furniture, toys, books, music, and more.

It's easy to find Kym's Kiddy Corner as you drive up 15th N.E. (north of Northgate Way), since the front yard has an eye-catching line-up of trikes, bikes, strollers, riding toys, and outdoor play equipment. More equipment and furniture is displayed on the porch area and in a full room inside. Kym's carries an assortment of packaged safety items by Safety 1st, as well as other new accessories and toys. They have several products by Fisher Price (booster seats, toys) and Little Tikes (potty seats for $18), umbrella strollers ($25) and double strollers ($70-$99). Prices for used swings range from $15-$40, high chairs from $13-$40, and playpens in the $14-35 range. This store carries cribs, too; there are at least 6 available to choose from.

The clothing selection at Kym's is excellent, with sizes from newborn to 14. There are lots of used clothes in good condition and reasonably priced. The store carries an assortment of new clothes too, including the locally popular Cotton Caboodle line and some very pretty dresses by Jo Lene starting at $40. Kym's Kiddy Corner will also buy or trade for your used baby and children's items. You get cash or store credit the same day for your brand-name clothes, furniture, toys or equipment.

Since Kym and her employees often bring their own children to work, the store is quite child-safe and family-friendly. The playroom in the back has toys and videos, so you can shop in relative peace while your child is occupied.

■ MERRY GO ROUND BABY NEWS
454-1610
11111 N.E. 8th St.
Bellevue, WA 98004
Hours: M-Sat.   10:00 a.m.-6:00 p.m.
       Th   until 8:00 p.m.
       Sun.   Noon-5:00 p.m.

Merry Go Round sells both clothing and baby products, making it convenient for parents to shop in one place. It offers a wide selection of cribs, strollers and car seats. Product lines include Simmons, Child Craft, Graco, Kolcraft, Aprica, Combi and more. Pricing is competitive—during my visit, several cribs were available in the $300 range.

Merry Go Round also carries a nice selection of infant and toddler clothing. The clothing selection had many brand name designers to choose from. Plan on spending $13 on up for an infant's outfit. The store had one of the widest selections of preemie outfits and accessories we found. Along the front wall were clothing, hats, and even Pampers diapers. They also had christening gowns for both boys and girls. One of my favorite brands for a girl's christening gown, Sweet Baby Jess, was available here. Merry Go Round is located near Bellevue Square and has been in business since 1947.

■ **TOYS R US**
771-4748
18601 Alderwood Mall Blvd.
Lynnwood, WA 98036

575-0780
16700 Southcenter Pkwy.
Tukwila, WA 98168

946-0433
31510 20th St.
Federal Way, WA 98023

453-1901
103 100th N.E.
Bellevue, WA 98004

353-8697
1325 S.E. Everett Mall Way
Everett, WA 98204
Hours: M-Sat.   9:30 a.m.-9:30 p.m.
            Sun.   10:00 a.m.-7:00 p.m.
Toys R Us carries a wide variety of baby items from diapers and formula to car seats and strollers to baby bottles and diaper bags. They offer about everything under the sun for your baby. Check out the baby registry, where you can register for all your baby needs. Baby product brands include Fisher Price, Graco, Kolcraft, Petrus, Century, Renolux, Evenflo, and Cosco. The only difficulty with carrying so many products is the large amount of space needed. Because of this, many of the products are overhead and difficult to reach. To "test-drive" those products you need to ask for staff assistance. Toys R Us carries a large supply of strollers, swings and car seats and a relatively small selection of cribs. To stay competitive, Toys R Us offers a price guarantee.

Besides products, Toys R Us also offers infant clothing and, of course, toys. The baby clothing section consists of sleepers, play and dress outfits, jackets,

swim suits and tons of socks. Playskool sleepers begin at $6 and play outfits average about $8. You'll also find a huge selection of toys that has everything from Barbie to Legos to mini kitchens and mini race cars. It is a smorgasbord of the latest commercial toys. The toy selection is truly overwhelming. With this in mind, once your child nears the age of two, shopping together at Toys R Us will be a challenge, so be prepared and beware.

MATERNITY STORES

■ **A PEA IN THE POD**
292-9200
Westlake Center
400 Pine
Seattle, WA 98101
Hours: M-Sat.   9:30 a.m.-9:00 p.m.
            (winter hours until 8:00 p.m.)
            Sun.   11:00 a.m.-7:00 p.m.
            (winter hours until 6:00 p.m)
This elegant maternity boutique believes you don't have to compromise fashion during pregnancy. A Pea in The Pod has a dynamic selection of tailored business suits, career and casual dresses which range from $68 to $185. The casual selection ranges from conservative to trendy.

The selection of special occasion evening wear features everything from simple black dresses to beaded evening gowns—all of which are gorgeous. A Pea In The Pod offers its own label, as well as other designer labels, in petite to larger sizes. One- and two-piece maternity swimsuits are available year-round starting at $58. The store also carries a variety of maternity lingerie.

There is a nice sitting area with toys, so husbands and children are made to feel welcome. A Pea in the Pod also has a personal shopping service and overnight shipping. Watch this store for sales. Mark-down merchandise may be discounted as much as 75%.

■ **BABY LOVE MATERNITY**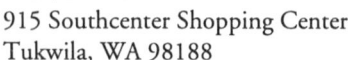
246-7111
915 Southcenter Shopping Center
Tukwila, WA 98188

362-1021
758 Northgate Mall
Seattle, WA 98125

776-1262
574 Alderwood Mall
Lynnwood, WA 98046

454-2122
231 Bellevue Square
Bellevue, WA 98004
Hours: Vary with each store.
              Same hours as mall(s).

Baby Love is the largest chain of maternity clothing in the Seattle area. It is also the oldest. Baby Love opened its doors in 1973 and has expanded its business since. Located conveniently in four major malls, customers can shop 7 days a week and evening hours. At Baby Love, you'll find a wide array of clothing and accessories. They offer clothing that is comfortable as well as career attire. Pricing is competitive with other large maternity stores. Career dresses starts around $70. Most dresses are very fashionable and fun. Casual clothing costs about $25 on up. And, for the budget conscious, a clearance rack offers excellent buys. Baby Love also offers a huge selection of undergarments, including hose, bras, and nursing wear. Most of the undergarments are behind the counter, so you'll need to ask a sales person for the merchandise. Also, Baby Love now rents hospital-grade Medela breast pumps.

■ **BIRTH AND BEYOND**
324-4831
2610 E. Madison St.
Seattle, WA 98112

Owned by Lyndsey Starkey, Birth and Beyond is truly a unique maternity store—unique in the fact that it does not carry maternity clothing, but instead just about anything else you may want during pregnancy and postpartum. You'll find a wide selection of nursing clothing, books, tapes, breast pumps, slings, music and much more at this sophisticated, yet friendly store. Besides offering products, Birth and Beyond also has childbirth classes, a resource lending library and much-appreciated personal attention to its customers. We also found many unique local products here. If you're pregnant, have a new baby or are just interested in learning more about childbirth, this store should be a definite stop.

■ **DESIGNER MATERNITY**
    FACTORY AND KIDS RACK
451-1945
11010 N.E. 8th St.
Bellevue, WA 98004
Hours: M-Sat.   10:00 a.m.-6:00 p.m.
              Sun.   Noon -5:00 p.m.

Only one block from Children's World and a few blocks from Bellevue Square Mall is a small "home"-like store that carries a wide variety of maternity wear.

    At first when you drive up to the store it seems a little unconventional, as the entrance is difficult to find. Once you enter the store, you'll find a nice variety of maternity clothing, with brands such as Hayley Michaels, One on the Way, Dressing for Two, and many others. Clothing ranges from the sophisticated to the fun and funky. Prices start at about $20 for most items and expect to find an average work dress starting at $50. The quality, however, at this store is still excellent— even though the prices may be lower. You'll also find one-on-one service as the owner, Denise, and her employees provide individual fashion coordinating for moms-to-be. During our visit, she offered many good suggestions from clothing to nursing bras. Best of all, they have a bathroom easily accessible for any pregnant woman—a definite plus in this book.

And, if you're looking for children's or infant clothing, this store offers a variety of apparel at 50-70% below retail. You'll find name brands, party dresses (they have some great velveteens) and daily wear at very affordable prices.

■ MIMI MATERNITY
637-8785
Bellevue Square
Bellevue, WA 98004
Hours: M -Sat. 9:30 a.m.-9:30 p.m.
           Sun   11:00 a.m.-6:00 p.m.

Mimi Maternity is owned by the same company as A Pea in the Pod. The difference you'll find between the two stores is Mimi is a little more contemporary and casual than A Pea in the Pod. The prices are also slightly lower. Quality, fun, and fashionable is the best way to describe this store. And, it is difficult to imagine the clothing in stock as maternity wear. It's like looking at all the most fashionable styles and realizing you don't have to miss out on the latest look even though you're pregnant. Items start at about $20 on up. Mimi also has nursing bras, underwear, and lingerie. I found the staff at Bellevue Square very knowledgeable and helpful. Also, look for a Mimi Maternity brochure that offers a $10 off coupon for any item of $50 or more.

■ MOTHERHOOD
454-1355
Bellevue Square
Bellevue, WA 98004
Hours: M-Sat.   9:30 a.m.-9:30 p.m.
           Sun.   11:00 a.m.-6:00 p.m.

Motherhood is conveniently located on the ground floor of Bellevue Square, two stores down from the Tugboat. As part of a national chain, it offers only the "Motherhood" label. There is a nice selection of casual and professional clothing mid-priced to upscale. Dresses range in price from $40 to $100, shorts and tops between $20 and $40, and pants and skirts from $20 to $50. The store also carries maternity undergarments including pantyhose and nursing bras.

During my visit, many items were on sale at substantial savings. A mailing list is available to keep customers informed about upcoming sales. The sales staff is very friendly, helpful and upbeat.

■ VILLAGE MATERNITY [Baby Pages]
523-5167
2635 N.E. University Village Mall
Seattle, WA 98105
Hours: M-F   10:00 a.m.-8:00 p.m.
           Sat.   10:00 a.m.-6:00 p.m.
           Sun.   11:00 a.m.-5:00 p.m.

Voted as best maternity store by Seattle's Child readers, Village Maternity is conveniently located in the University Village. Village Maternity prides itself in offering primarily 100% cotton clothing for both children and expectant mothers. In maternity wear, mothers can find stylish and contemporary clothing. Many of the items had a natural and comfortable feel. Sweaters, jumpers and business suits all offer an original "Seattle" feel. I also found nursing tops and one of my favorite brands, Japanese Weekend, at Village Maternity.

Formal Wear rentals are available for your special occasion. Pricing is very competitive.

For children's wear, the selection is a little bit smaller, but complete. All children's clothing is 100% cotton with most of the name brands you would expect. A variety of play and dress clothing is available for infants and toddlers.

DEPARTMENT/ DISCOUNT STORES

■ BEST PRODUCTS, CO., INC.
454-5696
888 116th N.E.
Bellevue, WA 98004

775-9311
19801 40th Ave. W.
Lynnwood, WA 98036

941-5000
2200 S. 320th
Federal Way, WA 98003

248-2377
240 Andover Park W.
Tukwila, WA 98188

258-4251
1001 N. Broadway
Everett, WA 98201
Hours: M-Sat.   10:00 a.m.-9:00 p.m.
        Sun.   11:00 a.m.-6:00 p.m.
Best Products offers a wide selection of baby products at competitive prices. You'll find Graco, Gerry, Cosco, Petrus, Kolcraft, and Fisher Price brands readily available. The store has a moderate supply of cribs (only seven at one store), but a larger supply of strollers. Many of the strollers, portable cribs, and swings are on display on high shelves over your head, so bring a friend to help if you want to try out your prospective purchase. Diaper bags, bumper pads, and crib sets are available. There is a wide selection of Playskool, Disney, and Fisher Price toys.

Best is primarily a self-service store. There is a special procedure for customers to follow when purchasing an item. If you need assistance in bringing items to your car, Best's staff will help. It has a good return and price guarantee policy. Be sure to save your receipt in order to take advantage of this policy.

■ THE BON MARCHE
455-2121
400 Bellevue Square
Bellevue, WA 98004
Hours: M-Sat.   9:30 a.m.- 9:30 p.m.
        Sun.   11:00 a.m.-6:00 p.m.

344-2121
1601 3rd Avenue
Seattle, WA 98101
Hours: M-Sat.   10:00 a.m.-7:00 p.m.
        Sun.   Noon-6:00 p.m.

712-6000
18700 Alderwood Mall Blvd.
Lynnwood, WA 98037
Hours: M-Sat.   10:00 a.m.-9:00 p.m.
        Sun.   11:00 a.m.-6:00 p.m.

529-6000
1901 S. Sea Tac Mall
Federal Way, WA 98003
Hours: M-Sat.   10:00 a.m-9:00 p.m.
        Sun.   11:00 a.m.-6:00 p.m.

440-6000
602 Northgate Mall
Seattle, WA 98125
Hours: M-Sat.   10:00 a.m-9:00 p.m.
        Sun.   11:00 a.m.-6:00 p.m.

656-6000
500 Southcenter Shopping Center
Tukwila, WA 98188
Hours: M-Sat. 10:00 a.m-9:00 p.m.
Sun. 11:00 a.m.-6:00 p.m.

710-6000
1502 S.E. Everett Mall Way
Everett, WA 98204
Hours: M-Sat. 10:00 a.m.-9:00 p.m.
Sun. 11:00 a.m.-6:00 p.m.

The Bon Marche's infants and toddlers clothing section offers the impression of pure class. It carries delightful children's wear from name brand manufacturers such as Carter's, Little Me, Dior and Baby b'Gosh. Prices vary depending on the manufacturer. The Bon Marche also has a nice selection of preemie wear and christening gowns. And when shopping during one of their fantastic sales, prices are very competitive with even some of the discount stores. Quality and elegance is the best way to remember their infants and toddlers department.

The Bon Marche carries maternity clothes at their stores in downtown Seattle, Northgate, Everett, and Alderwood. The maternity department has a nice selection of dresses, separates, swimsuits, sleepwear, rompers, and maternity hose. They carry both upscale and casual clothing, in a range of prices. A full price Hayley Michaels pant suit cost $114, and denim overalls and jumpers by J. Michele were in the $50-60 range. There were some great bargains on the sales rack though, with colorful sweaters originally priced at $43 discounted to $12, and a rayon romper by Oh!Mamma reduced from $98 to $24.

At the Downtown and Northgate Bon Marche, you can also visit Toytropolis or the "city of toys." And, this it is...stroll through the "zoo" for a look at the selection of stuffed animals—everything from the whimsical to wild! Whatever your desire, Toytropolis has much to offer. Some of the well known brands include Brio, Playmobil, Educational Insights, Parent's Magazine Developmental Toys and Ravensburger. Free gift wrapping, children's activities, and special events are also just a few of the unique features you'll find at Toytropolis.

■ COSTCO

542-0494
Aurora Village
Hwy. 99 & 205th N.E.
Edmonds, WA 98020

622-1144
4401 4th St.
Seattle, WA 98105

874-0878
35100 Enchanted Pkwy.
Federal Way, WA 98023

828-6767
8629 120th N.E.
Kirkland, WA 98034

775-2577
19015 Hwy. 99
Lynnwood, WA 98036

575-3311
1160 Saxon Dr.
Tukwila, WA 98188

313-0964
1801 10th Ave. N.W.
Issaquah, WA 98027
Hours: M-F 11:00 a.m.-8:30 p.m.
Sat. 9:30 a.m.-6:00 p.m.
Sun. 10:00 a.m.-5:00 p.m.

This membership-only store is an excellent place to find bargains. Unfortunately, however, it does not always carry the same brands and so you never know what you'll find from one visit to the next. You also cannot depend on any sales help in making your baby product purchases. Costco usually does carry Huggies diapers in large packages of 160 in size medium and 120 in the large size. Also, Baby Fresh diaper wipes are often in stock. Products such as strollers and car seats usually can be found but the selection is limited to a few brands, including Baby Trend, Emmaljunga, Century and Gerry. There is also a good selection of clothing that includes the locally-made Cotton Caboodle, OshKosh b'Gosh, and Carter plush. Books are always a great bargain here. This section includes tape cassettes, and at times, crayons, paints, and markers. The toys are sometimes plentiful, especially during the summer and winter holiday seasons, but again, it is hit and miss.

Costco prices often beat any items you may find on sale at other stores. Check into a membership.

■ FRED MEYER

931-5550
801 Auburn Way N.
Auburn, WA 98002

865-8560
2041 148th N.E.
Bellevue, WA 98007

433-6411
14300 1st Ave. S.
Burien, WA 98168

348-8400
8530 Evergreen Way
Everett, WA 98208

952-0100
33702 21st Ave. S.W.
Federal Way, WA 98023

859-5500
10201 S.E. 240th
Kent, WA 98031

820-3200
12221 120th Ave. N.E.
Kirkland, WA 98034

670-0200
4615-A 196th S.W.
Lynnwood, WA 98036

840-8150
1100 N. Meridian St.
Puyallup, WA 98371

235-5350
17801 108th Ave. S.E.
Renton, WA 98055

328-6920
417 Broadway E.
Seattle, WA 98102

784-9600
100 N.W. 85th (Greenwood)
Seattle, WA 98117

546-0720
18325 Aurora Ave. N.
Seattle, WA 98133

440-2400
13000 Lake City Way N.E.
Seattle, WA 98125
Hours: Most stores,
           M-Sun. 7:00 a.m.-11:00 p.m.
Fred Meyer is the local leader in "one-stop" shopping, since nearly all of their stores include a full grocery store. In recent years they've made shopping even easier, since items purchased in any department can be paid for at one checkout line. They have a full line of baby products, including furniture, strollers, car seats, swings, monitors, toys, books, and safety items. The infants' and children's clothing departments offer a good variety

of affordable choices, from brand names like Gerber Babies to their own line, Fred Bear. Many of the larger stores also have a maternity department too, with a selection of apparel for expecting moms.

Fred Meyer discounts prices in all of their departments and has frequent sales and temporary price reductions. While it's certainly possible to find an individual item at a lower price somewhere else in town, it's unlikely that you'll find such a range of choices and overall low prices at any other single store.

Besides basic groceries, Fred Meyer was one of the first local grocery chains to offer a natural foods section—a trend that many other stores have followed. Most Fred Meyer's now have in-store delicatessens and bakeries. And five of the stores—Auburn, Bellevue, Federal Way, Puyallup, and Renton—have a family-friendly feature called "Freddy's Playland." It's an instore play area where you can drop off your preschoolers (2-6 yrs.) for up to one hour while you shop. There's no charge for this service and safety and health rules are strictly enforced. Parents and their kids get numbered ID bracelets and parents also get a pager so they can be contacted if needed.

■ KMART
228-5840
440 Rainier Ave. S.
Renton, WA 98055

363-6319
13200 Aurora Ave. N.
Seattle, WA 98133

747-4300
15015 Main St.
Bellevue, WA 98007

774-7726
22511 Hwy. 99
Edmonds, WA 98020

353-8103
8102 Evergreen Way
Everett, WA 98203

941-3820
1207 S. 320th
Federal Way, WA 98063

852-9071
24800 West Valley Highway
Kent, WA 98032

767-7004
7345 Delridge Way S.
Seattle, WA 98106
Hours: Daily   8:00 a.m.-9:00 p.m.
K-Mart is among the lowest priced local stores for maternity and infant wear. The maternity section has a few fashionable outfits (the New Edition line) for under $20 with most tops and pants available for under $10. Nursing bras and maternity underwear are located in this section and priced at $6 each. Depending on what store you visit, the merchandise and store appearance differs.

Infant attire ranges in price from $3 to $8. The store has a nice selection of clothing for newborns and also offers a large section containing bottles, rattles, bibs, cotton diapers, blankets and comforters.

The baby product selection equals that of other discount stores and is very well-priced. Evenflo, Fisher Price, Graco and Gerry were a few of the brands in stock. A Jenny Lind crib can be purchased for about $100 and many other popular products are available at close to the lowest prices in town.

❧ *Call ahead to confirm hours and locations.*

■ LAMONTS

771-6497
3100 184th St. S.W.
Lynnwood, WA 98037
Hours: M-Sat. 9:30 a.m.-9:30 p.m.
       Sun. 11:00 a.m.-6:00 p.m.

644-2941
15600 N.E. 8th
Bellevue, WA 98008
Hours: M-Sat. 10:00 a.m.-9:00 p.m.
       Sun. 11:00 a.m-6:00 p.m.

433-0676
460 S.W. 152nd
Burien, WA 98166
Hours: M-Sat. 10:00 a.m.-9:00 p.m.
       Sun. 11:00 a.m.-5:00 p.m.

644-2921
4001 Factoria Square Mall
Bellevue, WA 98006
Hours: M-Sat. 10:00 a.m.-9:00 p.m.
       Sun. 11:00 a.m.-6:00 p.m.

367-7716
Lake Forest Park
17171 Bothell Way N.E.
Seattle, WA 98155
Hours: M-Sat. 10:00 a.m.-9:00 p.m.
       Sun. 11:00 a.m.-5:00 p.m.

367-7690
900 Northgate Plaza
Seattle, WA 98125
Hours: M-Sat. 9:30 a.m.-9:30 p.m.
       Sun. 11:00 a.m.-6:00 p.m.

839-8950
2001 S. 320th
Federal Way, WA 98003
Hours: M-Sat. 10:00 a.m.-9:00 p.m.
       Sun. 11:00 a.m.-5:00 p.m.

821-7788
12601 120th N.E.
Kirkland, WA 98034

Hours: M-Sat. 10:00 a.m.-9:00 p.m.
       Sun. 11:00 a.m.-6:00 p.m.

938-4116
2600 S.W. Barton
Seattle, WA 98126
Hours: M-Sat. 10:00 a.m.-9:00 p.m.
       Sun. 11:00 a.m.-5:00 p.m.

557-6550
775 N.W. Gilman Blvd.
Issaquah, WA 98027
Hours: M-Sat. 10:00 a.m.-9:00 p.m.
       Sun. 11:00 a.m.-6:00 p.m.

Lamonts offers one of the nicest and most affordable selections of children's clothing around. During several visits, I took advantage of sale items on infants' wear. When on sale, basic clothing such as leggings and T-shirts are about as affordable as anywhere else in the city. They carry name brands such as Hush Puppies, OshKosh b'Gosh and Carter's. In fact, they offer a huge display of Carter's wear that includes T-shirts, sleep wear and blankets. This is a good place to shop for babies and children as it offers everything from play clothes to dress wear and the prices are great. Lamonts also offers a small selection of Carter's preemie wear starting at $10.

■ MARSHALL'S DEPARTMENT STORES

575-0141
17900 Southcenter Pkwy, Ste. 154
Tukwila, WA 98188

367-8520
15801 Westminister Way N.
Seattle, WA 98155

771-6045
3205 Alderwood Mall Blvd.
Lynnwood, WA 98036

644-2429
2150 148th Ave. N.E.
Redmond, WA 98052-5534
Hours: M-Sat.   10:00 a.m.-9:00 p.m.
　　　　Sun.   11:00 a.m.-6:00 p.m.
Marshall's infant/toddler section is well-marked with signs which are easily noticeable. Although the selection is limited, the prices are excellent. You will find many name brands that elsewhere may cost at least 20% more. Marshall's also has a small maternity clothing selection. You can count on a bargain when shopping at Marshall's.

■ MERVYN'S
941-8800
2201 S. 320th
Federal Way, WA 98003

672-7765
3301 184th S.W.
Lynnwood, WA 98037

643-6554
4126 124th S.E.
Bellevue, WA 98006

439-1919
1100 Southcenter Shopping Center
Tukwila, WA 98188

558-9500
17601 N.E. Union Hill Road
Redmond, WA 98052
Hours: M-F   10:00 a.m.-9:30 p.m.
　　　　Sat.   9:00 a.m.-9:30 p.m.
　　　　Sun.   10:00 a.m.-7:00 p.m.
Mervyn's is famous for its baby clothing sales. When a sale pops up, people line up outside the store's doors because of the quality of the merchandise that is discounted. OshKosh b'Gosh and Sprockets are just two of the lines Mervyn's carries. The Sprockets line is great for the necessary T-shirts, onesies, and jumpers. You

can buy clothing at Mervyn's from $8 on up. The infant department also has crib coordinates, layette items, stuffed animals and infant shoes.

■ NORDSTROM
628-2111
1501 5th
Seattle, WA 98101
Hours: M-Sat.   9:30 a.m.-8:00 p.m.
　　　　Sun.   11:00 a.m.-6:00 p.m.

246-0400
100 Southcenter Shopping Center
Tukwila, WA 98188
Hours: M-Sat.   9:30 a.m.-9:30 p.m.
　　　　Sun.   11:00 a.m.-6:00 p.m.

364-8800
715 Northgate Mall
Seattle, WA 98125
Hours: M-Sat.   9:30 a.m.-9:30 p.m.
　　　　Sun.   11:00 a.m.-6:00 p.m.

455-5800
100 Bellevue Square
Bellevue, WA 98004
Hours: M-Sat.   9:30 a.m.-9:30 p.m.
　　　　Sun.   11:00 a.m.-6:00 p.m.

771-5755
Alderwood Mall
2800 184th S.W.
Lynnwood, WA 98037
Hours: M-Sat.   9:30 a.m.-9:30 p.m.
　　　　Sun.   11:00 a.m.-6:00 p.m.
At Nordstrom, service and presentation are as close to perfection as you can find in a large department store. Seattle natives know the excellent reputation Nordstrom has built and maintained. The children's department is no exception. The selection is ample and the quality very good. Nordstrom offers its own lines—Basically Nordstrom and Baby N Hand (along with other name brands.) It also offers

everything from custom bedding to outerwear to toys. Voted by Seattle's Child as the best place to buy shoes, you'll find a wide array of styles and selection of your favorite brands that should last, at competitive prices.

I found Nordstrom a favorite place for special gift items. And, prices may surprise you. Even the most budget-conscious person can find something in their price range, such as soft and comfortable footed pajamas for only $9. Employees do a nice job of gift-wrapping at no extra cost, which is great when you're shopping for presents. A Seattle favorite, Nordstrom is a wonderful place to shop—sale or no sale!

■ JC PENNEY CO., INC.
771-9555
18601 33rd Ave. W.
Lynnwood, WA 98037
Hours: M-Sat.   10:00 a.m.-9:30 p.m.
       Sun.   11:00 a.m.-6:00 p.m.

454-8599
300 Bellevue Square
Bellevue, WA 98004
Hours: M-Sat.   9:30 a.m.-9:30 p.m.
       Sun.   11:00 a.m.-6:00 p.m.

361-2500
475 Northgate Mall
Seattle, WA 98125
Hours: M-Sat.   10:00 a.m.-9:30 p.m.
       Sun.   11:00 a.m.-6:00 p.m.

246-0850
1200 Southcenter Shopping Center
Tukwila, WA 98188
Hours: M-Sat.   10:00 a.m.-9:30 p.m.
       Sun.   11:00 a.m.-6:00 p.m.

852-3260
403 W. Meeker
Kent, WA 98031
Hours: M-F   10:00 a.m.-8:00 p.m.
       Sat.   10:00 a.m.-6:00 p.m.
       Sun.   11:00 a.m.-5:00 p.m.

Penney's has a nice selection of maternity and children's wear. Mid-priced maternity clothes are available with casual jumpers starting at $36 and career dresses starting at $64. They also have name-brand jeans and other casual attire that start at $20. For summer, they carry several cute floral outfits and Cherokee-brand relaxing wear. In the fall, the store offers corduroy jumpers and paisley patterns. Penney's also has its own line called Maternity Dividends. The maternity section has the basics and then some.

The infants' and toddlers' area features clothing, baby products, and a gift section. The clothing includes name brands such as Sesame Street and Carter's, as well as Penney's own line, Toddletime. A few preemie and christening outfits are also offered. A small selection of baby products are available. Books, toys, and stuffed animals are also in this department. Penny's offers a gift registry as well.

The Penney's store clerk reminded me the store has a catalog that offers a wide selection of merchandise. Delivery is available.

■ ROSS DRESS FOR LESS
575-0110
17672 Southcenter Pkwy.
Tukwila, WA 98188

644-2433
14327 N.E. 20th
Bellevue, WA 98007

941-2122
32075 Pacific Hwy S.
Federal Way, WA 98003

367-6030
13201-B Aurora Ave. N.
Seattle, WA 98133

623-6781
1418 3rd Ave.
Seattle, WA 98101

313-9616
975 N.E. Gilman Blvd. #D
Issaquah, WA 98027
Hours: M-Sat.   9:30 a.m.-9:00 p.m.
        Sun.   11:00 a.m.-6:00 p.m.
Ross carries brand-name clothing for a very reasonable price. You can find OshKosh b'Gosh, Levi's, Carter's and more at discounted prices. Girls' dresses can be found for under $10 and overalls are sold for about $15. The store also carries diaper bags, a few baby items, and infants' and children's shoes. Ross is one of the easier discount stores to shop at because each department is very organized and clearly labeled. Some Ross stores also carry a few reduced-priced maternity items.

■ **TJ MAXX**
363-9511
11029 Roosevelt Way N.E.
Seattle, WA 98125

946-2887
1910 S. 320th
Federal Way, WA 98063
Hours: M-Sat.   9:30 a.m.-9:30 p.m.
        Sun.   11:00 a.m.-7:00 p.m.
T.J. Maxx is a brand name discount store that offers an infants' and children's department located toward the back of the store. Prices here are very good, although their selection is limited to stock on hand.

This is a good place to shop when you have the time to go through the racks. It is also the kind of store you'll want to visit frequently, since the merchandise is always changing. Sock bins have great, durable OshKosh b'Gosh socks for at least half price.

■ **TARGET**
670-1435
18305 Alderwood Mall Blvd.
Lynnwood, WA 98036

575-0682
301 S. Strander Blvd.
Tukwila, WA 98188

932-1153
2800 S.W. Barton
Seattle, WA 98126

562-0830
4053 Factoria Square Mall S.E.
Bellevue, WA 98006

353-3167
405 S.E. Everett Mall Way
Everett, WA 98208

850-9710
26301 104th Ave. S.E.
Kent, WA 98031

556-9533
17700 N.E. 76th St.
Redmond, WA 98052

392-3357
755 N.W. Gilman Blvd.
Issaquah, WA 98027
Hours: M-Sun.   8:00 a.m.-10:00 p.m.
A wide array of infants' and children's clothing and maternity wear await you at Target. In addition, you'll find a nice selection of baby products. As a discount store, Target's prices are reasonable, and the quality is good. Target carries a nice

selection of casual maternity wear, focussing on big shirts and stretch pants. Most shirts are under $12 and you could put together an outfit for close to $20.

In terms of infant and layette clothing, Target's baby department has an abundance of items. Most run between $3 and $14. Target also carries a large selection of bottles, rattles, cups and other baby necessities. The store has socks, shoes, tights, and booties as well. Prices on disposable diapers, baby wipes, and baby formula are close to the best in town. Cloth diapers, wraps and plastic pants are also available. Parenting and children's books are discounted by 10 percent.

Target offers a gift registry service for new parents. Everything's computerized. Parents-to-be register at the computer that's at the guest service desk and are given a bar-code scanning tool so they can tour the store and scan in to their wish list any items they need.

Target's mid-sized baby product department includes items by Fisher Price, Gerry, Cosco, Graco, Evenflo, Playskool, and Little Tikes. Most of the swings, strollers, cribs, and walkers are on a shelf overhead, making it difficult to test them. Overall, Target has much to offer the new parent in quality, selection, and price.

CHILDREN'S CLOTHING STORES

■ **BABY ME**
433-1195
Southcenter Shopping Center
Tukwila, WA 98188

471-7708
4502 S. Steele #1101
Tacoma, WA 98409
Hours: M-Sat.   10:00 a.m.-9:30 p.m.
    Sun.   11:00 a.m.-6:00 p.m.

Baby Me operates from a booth in the mall near Nordstrom, as well as a larger store in Tacoma, with an expanded product line. They offer their own line of colorful, handmade cotton clothing in unique designs sold only in their stores. Lines offered include Allison Rose, Heartstrings, and Le Top. The clothes are very classy, but also affordable. This is a great place to purchase coordinating outfits for siblings! The store also carries hats by PeekaBoo Creations and booties by Mullin Square, as well as other lots of other wonderful accessories and infant toys. The Tacoma store, recently remodeled, is well worth a trip.

■ **BOSTON STREET BABY STORE**
728-1490
101 Stewart St.
Seattle, WA 98101
Hours: Daily   10:00 a.m.-6:00 p.m.

634-0580
Wallingford Center
1815 N. 45th
Seattle, WA 98103
Hours: M-F   10:00 a.m.-8:00 p.m.
   Sat.   9:30 a.m.-6:00 p.m.
   Sun.   10:00 a.m.-5:00 p.m.

You won't find Boston Street Baby Store on Boston Street—their two stores are in Wallingford and downtown near the Pike Place Market. What you will find at both stores is colors—bright, striking, and, as one salesperson put it, "sensory-stimulating." Whether it's clothing, accessories, bedding, or toys you're looking for, you're guaranteed to find some of the most dazzling choices here. Items range from affordable and casual, such as the always-popular Cotton Caboodle line, to dressy designer styles, like a girls crinkle dress by Mousefeathers ($88). Sizes run from preemie to 14 and there's a good representation of local designers' works, such as the Juliani Children's Wear line. One of the most colorful and intriguing lines I noticed was Buddha Baby's ethnically-inspired clothes costing $25 and up. Besides clothes, Boston Street also carries strollers (Perego and Emmaljunga), baby slings, lots of hats and other accessories, and locally-made baby quilts.

■ **BRAT PACK**
784-2442
2240 N.W. Market
Seattle, WA 98107
Hours: M-F   10:00 a.m.-6:00 p.m.
        Sat.   10:00 a.m.-5:00 p.m.
883-1006
16564 Cleveland St., Ste. P
Redmond, WA 98052
Hours: M-F   10:00 a.m.-6:00 p.m.
        Th   until 7:00 p.m.
        Sat.   10:00 a.m.-5:00 p.m.
The Brat Pack stores have an excellent selection of baby products and children's clothes. A wide variety of apparel includes styles by Esprit, Le Top, Flapdoodles, Sweet Potatoes, Just Kidd'n, Heartstrings, and Zoodles. With so many different brands, there's plenty of play clothes and dressy clothes to choose from. Sizes go from preemie to 14, and prices are moderate to upscale, with a typical baby outfit starting at about $20. Like most of the other children's clothing stores, Brat Pack offers much more than just clothes. Additional items include hats, backpacks, slippers, stuffed animals, toys, cups, frames, lamps, bedding, baby supplies and gifts. A new addition is the children's haircutting salon. A child can get a haircut for $11.50 and watch videos, play with toys, or blow bubbles at the same time. The staff is very helpful here and they mentioned that the baby department is being expanded to include more bedding and related items.

■ **COTTON CABOODLE**
282-2701
203 W. Thomas
Seattle, WA 98119
Hours: T-Sat.   10:00 a.m.-4:00 p.m.
This is the place to shop if you're a Cotton Caboodle fan looking for a bargain. Located on lower Queen Anne next to the Cotton Caboodle factory, the outlet store sells overstocks far below retail price. On one visit, there was a full rack of half-off items, as well as a container of dresses marked down to $3 and $5, and shorts for $2.50. A cute collar dress was $17 and jumpers were marked down to $8.50. Although merchandise changes seasonally, you'll always find plenty of the basics—knit shirts, pants, tops, bloomers, and jumpers.

■ **COUNTRY CRADLE**
486-7617
23718 Bothell-Everett Hwy. #D
Bothell, WA 98021
Hours: M-Sat.   10:00 a.m.-6:00 p.m.
         Sun.   11:00 a.m.-5:00 p.m.
Country Cradle is located in Country Village, an assortment of wonderful little shops in one of the prettiest shopping places around. The store is in the row of buildings directly facing the Bothell-Everett Highway. On good-weather days, you'll often find a rack or two of clothes outside the door, beckoning you in. Inside, the store is fairly evenly split between baby and toddler sizes on one side, and preschool up to size 14 on the other side.

A large selection of baby products includes bedding, bibs, diaper bags, shoes, toys, stuffed animals, and books. Cute accessories are offered too—lots of hats and some darling baby sunglasses in the shape of dinosaurs or animals for $5.50. The store carries preemie sizes, with outfits by Little Me costing $16 and up. A nice selection of christening apparel for boys and girls is available, starting at $34 for a boy's outfit by Alexis. Brands carried in infant and toddler size clothes include Mini Bum Equipment, Le Top, Sweet Potatoes, and Zutano, which offers colorful knit coordinates at very moderate prices.

Besides Country Cradle, plan on exploring the quaint shops at Country Village, where children will enjoy feeding the geese and ducks, running after the roosters, crossing the foot bridge, and playing on the playground equipment. Also not to be missed is the Toys That Teach store and doll store (complete with a doll hospital) next door.

✒ Call ahead to confirm hours and locations.

■ **THE DISNEY STORE**
622-3323
Westlake Center
400 Pine St. #238
Seattle, WA 98101
Hours: M-F   10:00 a.m. - 9:00 p.m.
         Sat.   9:00 a.m.-7:00 p.m.
         Sun.   11:00 a.m. - 6:00 p.m.

241-8922
846 Southcenter Shopping Center
Tukwila, WA 98188
Hours: Mall hours

451-0540
148 Bellevue Square
Bellevue, WA 98004
Hours: Mall hours

368-2656
Northgate Mall
Seattle, WA 98125
Hours: Mall hours
A fun place to shop, like a little taste of Disneyland right in your own backyard. The window displays are fun and attractive and movie screens show favorite Disney shows while you shop. Children love to go here, which is both good and bad! The store sells clothing items, all depicting some Disney character or scene, and a large selection of gift items and Disney memorabilia. Everything from Dalmatian pencils to Mickey Mouse ties can be found. T-shirts start at $12 and pajamas at around $20.

■ **EDEN WEAR**
775-6546
23632 Hwy. 99 #217
Edmonds, WA 98026
Eden Wear makes handcrafted clothing from cotton fabric that is certified organic or transitional organic. They'll send you a catalog that includes their basic styles:

gowns, jumpers and jumpsuits, tops and bottoms, T-shirt dresses, blankets, baby slings, and even styles for moms. They also include fabric samples. Prices are reasonable: $11 for a long-sleeve T-shirt, $18 for french terry sweatshirt or sweat pants, $28 for the child's T-shirt dress in floral jersey. In-stock items are shipped within 48 hours.

■ **FLEECE FARM**
392-5369 or 800-776-5319
3020 Issaquah Pine Lake Rd. #91
Issaquah, WA 98029
Hours:　Daily　9:00 a.m.-5:00 p.m.
　　　　　　　　(phone orders)
Fleece Farm is a local mail order company that sells a full line of colorful and comfortable 100% cotton clothes for kids and moms. Besides mail order, they also do home parties, where the hostess can earn Fleece Farm clothes. Their clothing has different screen print designs which can be placed on T-shirts, sweat shirts, dresses and more. The designs are very high quality, with such names as Cats 'n' Hats, Horse Haven, Ballet Class, and Polar Bear Nites—29 designs total in the spring/ summer catalog. Especially for newborn babies is the "baby sac" style, with hood, long sleeves, and drawstrings at the bottom; it costs $22.95. Also for babies are knit caps in solid colors for $6.50, and a bubble style jersey playsuit for $24.95. Fleece Farm's designs are available in infant sizes all the way up through adults' extra-large, making these great for family matching outfits.

The catalog is interspersed with advice and information on cotton care, and explains that the reason many of the items are on white cotton is so they can be bleached. Especially helpful is the fact that bleaching won't damage the colorful screen-printed designs.

■ **GAP KIDS**
246-9934
1052 Southcenter Shopping Center
Tukwila, WA 98188
Hours:　M-Sat.　10:00 a.m.-9:30 p.m.
　　　　　Sun.　11:00 a.m.-6:00 p.m.

625-1470
4th & Pine
Seattle, WA 98101
Hours:　M-Sat.　9:30 a.m.-7:30 p.m.
　　　　　Sun.　11:00 a.m.-6:00 p.m.
525-2146
2730 N.E. University Village, Bldg. D
Seattle, WA 98105
Hours:　M-Sat.　10:00 a.m.-9:00 p.m.
　　　　　Sun.　11:00 a.m.-6:00 p.m.
454-1539
Bellevue Square
Bellevue, WA 98004
Hours:　M-Sat.　9:30 a.m.-9:30 p.m.
　　　　　Sun.　11:00 a.m.-6:00 p.m.
Not unlike the regular Gap, Gap Kids carries infant and toddler clothing with a preppie-look including jeans, jean jackets, button-down shirts, and t-shirts. The style is comfortable and looks great on kids. Belts, socks, and hair accessories are available to finish off the outfit. In the back of the store are sale items where you can really find a good bargain. The Gap offers sturdy, high quality clothing.

■ GYMBOREE

450-9460
Bellevue Square
Bellevue, WA 98004

771-4558
Alderwood Mall
Lynnwood, WA 98037
Hours: Mall hours

Gymboree is a franchise that carries its own label. The styles are simple and comfortable. Most of the clothing is 100% cotton. Gymboree has its own style of mix-and-match clothing utilizing both primary colors and pastels. Sale items are in the back of the store and you'll find bargains here: 25 to 50 percent off. Some toy items and Gymboree videotapes are also sold here. The help is friendly and helpful, often willing to blow bubbles to amuse your child while you are shopping. You can expect to spend about $14 for leggings and $20 for a sweatshirt.

■ INFANT OUTFITTERS

283-8042 or 800-OUTFITS
224 W. Galer
Seattle, WA 98119
Hours: T-Sat.   10:00 a.m.-4:00 p.m.

Gwen Evans started her Infant Outfitters line of baby and toddler clothes in 1984 when her first child was born, and her business has continued to grow since then. Now with a nationwide following, the line is sold locally at several children's boutique stores as well. The popular playclothes in sizes newborn to 4 are available in over 20 different designs and lots of stunning and playful fabrics. Prices for the reversible and nonreversible items start at around $6.95 for a hat and $14.95 for a shirt.

At the retail design studio on Queen Anne, you can come in and personally select fabrics and styles to have custom made, or you can choose from the many one-of-a-kind items available on the racks. There's plenty to choose from, not only in the infant/toddler line, but in two new lines for older children too. Sophie's Choice features dramatic, yet practical dresses, skirts, vests, jumpers, leggings, and hats for girls ages 2-10. Unusual fabrics, top-quality materials (cotton and washable silk) and fun dress-up styles make this a popular line. Prices range from $20-$80 for most items.

For boys, the Zack's Back line offers casual, loose-fitting playclothes to mix and match. Fabrics include chambray and plaids, denims, and plaid flannels. Prices in this line range from $15-$40 (more for dressy items, jackets, etc.). Considering that everything is hand sewn, these are extremely affordable prices. If you can't visit the studio or want to share these great designs with friends and families out of town, call to request a catalog and/or the Infant Outfitters newsletter to keep up with the latest happenings. Gwen will even send you drawings and fabric swatches and work with you to create a special outfit for your special child.

■ THE JOY OF CHILDREN

933-1506
7011 California Ave. S.W.
Seattle, WA 98126
Hours: M-Sat.   9:00 a.m.-6:00 p.m.

This West Seattle store carries new clothing in popular lines, including Le Top, Wee Clancy, Poco Poco, Maddie Jane, Allison Ann, JoLene, After the Stork, Samara, Curious George by Loo Na, Golden Rainbow, and New Potatoes. The styles are great—classic with wonderful matching accessories. When we visited, a wonderful Wee Clancy outfit included a birdhouse character print dress with matching hat and wooden birdhouse necklace on a rope, for $31. The store also has two walls of clean and stylish consignment clothes and other consigned items. We found an $18 Gap Kids hat for just $4. Merchandise ranges from casual to very fancy, and includes quilts, swings, rocking horses, videos and tapes, and Boppy nursing pillows. Several hand-painted, wooden rocking horse zebras were being sold here for $200 and up, and were pronounced "very cool" by one of our researchers!

■ JULIANI CHILDREN'S WEAR
783-8972
Hours: Call for a studio appointment
Grasa Adler sells her handcrafted children's clothing at several local clothing stores, as well as nationally and at arts and crafts fairs. She uses incredibly colorful fabrics with wonderful patterns for kids, including beach scenes, fish, dolphins, jungle animals, cowboys, farm scenes, celestial designs, and a darling kitten pattern. My personal favorite is a striking sunflower fabric. Her designs are very unique and reflect her Brazilian heritage. A swingy collar dress with a scalloped hem is a good example of that influence. Other items include reversible rompers, jumpers, hats, pants, shirts, dresses, and T-shirts with fabric insets that match other separates. Prices are moderate, considering the amount of labor and care that go into handcrafted work like this. Grasa has a high level of creativity and skill; one boutique store manager noted that for sewing quality her garments are some of the best handcrafted ones available. Because this is basically a

one-woman operation, Grasa schedules personal appointments in advance. There's usually lots of merchandise to select from in sizes newborn to 6 and of course she'll take custom orders as well.

■ KIDGEAR
624-0756
1420 5th Ave., Ste. 219
Seattle, WA 98101
Hours: M-W 10:00 a.m.-6:30 p.m.
        Th-F 10:00 a.m.-7:00 p.m.
        Sat. 10:00 a.m.-6:30 p.m.
KidGear is located on the second floor of the City Centre Building (across from the Sheraton downtown). Unique is the best word to describe this store; you'll find things here that you won't find in any other children's store in the Seattle area. Although you'll see some recognizable brands like Flapdoodles and Baby Guess, the emphasis is on original clothes by individual designers. KidGear's focus is to provide customers with clothing and accessories that are high quality and stylish, very unique, yet functional and lasting for kid wear. The clothing is attractively displayed with coordinating accessories, so you can easily put together a complete outfit for your little one. Sizes range from newborn to 14. Prices are mid-priced to upscale, although it's usually easy to find an outfit on sale for less than $25. Besides offering many choices in both play and dress-up clothes, the infants and toddlers department has a good selection of baby toys, accessories, parenting and baby books. They carry furniture too—the line of custom made wood items includes a children's table and chair set, rocking horse, toy trunk, and doll beds and chairs. You can also find the Emmaljunga stroller line at

KidGear and as a major dealer for the line, they have items in-stock and available for purchase (some stores require special orders). One of the most unique and practical items at KidGear is the Sit 'n' Stroll, a combination car seat and stroller for children newborn to 3 years old. Priced at $149, it's FAA approved for use on airplanes, and is very easy to change from seat to stroller and back again. KidGear also operates a factory outlet, with most items sold below or at wholesale price. They carry sizes newborn-7. The outlet center is located in a residential neighborhood in Seattle's northend; call 361-4675 for directions.

■ KID'S COTTAGE
481-2106
13300 N.E. 175th St., Ste. 1
Woodinville, WA 98072
Hours: M-Sat. 10:00 a.m.-5:00 p.m.
As you first enter the store, you'll see clothes and quite a few accessories for babies, including lots of rattles, toys, stuffed animals, dolls, and bibs. A product that looks especially practical is the Boppy Support Pillow ($39.99).

There's a nice selection of new clothes, with brands like Sweet Potatoes and Little Me. Pajamas by Skivvy Doodle that are 100% cotton are the current fastest moving item. Prices are moderate for these lines—infant sleepers and play outfits start in the $20 range. The size range is considerable too—newborn to 14 (girls) and to 16 (boys). This store has a consignment room where consignment clothes and baby equipment are on display. Baby carriers, strollers, and cribs were all available when we visited, and the condition of all consignment items was quite good. The store offers complimentary gift wrap and the staff is friendly and helpful.

■ KID'S MART
939-4978
1101 Super Mall Way #1261
Auburn, WA 98007
Hours: M-Sat. 9:30 a.m.-9:30 p.m.
           Sun.   10:00 a.m.-6:00 p.m.

839-6306
32041 Pacific Hwy. S.
Federal Way, WA 98003
Hours: M-F   10:00 a.m.-9:00 p.m.
           Sat.   9:30 a.m.-7:00 p.m.
           Sun.   11:00 a.m.-6:00 p.m.

562-1495 - (Outlet Store)
4068 128th S.E.
Bellevue, WA 98006
Hours: M-Sat. 10:00 a.m.-6:00 p.m.
           Sun.   11:00 a.m.-6:00 p.m.
Kid's Mart has low to moderate prices with many sale items. It carries Way Out Wear that starts at $5.99 and Cherokee T-shirts for $9.99. The store also offers Tiger Pals, an excellent durable infants' brand (but a little more costly) with merchandise beginning at about $12.99. Kid's Mart clothing is clearly sorted with boys' on one side and girls' on the other. It's a great place to buy both play and dress clothing for your child.

■ KINDER BRITCHES *Baby Pages*
778-7600
422 Main St.
Edmonds, WA 98020
Hours: M-F   10:00 a.m.-6:00 p.m.
           Sat.   10:00 a.m.-5:30 p.m.
           Sun.   Noon-4:00 p.m.
Located downtown at the fountain, Kinder Britches offers a full range of children's wear and accessories. Sizes range from preemie to 8 (boys) and preemie to 14 (girls). They have a good mix of both casual and dressy clothes. Unique and fun

specialty lines mingle with quality basics such as Esprit and Guess, and some of the dressier lines include: Biscotti, Allison Rose, and Tailfeathers for girls and Kitestrings and Golden Rainbow for boys. They offer a full line of specialty preemie clothes by Eensie Esse, several quality all-cotton baby lines, hand-smocked booties and bonnets, and a fine selection of christening outfits priced from $45 to $85. Kinder Britches is a registered dealer of the Baby Jogger stroller and has them priced competitively. Toys, fanny packs and backpack diaper bags, Lamby Nursery lambskins, fun hats, a great play area for kids, customer service, and free gift wrap are also found at Kinder Britches.

Baby gifts, crib blankets, comforters, and other gift items and accessories are also available at Kinder Britches.

■ LA PRECIOSA BOUTIQUE
246-9318
221 S.W. 152nd St.
Burien, WA 98144
Hours: M-Sat. 10:00 a.m.-6:00 p.m.

Located in Burien, this store specializes in special occasion clothes, many imported from Central America. Dresses start at $30 and feature lots of lace and ruffles. There's a good selection of hats, some accessories, and some playclothes too. A three-piece outfit by Dorissa (from El Salvador) included a top, pants, and headband and was sale-priced at $35. Sizes are newborn-14. This is a good place to look for christening clothes and they have special occasion clothes for adults as well. There wasn't a children's play area here, which would be helpful considering the great temptation of little ones to touch all those fancy fabrics. The store also carries some bedding for babies, including a practical and affordable "baby mink blanket" from Mexico for $18 and a smaller baby bag for $13.50.

■ LIL' PEOPLE
455-4967
Bellevue Square, Space #115A
Bellevue, WA 98004
Hours: M-Sat. 9:30 a.m.-9:30 p.m.
        Sun. 11:00 a.m.-6:00 p.m.

623-4463
Westlake Center
400 Pine St. #324
Seattle, WA 98101
Hours: M-Sat. 10:00 a.m.-8:00 p.m.
        Sun. 11:00 a.m.-6:00 p.m.

"Cozy cotton artwear" is what Lil' People's business card says, and that's certainly reflected in the fun variety of colorful clothes and accessories offered here. The store carries its own line of prewashed and garment-dyed knits, available in a wide selection of colors. They also feature original prints and designs by their own artists. Besides their own line, Lil' People carries comfortable cotton knits by Flaphappy and dresses by Mousefeathers. Other choices include jumpers, pants, vests and stylish tops by Echo Field, Rumbletumble, Warm Heart, Infant Outfitters, and Just Kidd'n. The selection of accessories is astounding, with a great assortment of socks, lots and lots of hats, jewelry, suspenders, ties, hairbows, wrist rattles, and more. The "artwear" influence is definitely reflected in these accessories, as well as in special items like the corduroy TV booties with kitty faces (just $7 a pair). Dinosaur water bottles are sure to be a hit with the toddler/preschool set, as will the many stuffed animals, and other toys.

■ **ME 'N' MOMS**
524-9344
Roosevelt Square
1021 N.E. 65th St.
Seattle, WA 98115
Hours: M-F   9:30 a.m.-8:00 p.m.
            Sat.-Sun.10:00 a.m.-5:00 p.m.
Me 'n' Moms carries colorful and comfortable children's clothing, with a strong emphasis on knits. The store features popular brands like LeTop, Marimekko, Fresh Produce, and Flapdoodles. Items are mid-priced, with many infants' coordinated play sets in the $20-$30 range. That's if you pay full price—there's also a large section in the back called Backroom Bargains where regular merchandise has been discounted 25-50%. For even lower prices, look through the consignment section, where a play outfit in good condition can usually be found for $6-$12. The store has a play area for kids, and sells an assortment of baby products and accessories including toys, bibs, and hats.

■ **MOONBEAMS**
391-4688
Gilman Village
317 N.W. Gilman Blvd., Ste. 5
Issaquah, WA 98027
Hours: M-W, Sat.10:00 a.m.-6:00 p.m.
            Th, F   10:00 a.m.-8:00 p.m.
            Sun.   Noon-5:00 p.m.
Moonbeams is located in the charming Gilman Village. If you haven't visited this shopping area, you'll find a collection of about 40 restored homes. One of the stores is Moonbeams, a European boutique which offers unique and exclusive children's clothing from size preemie to 4T. Infants' outfits range from $25 to $200. You can find brands such as Mini Man, Deux Par Deux, as well as some classic Winnie the Pooh lines. To coordinate your baby's outfit, Moonbeams offers accessories such as hats, shoes, socks and hairbands. The store itself is bright and airy with a definite boutique feel. A separate children's play area offers toys and videos. Moonbeams offers gift certificates and free gift wrapping.

■ **ORIGINAL CHILDREN'S SHOP**
328-7121
4114 E. Madison
Seattle, WA 98112
Hours: M-F   10:00 a.m.-5:30 p.m.
            Sat.   10:00 a.m.-5:00 p.m.
Located in the Madison Park area, Original Children's Shop is a well-stocked children's boutique. They carry lots of cute styles from popular brands like LeTop, Echo Fields, Bambine Penguini, Little Me, Just Ducky, Patsy Aiken, and Julian's. There's a big selection of Flaphappy hats for $10, and affordable knit tops by Zutano Baby. The store carries preemie sizes and christening gowns too. Most lines are priced at 10% less than retail. Besides clothing, the shop has a full assortment of baby accessories, including infant headrests by Nojo, cute and comfy Padders baby shoes, toys, diaper bags, soft books, and soft sculpture toys that we haven't seen in other stores.

■ **THE SHOE ZOO**
525-2770
2675 N.E. University Village Mall
Seattle, WA 98105
Hours: M-F   10:00 a.m.-8:00 p.m.
        Sat.   10:00 a.m.-6:00 p.m.
        Sun.   11:00 a.m.-5:00 p.m.

392-8211
240 N.W. Gilman Blvd.
Issaquah, WA 98027
Hours: M-Sat. 10:00 a.m.-6:00 p.m.
        Sun.   Noon-5:00 p.m.

The Shoe Zoo is conveniently located across from Kids Club in University Village Mall for Seattle shoppers and at Gilman Station (under the clock tower) in Issaquah for Eastsiders. They carry a large selection of shoes for infants to preteens. Parents can find brands such as Stride Rite, Toddler University, Keds, and Nike at the Shoe Zoo. They offer a great selection available for any occasion. Regularly priced shoes will cost about $35 to $45. And, if you buy at least one pair of shoes a year that is regularly priced, you will receive a 15% discount on your child's birthday. The Shoe Zoo is also very well equipped with accessory items such as socks, backpacks, slippers and hats. You'll find great service at this store which makes it a fun shopping experience for kids and parents.

■ **SMALL FRY**
283-4556
3209 W. McGraw
Seattle, WA 98199
Hours: M   10:00 a.m.-5:00 p.m.
        T-F   10:00 a.m.-6:00 p.m.
        Sat.   10:00 a.m.-5:00 p.m.
        Sun.   Noon-4:00 p.m.

This Magnolia children's shop has a distinctly neighborhood feel, offering personalized service and an excellent selection of apparel, accessories, and gift items. They carry many popular children's lines, including Marimekko, Flaphappy, Fresh Produce, Cotton Caboodle, Zutano, and City Lights. There's always a full selection of darling dresses by Mousefeathers and 100% cotton infant apparel by Sara's Prints. Clothing sizes run from infant to 14. Shoes in infant sizes are available, and larger sizes are often offered in seasonal items like sandals and boots. Small Fry has a good selection of picture frames and dresser decorations, and also carries a line of Beatrix Potter items. There's lots of toys, accessories (plenty of hats!), and unique gift possibilities. Some cute and comfy leather baby booties, lined with flannel, were just $17.95 and would certainly be a treasured baby gift. The store also carries some local baby products, including Teddy Toes baby blankets. And you can't miss their great selection of Magnolia T-shirts on display throughout the store!

■ **STARS CHILDREN'S WEAR**
392-2900
55 N.E. Gilman Blvd.
Issaquah, WA 98027
Hours: M-F   9:00 a.m.-9:00 p.m.
        Sat.   10:00 a.m.-6:00 p.m.
        Sun.   11:00 a.m.-6:00 p.m.

575-2625
17550 Southcenter Pkwy.
Tukwila, WA 98188
Hours: M-F   9:30 a.m.-9:00 p.m.
        Sat.   9:30 a.m.-7:00 p.m.
        Sun.   11:00 a.m.-6:00 p.m.

Stars is a children's superstore, featuring a huge selection of high quality brand name clothing, accessories, layette, toys and books for children of all ages. More than

500 manufacturers are represented, with a great mix of moderate-priced to better labels. Their clothing is not factory seconds. Clothing styles are up-to-date and quality is excellent. Sizes run from preemies up to 14 in girls and 20 in boys. A full selection of christening apparel is available, as well as practically anything else you might want for your baby. There are baby toys, stuffed animals, cards, gifts, books, music, and accessories. Their Great Wall of Socks features more than 16,000 pairs. And if just shopping in such a store isn't fun enough, Stars also offers free family entertainment on the weekends. Music, storytellers, puppet shows, juggling, and balloon artists are some of the fun that awaits you here. Because they're so big (stocking more children's clothes and accessories than any other store in the western U.S.), they can offer prices 20-40% lower than the competition. With more than 25,000 square feet, the store is easy to maneuver even with a shopping cart or stroller in their wide aisles and well-organized sections.

■ WARNER BROTHERS STUDIO STORE

646-8738
1050 Bellevue Square
Bellevue, WA 98006
Hours: Mall hours
The Warner Brothers Studio Store is filled with—you guessed it—Warner Brothers' character clothing and items. Tweety Bird, Batman and Robin, Bugs Bunny and more await you at this lively store! Prices are what you would expect from a specialty store with clothing around $16 on up. There is also unique memorabilia and items that you could not buy elsewhere. Like the other character stores, Warner Brothers is a fun place to shop!

RESALE STORES

■ A TO Z CHILDREN'S CONSIGNMENT

325-9903
2812 E. Madison #3
Seattle, WA 98112
Hours: T-Sat.   10:00 a.m.-5:00 p.m.
         Sun.   Noon-4:00 p.m.
A to Z is located in a lovely courtyard set back from the north side of Madison Street—look for the old-fashioned baby buggy filled with plants outside. There's an excellent selection of both children's and maternity consignment wear, as well as some new merchandise. The consignment clothes are in great condition and children's outfits average in the $5-$10 range. The maternity section offers many choices too, with barely-used dresses in both casual and career styles ranging in price from $8-$60, most between $20-$40. Besides consignment clothes, the store carries new maternity clothes, including Maternity Blues denim nursing tops ($39.95) and knit maternity shorts ($14.75). There's a large section of Discreet Wear solid-color leggings and stretch pants in ribbed and textured knits for $12.95. A to Z has a well-stocked center display of nursing supplies, including videos, books, nursing pillows, breast pumps, and more. (The owner noted that they strongly support breastfeeding.) Other new merchandise includes lots of cute kids' hats by Laarni starting at $9.95, a double sling Baby Bundler baby carrier, books, and accessories. Upstairs is more consignment merchandise—clothes in children's sizes 4-12, toys, and books. You also may find some equipment such as strollers and swings, and a small supply of bedding.

■ **ABOUT FACE CONSIGNMENTS**
771-4190
7300 196th St. S.W.
Lynnwood, WA 98046
Hours: T-Sat.   10:30 a.m.-4:30 p.m.
About Face is west of Highway 99 on
196th S.W. The store offers both maternity and children's wear. The maternity
clothes are a good mix of casual and career
wear. Several denim jumpsuits were on
display when we visited, as well as dresses,
sweaters, tops, pants, and shorts. They
sell new maternity items too, including
Discreet Wear nursing tops, which they
sell at just over wholesale price. The
children's department has a complete selection of affordable clothes for babies
and children. Sleepers average $2.50-
$4.50, dresses $6, rompers $4, and we
spotted a pair of nearly-new pink OshKosh
b'Gosh overalls for $5.50. A small selec-
tion of equipment is usually available;
items like swings and strollers are sometimes offered. Bedding items are also carried. The staff at About Face is very
helpful and considerate, and the store
provides a small, well-organized play area
for kids.

■ **BABY EXPRESS**
337-3739
13416 Bothell-Everett Hwy.
Mill Creek, WA 98012
Hours: M-Sat.   10:00 a.m.-6:00 p.m.
         Sun.   Noon-5:00 p.m.
Baby Express is located at Gateway Center at Murphy's corner, Mill Creek. The
store opened in fall 1995 and carries a
variety of both new and pre-owned clothing in children's sizes newborn-8. New
clothing lines included Alexis, New Potatoes, Parigi, and Peaches n' Cream. The
store carries a full line of Winnie-the-

Pooh items, as well as NoJo and Dex
products. They also carry a wide selection
of christening gowns in the $20-$30 range
and carry some premature clothing too.
In addition, they sell maternity clothing,
toys, gifts, shoes, baby equipment, and
furniture. Cribs are available from $30-
$425; new all-terrain strollers by J Mason
cost around $100. The store looks so
attractive and "boutique"-like from the
outside, that customers have told owners
Paulina and Genifer that they hesitated
coming in at first, because they thought
the merchandise would be expensive. But
the focus here is definitely on quality,
affordable used items. Some added bo-
nuses include free gift wrapping, shower
registry, and a kids' play area with toys
and videos. Consignment records are all
computerized too.

■ **BOOTYLAND**
328-0636
1321 East Pine
Seattle, WA 98122
Hours: M-Sat.   10:00 a.m.-6:00 p.m.
Bootyland is a fun and fashionable baby
store, owned and operated by two mothers in the Capitol Hill area. The store
carries both new and used items for infants through size 7. Bootyland is very
clean and organized, and offers a wide
supply of merchandise from books to
clothing to products. We also found several unusual local products at Bootyland
and a great selection of tie-dye clothing,
handmade hats, and used baby carriers.
Prices begin at about $2 for infant cloth-
ing. Bootyland has a great area for your
children to play while you shop! One
Seattle mom wrote and requested that we
review Bootyland to share this unique
store with other readers. That is loyal
support!

■ **FIFTH AVENUE KIDS**
526-5683
8312 5th Ave. N.E.
Seattle, WA 98115
Hours: T   10:00 a.m.-5:00 p.m.
        W   11:00 a.m.-6:00 p.m.
        Th   Noon-8:00 p.m.
        F-Sat.   11:00 a.m.-5:00 p.m.

Fifth Avenue Kids opened in 1993 and has quickly become an excellent northend shopping option for children's clothes. The name alone makes it easy to find and the line-up of baby equipment outside certainly helps too! Depending on when you visit, you may see strollers, playpens, rocking chairs, tables, and outdoor play toys. Inside, there's a good selection of both new and gently used clothing. New clothes include the popular Cotton Caboodle line of knits. Clothing sizes range from newborn to 6 and consignment clothing is in very good condition and affordably priced. Some accessories and toys are available, too.

■ **FINER CONSIGNER**
522-7441
6407 Roosevelt Way N.E.
Seattle, WA 98115
Hours: T-Sat.   10:00 a.m.-6:00 p.m.

Located across the street from Roosevelt Square, Finer Consigner opened in 1993. Although the store isn't too big, they do carry an assortment of both children's and maternity wear. Prices are good here, with maternity jumpers and dresses in the $10-$20 range and some Discreet Wear tops (in great condition!) for just $11 when we visited. Children's clothes offer the greatest choices in the newborn-24 months section, although the selection in larger sizes is sure to grow as the children of regular customers do too. Prices were

very inexpensive, about $1-$5 for play clothes, and some snow suits for $16-$18 were available too. A new, handmade white crocheted sweater with matching cap was just $8. If you're in the neighborhood, this store is worth a stop!

■ **FORGET-ME-NOT**
789-6463
5918 Phinney Ave. N.
Seattle, WA 98103
Hours: M-Sat.   10:00 a.m.-6:00 p.m.
        Sun.   Noon-5:00 p.m.

Forget-Me-Not is a delightful new and gently used clothing store. They also have a full selection of used toys and equipment such as strollers, high chairs, swings, car seats and carriers, and playpens. Prices are good—swings for $12, high chairs for $40, etc. Forget-Me-Not also carries a bright and lively selection of new clothing. Play clothes, dresses and accessories are attractively displayed. There's a big play room for kids so you can shop at a more leisurely pace. What makes this store especially unique is their assortment of collectibles—antique toys, prams, sleds, and children's furniture are attractively displayed throughout the store. For parents in their 30's, you'll find many items from your childhood. I was especially impressed with the Holly Hobby kitchen—it brought back many memories. Also, their location near the zoo and one block north of Woodland Park makes this a convenient and fun shopping destination.

■ **FUNKY JANE'S**
937-2637
4738 42nd Ave. S.W.
Seattle, WA 98116
Hours: M-F   10:00 a.m.-8:00 p.m.
        Sat.   10:00 a.m.-6:00 p.m.
        Sun.   Noon-5:00 p.m.
Funky Jane's is located in West Seattle in Jefferson Square (look for the adjacent Safeway store). The emphasis in this large store is on women's wear and you'll find a striking display of stylish clothes and accessories as you enter. Head toward the back right and there's a good-sized section of consigned children's wear in sizes newborn-6X. The condition of clothes is good, and prices are in the $2-$10 range. On the maternity racks, you'll find jeans for around $10 and dresses and jumpers from $20-$30.

■ **GOOD AS NEW**
878-5036
21927 Marine View Dr. S.
Des Moines, WA 98198
Hours: M-Sat.   10:00 a.m.-5:00 p.m.
Good as New carries good quality used children's and maternity clothing, as well as some new and handcrafted items. Kids clothes go up to size 7 for boys and 14 for girls, and there's a big selection of outfits for $3 and up. The maternity clothes are in excellent condition, with lots of career and casual dresses from $25-$40. The store also offers a selection of toys, books, a few car seats, baby equipment, and other accessories.

✿ *Call ahead to confirm hours and locations.*

■ **HEAVEN SENT**
946-2229
1200 S. 324th, Ste. 5
Federal Way, WA 98003
Hours: M-F   10:00 a.m.-6:00 p.m.
        Sat.   10:00 a.m.-5:00 p.m.
Heaven Sent has a great selection of resale items. Clothes are on racks along the walls and on circle racks in the middle of the store, and the store makes good use of their space with a very well-organized layout. Besides clothes, they carry practically everything you might need for baby: car seats, swings, front and back carriers, jump-ups, bottles, bibs, strollers, bassinets, cribs, mobiles, and wall decorations. They also have a good selection of toys, games, dolls, and play furniture. Prices are very affordable; cribs range from $60-$200, pairs of socks start at 40 cents, and some nice, good quality boys' suits (complete with cummerbunds or vests) cost less than $11.

■ **JUST FOR YOU**
542-3993
1114 N. 183rd
Seattle, WA 98133
Hours: M-F   9:30 a.m.-7:00 p.m.
        Sat.   10:00 a.m.-5:00 p.m.
In business since 1981, Just for You is one of several consignment shops in the Seattle area that you shouldn't "street-appraise." Tucked in an L-shaped strip mall that's fronted by a QFC store, the shop is on the south-facing side, next to a hobby shop. Behind its unassuming front is a well-stocked two-level store. On the first floor, there's a large section of new handcrafted items, including clothing and accessories, and large supply of inexpensive toys. Consigned clothes are reasonably priced, with a very large variety of all items from sleepwear to dress clothes in

sizes newborn to 14 (girls) and 16 (boys). We found not only good prices, but also great brands and quality. Just for You carries Daisy Kingdom, Gymboree, Baby Gap—both new and used. Upstairs is where the baby products are. And, there is also an ample supply. We found swings, strollers, carriers, high chairs and much more in this section. Prices, again, were very reasonable. If you're looking for maternity clothing, Just for You carries a large section with mostly casual clothes and some career dresses. The store also sells large outside play equipment such as slides, activity areas, swings and sand boxes. Their selection may vary on these items, so call ahead to find out what is available. You may also find bottles, breast pumps, books, toys, rollerskates, shoes,games and videos. Plan some time at this store to check out all of the merchandise. And, if you have young children there is a play area complete with a TV and videos.

■ KIDS BY GOSH
432-9336
22035 S.E. Wax Rd.
Maple Valley, WA 98038
Hours: M-F   10:00 a.m.-6:00 p.m.
           Sat.   10:00 a.m.-5:00 p.m.
           Sun.   Noon-5:00 p.m.
Kids By Gosh offers everything under the sun for kids! They carry hard-to-find christening gowns and premature baby clothing, and sell both new and used clothes. Brands include OshKosh b'Gosh, JoLene, Peaches & Cream, Plum Pudding, B.U.M., Esprit, HealthTex, Disney, Weather Tamer, and Beatrix Potter. The store is very well-organized, with walls filled with shelves and hangers of new baby clothes, hats, shoes, socks, and other accessories. Besides things to wear, they have baby furniture, toys, games, puzzles, lullabye tapes, and much more. Prices range from $2.98 and up, and in the consignment area for 98 cents and up. The staff here is friendly and there's a play area for kids, so you can take your time shopping.

■ KIDS ON 45TH
633-5437
1720 N. 45th St.
Seattle, WA 98103
Hours: M-Sat.   10:00 a.m.-6:00 p.m.
         Sun.   11:00 a.m.-5:00 p.m.
Kids on 45th carries a wide variety of products for babies and children. The front part of the store offers new clothes, with an extra large selection of their own line of cotton basics, affordably priced from $7-$20. This line is very popular, as is the consignment section which offers clothing and other products. On one visit there were several gently used swings, strollers, and car seats for sale. The consignment clothing is well-organized and displayed, with separate racks for dresses, pants, tops, shirts, overalls, coats, and shorts. There's also a big selection of velcro-fastening diaper covers selling for about $2 each. A dollar rack offers even more bargains on children's clothes. The store sells new baby accessories too. One that looked quite practical was a plastic bib by Roo! that's dishwasher safe and just $4.95.

■ KIDS PLUS
743-4171
16725 52nd W.
Lynnwood, WA 98037
Hours: T-F 10:00 a.m.-6:00 p.m.
        W   10:00 a.m.-5:00 p.m.
        Sat. 11:00 a.m.-5:00 p.m.

Almost all of what Kids Plus sells is resale, although they did have one small rack of new items when we visited, with dresses by JoLene. They carry lots of children's clothing in fair to good condition, with very affordable prices—it's easy to find basic play outfits in the $4-$5 range. The store has toys, books, greeting cards, maternity wear, and several cribs, ranging in price from around $70-$200. They also carry Motiv's "Joggette" jogging stroller, priced at around $100 for a new one.

■ KIDSIGNMENT
861-9548
164th & 83rd
Redmond, WA 98052
Hours: M   10:00 a.m.-5:00 p.m.
        T-F 10:00 a.m.-6:00 p.m.
        Sat. 10:00 a.m.-4:00 p.m.

This children's consignment store recently moved in with the Consignment Crate, a shop that's been in Redmond for about 3 years. It's located in a house, which makes it a comfortable place to shop. In addition, there's a hair salon upstairs and a play area where parents can see their children while they shop. The store's focus is on quality, pre-owned clothing, so they don't carry furniture or baby equipment. Sizes go up to 6X for kids. They also carry maternity wear. Name brands are prevalent here; the store's owner places a high priority on selling quality, gently used wear. Oshkosh overalls cost around $5-$7, Gymboree items are $10-$16.

■ LABELS
781-1194
7212 Greenwood Ave. N.
Seattle, WA 98103
Hours: T-Sat. 10:00 a.m.-6:00 p.m.
        Th   10:00 a.m.-8:00 p.m.
        Sun.   Noon-5:00 p.m.

Labels is a small store but offers some of the most stylish choices in regular women's wear, including some European and better labels. The emphasis on fashionable clothing can be found in the maternity section too, where choices in dresses included several in the Motherhood line for $24-$28. Sundresses were being offered for under $20 and all clothes were in excellent condition. The children's section includes a nice assortment of outfits, most in the $4-$5 range, and there are also plenty of socks, bibs, hats, and other accessories. Kids will stay occupied in the store's play kitchen area while you shop.

■ LI'L ONE'S RERUNS
368-5484
910 N.E. 185th St.
Shoreline, WA 98155
Hours: Call for current hours

Li'l One's Reruns in Shoreline is one of the newest consignment stores in the greater Seattle area, having just opened in late 1995, but you might find that hard to believe upon visiting! The store has lots and lots of merchandise already, and it's all very attractively displayed in this colorful, bright store. The building was once a 7-11 administrative office, then a youth center. When the store's owner, Lisa Pyper, took over the site, it was with the goal of providing a place where families from nearby neighborhoods could walk, then spend an afternoon shopping and enjoying a latte, while their kids play in the store's play area. Even without major advertising, the store began to serve this "community center" function in its first few months of operation. No doubt the espresso stand out front has been a big draw, as well as the rainbow-colored fabric panels on the store's windows. The rainbow theme continues inside, with fabric panels suspended from the ceiling, and lively murals on the walls. The kids' play area is a large raised stage, visible throughout the store. Another community-related service that Lisa offers is a bulletin board where parents can sell or exchange large items, such as outdoor play equipment. A homeschooling network is also planned, so that local homeschooling families can connect and exchange or sell curriculum materials, plan shared activities, etc. The store's merchandise is quite varied, with an excellent range of sizes in both girls and boys clothes. Some locally-made new, handcrafted items are also available. Equipment such as strollers ($30), car seats ($20-$30), and cribs are for sale, as well as new Dorling Kindersley books, used books, toys, stuffed animals, accessories, and much more.

■ **LITTLE MUNCHKINS**
244-0616
13635 1st Ave. S.
Burien, WA 98166
Hours: M-Sat.   10:00 a.m.-6:00 p.m.
Little Munchkins is in Burien, where Suzi Q's Consignment Store used to be. The new owners will buy used baby clothes and products as well as trade for store credit. The store is very nicely organized, with separate racks for dresses, pants, shirts, rompers, overalls, jumpers, etc. This makes shopping much easier and

less time-consuming. Sizes range from preemie to 6X. Clothing quality is very good and prices are affordable—OshKosh b'Gosh overalls go for about $7, almost-new dresses for $6 and up. A bargain rack offers items for 50 cents.

There's a good selection of rattles, baby and children's toys (Cabbage Patch dolls for $7!), and lots of shoes. Baby equipment includes strollers, cribs, car seats, bassinets, and playpens. We also saw Snugli baby carriers ($15.95) and a nice assortment of bedding. They also offers their own line of handmade dresses, pants, and diaper wraps in cottons and knits. The staff is quite friendly and helpful, and there's a play area for children.

■ **LITTLE TROOPERS**
486-2081
6522 N.E. Bothell Way
Seattle, WA 98155
Hours: M-F   10:00 a.m.-6:00 p.m.
        Sat.   10:00 a.m.-4:00 p.m.
Little Troopers is in the Kenmore area in a strip mall off Bothell Way. This is a great place if you're a bargain hunter, as you will find plenty to choose from here. We were especially impressed with the large selection of toys and stuffed animals at amazingly low prices. The consignment clothes are generally in very good condition and there's a nice variety of items in sizes to 12. The baby and toddler section has a lot of clothes, bedding, and accessories like diaper bags. The store also sells used shoes, videos, and books. Equipment like strollers, cribs, high chairs, and car seats are available from time to time, but usually go fast since the prices are so good. New items for sale include socks, hats, headbands, and other clothing accessories. Little Troopers has a small play area for kids.

■ **LOLLIPOPS**
243-1795
2038 S.W. 152nd
Burien, WA 98148
Hours: M-Sat. 10:00 a.m.-5:30 p.m.
Lollipops is the only consignment shop we visited that carried clothes for the entire family. The selection of children's clothes is quite good, and condition of clothing ranges from fair to excellent. The merchandise is sorted by items within each size, so it's easy to see all the size 2T jumpers at once, rather than raking through the racks. When we visited, there was a large selection of baby dresses in practically brand-new condition, most for $5 or less. The maternity section wasn't too big, but prices again were quite good with dresses, denim jumpers, and pants for $10 or less. The store carries baby equipment including toddler beds, swings, strollers, and car seats. There's some baby bedding too, and a wall of plastic stacking baskets—each clearly labeled and filled with toys, books, dolls, doll clothes, diaper wraps, and more.

■ **MOM'S N TOT'S**
451-4439
137 106th Ave. N.E.
Bellevue, WA 98006
Hours: M-F   10:00 a.m.-5:00 p.m.
        Sat.   10:30 a.m.-5:30 p.m.
Mom's n Tot's, located in Bellevue on 106th N.E. and Main Street, has been in business on the eastside for more than 10 years. They carry a wide selection of business and casual maternity wear for moms and a first-class clothing selection for tots in sizes from birth to 12 years. The store is clean and well-organized with a variety of toys, books, shoes, bedding and furniture, as well as consignment clothing.

Ample parking in the mall setting makes it a very convenient place to shop. Each month, Mom's n Tot's features 20% off on selected items with a color ticket for easy bargain hunting. It's a great store to find super buys.

■ **ONCE UPON A CHILD**
774-8393
3225 Alderwood Mall Blvd., Ste. E
Lynnwood, WA 98036
Hours: M-F   10:00 a.m.-7:00 p.m.
        Sat.   10:00 a.m.-6:00 p.m.
        Sun.   11:00 a.m.-5:00 p.m.
Unlike any other resale store in the area, Once Upon a Child is a franchise. The store offers both new and gently used merchandise, and the quality of the used items is so good that we had to check the labels ("new" items are marked as such) to tell the difference. The resale items here are not on consignment—the store purchases items for cash. They'll buy clothing, books, toys, puzzles, cribs and bedding, equipment, furniture, room decor and more; the main requirement is that the kids' stuff you want to sell be in great condition. The store offers some items that can be hard to find, including christening gowns by Tiny Star (several new ones in the $30-$35 range) and premature baby clothing. They carry many name brands, including Baby Gap, Gymboree, OshKosh, and more. A Gymboree boys shortalls with matching hat was selling for $12, girls Oshkosh overalls for $6, and a Pacific Trail ski jacket for $15. They also have a great selection of hats, Safety 1st safety accessories, books, cribs, bedding, toys, shoes, strollers, car seats, high chairs, gates, and other equipment. As a franchise, the store is part of a national buying unit that can give them volume discounts.

During the holidays, the new toys they sell are priced at or below the Toys R Us prices up the street. Shopping here is definitely a great option to the big-store, big-crowds shopping you'll find nearby.

■ THE OTHER PLACE
527-0766
8320 5th Ave. N.E.
Seattle, WA 98115
Hours: M-Sat. 10:30 a.m.-5:30 p.m.
        Th   10:30 a.m.-8:00 p.m.
The Other Place mainly carries women's wear, but there's usually at least one rack of maternity clothing. It's worth a stop if you're close by—the store is just up a few doors from Fifth Avenue Kids.

■ PEEK-A-BOO'S
440-1795
Ballinger Village
20032 Ballinger Way N.E.
Seattle, WA 98155
Hours: T-Sat. 11:00 a.m.-6:00 p.m.
Peek-A-Boo's consignment store opened in late 1995 in Ballinger Village, just next to Terrace Pharmacy. They didn't have a lot of merchandise yet when we visited but the items they did have were very affordable, making this a good shopping option for purchasing some of baby's basic clothing needs. T-shirts and onesies cost between 50 cents and a dollar. Girls' dresses and overalls were priced at around $6. A few cribs ($75-$120) and high chairs ($20 and up) were for sale, as well as some toys and books. One rack had new items, including velvet Jo Lene dresses for $20 and up, and Carter's jackets for $16. The store is large (2,000 square feet) and they have a children's play area in back.

■ RAINBOW BOUTIQUE
522-1213
9518 Roosevelt Way N.E.
Seattle, WA 98115
Hours: M-F   10:00 a.m.-5:30 p.m.
        Sat.   10:00 a.m.-4:00 p.m.
Located in an older strip mall on the east side of Roosevelt Way, you'll recognize Rainbow Boutique by its colorful rainbow sign. From the outside the store looks small but once you enter you're in for a surprise. Since the store recently expanded, there are now four full rooms of clothing, accessories, toys, equipment, and other baby supplies. The first room is filled with racks of high quality children's wear (newborn to size 10) and merchandise is in premium condition. There's a play area for children in this section, as well as a dressing room just for kids. Beyond the children's section is the toys and equipment room, with a sign at the entrance advising parents not to let kids play with the toys that are for sale. (Rainbow Boutique places a high priority on keeping consignors' merchandise in good condition.) There's a wide variety of books and videos, toys, stuffed animals, bedding, strollers, car seats, baby carriers, and cribs for sale.

A large section of women's wear offers stylish choices for after baby is born. In this area you'll especially notice the store's boutique feel, with fully accessorized outfits professionally displayed. There's a dressing room in the women's section too. And yet another dressing room is located in the maternity section, along with a play area and playpen. Maternity wear includes a full selection of shorts, pants, dresses, tops, jumpsuits, and other seasonal items. Prices are moderate—denim overalls for $20, dresses for $15-$20, new ribbed knit stretch pants for

$12.95—and quality on all items is excellent. On the price tags the store labels the fabric type (rayon, cotton, handmade, etc.), another nice touch. Rainbow Boutique is an immaculate, well-organized store that manages to have both a classy and friendly feel at the same time. No wonder they've been in business for more than a decade, with loyal customers and consignors throughout King County and beyond.

■ RE-DRESS
746-7984
513 156th S.E.
Bellevue, WA 98007
Hours: M-F   10:30 a.m.-6:00 p.m.
       Th   until 8:00 p.m.
       Sat.   10:30 a.m.-5:00 p.m.
       Sun.   Noon-5:00 p.m.

Re-Dress is located in the Lake Hills Shopping Center, near QFC. The main focus for Re-Dress has been women's clothing but it has recently expanded to include maternity and children's clothes. Kids' sizes range from newborn to size 14. The management strives to keep prices low for excellent quality, name-brand clothing such as Motherhood Maternity, Carter's, Guess for Kids, Baby Guess, Baby Gap, OshKosh, and more. The store is very clean and well-organized, and stroller accessible. The sales staff is very friendly and helpful in choosing maternity wear for business, casual, and evening attire.

■ SARAH'S HOPE CHEST, LTD.
281-5709
2123 Queen Anne Ave. N.
Seattle, WA 98109
Hours: T-Sat.   10:00 a.m.-6:30 p.m.

On the top of Queen Anne hill, Sarah's Hope Chest is a charming addition to the Queen Anne shopping scene. This store has quickly gained a popular following. One likely reason is the wide selection of affordable used clothing, in sizes from newborn to 14 and women's maternity wear. Most children's items cost from $2-$6—such as overalls for $4.50, dresses from $5-$6, and rompers for $3.50. There's a 50% off rack for even better bargains. Other used items for sale include car seats, strollers, bedding, bikes, games, toys and books. What makes Sarah's Hope Chest especially distinctive is its incredible variety of new clothing, consigned to the store by local designers and handcrafters. Unique designs, colorful and intriguing fabrics, and a good range of casual and dressy items are attractively displayed. Although lines will vary depending on when you visit, some that stood out when we visted were reversible clothing by Juliani, Laarni, and Wiggle Wear, the big selection of knit separates by Mr. Baby Wear, and handmade polar fleece wear. Sarah's Hope Chest definitely offers something for everyone!

■ **SATURDAY'S CHILD CONSIGNMENTS**
486-6716
18012 Bothell-Everett Hwy.
Bothell, WA 98012
Hours: M-F   10:30 a.m.-5:30 p.m.
        Sat.   10:00 a.m.-5:00 p.m.
        Sun.   Noon-4:00 p.m.

Saturday's Child is located near Mill Creek, just east of the 164th S.W. exit from I-5, on the Bothell-Everett Highway. It's a large store with lots of clothes—both new and handcrafted as well as consigned—for boys and girls up to size 14. The prices and quality of the used clothing are quite good. Many clothing items for babies and toddlers are in the $3-$5 range. The store also carries a full assortment of baby furniture and equipment, including swings, strollers, and playpens, as well as some bedding, accessories, and toys. There's a full wall of new Safety 1st baby safety items and the store sells popular children's videos (new) at a discount. There's a nice selection of handcrafted clothing too—we noticed a delightful reversible jumper by Garments of Praise for just $14.50.

■ **THE TREE HOUSE CHILDREN'S SHOP**
885-1145
Redmond Center
15742 Redmond Way
Redmond, WA 98052
Hours: M-F   9:00 a.m.-6:00 p.m.
        Th.   10:00 a.m.-8:00 p.m.
        Sat.   10:00 a.m.-5:00 p.m.
        Sun.   1:00 p.m.-5:00 p.m.

The Tree House is a very unique shop because it offers an especially large selection of both new (about one-third of the inventory) and used/consignment (about two-thirds the inventory) clothing. They've been in business for more than 15 years and have a loyal following. With 3,000 square feet, there's lots of room for merchandise, and it's very nicely organized and displayed. You'll find an extensive section of new baby clothes and accessories to your right as you enter the door. Prices are very moderate. Even preemie clothes, which sometimes carry a premium price at other stores, are available starting at $10 for a Carter's outfit with hat. Other clothing lines include Spumoni, Le Top, OshKosh b'Gosh and Baby b'Gosh, Little Me, Marimekko, and French Toast. Sizes go up to 14. Plenty of baby accessories and supplies are available, including diaper covers, TV booties, hats, and a big selection of rain boots ($6.99). The consignment section is large, with rows and rows of infant and toddler wear, most in good to almost-new condition. Expect to pay about $5 and up for a play outfit. There's also a round rack of consigned maternity clothes, mostly casual wear with pants and jeans for $4-$10 and a few nice dresses in the $8-$20 range. Kids will love the play area at The Tree House, since it features a Little Tikes Gym to climb and play on. And when your daughter reaches school age, you'll find a full supply of Brownie and Girl Scout uniforms here too.

■ **TWICE AROUND THE BLOCK**
783-6498
2406 N.W. 80th
Seattle, WA 98117
Hours: M-F   Noon-4:30 p.m.
        Sat.   10:00 a.m.-6:00 p.m.

This small consignment store is in the Crown Hill/Ballard area of Seattle. Most of what they carry is clothes (both children's and adults), although there are a few baby equipment items in stock, such as car seats. We also saw some toys and books and a few accessories for sale.

■ THE UNICORN BOUTIQUE
823-4868
12537 116th Ave. N.E.
Kirkland, WA 98034
Hours: T-Sat.   10:30 a.m.-5:00 p.m.
The Unicorn Boutique is across from Drug Emporium in the Totem Lake West shopping area. The store offers consignment clothing in women's, children's, and maternity sizes. The maternity rack has some nice jumpers and dresses for $10-$15, mostly in casual looks. There's a large selection of children's wear and prices are very good, averaging $3-$5. The store also carries some new children's wear by Peekaboo in colorful cotton and knits. Shirts start at $6, pants at $9, and rompers at $16. Besides clothing, you'll find a wide assortment of toys, accessories, socks, hats, baby shoes, stuffed animals, mobiles, books, videos, and small furniture items.

OUTLET MALLS

■ FACTORY STORES OF AMERICA OUTLET CENTER
888-4505
North Bend, WA 98045
Hours: M-Sat.   10:00 a.m.-7:00 p.m.
        Sun.   10:00 a.m.-6:00 p.m.
The outlet center in North Bend is right off I-90's exit 31, making this the closest outlet mall from Seattle's eastside. Children's stores include OshKosh b'Gosh and Healthtex. If you time your visit towards the end of the season, you'll often find outstanding bargains.

■ PACIFIC EDGE OUTLET CENTER
(360) 757-3549
Burlington, WA 98233
Hours: Mon.-Sat.10:00 a.m.-9:00 p.m.
        Sun.   10:00 a.m.-6:00 p.m.
This outlet center is located 60 miles north of Seattle, off I-5 at exit 229. Genuine Kids, a division of OshKosh, is one of the children's clothing merchants here. They carry clothes beginning with infant size, all the way through girls 16 and boys 20. There's also a Carter's Childrenswear outlet here.

■ SUPERMALL OF THE GREAT NORTHWEST
800-SAY-VALU
Auburn, WA 98001
Hours: M-Sat.   9:30 a.m.-9:30 p.m.
        Sun.   11:00 a.m.-6:00 p.m.
The new SuperMall is easy to find at Highways 167 and 18; just look for the traffic! The largest outlet mall in Washington state, it boasts over 100 stores. For infants' and children's wear, there's Kids Mart, Carter's Childrenswear, Burlington Coat Factory, and Marshall's. The mall is very family-friendly, with plenty of amenities and special events to encourage families to stay and shop awhile. There's even a designated area for nursing your baby. Their four themed areas include the Great Outdoors Court, Aviation Court, Train Court (with an 1884 locomotive on display), and Carousel Court (complete with a working carousel).

DIAPER SERVICES

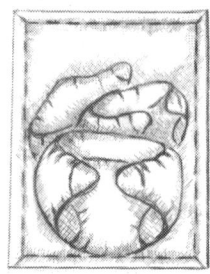

With most of us environmentally conscious today, diaper services are offering parents an alternative for keeping their babies dry. In the Seattle area there are several excellent diaper services available.

In researching diaper services, we found most operate similarly. Compare the prices and services of each and make sure the company you choose meets your needs.

- If you like planning ahead, you may order diapers one month before your baby's due date. Diapers should be delivered a week ahead of time.

- With some services, it takes about a week from the time you request service to the time you receive your first diaper delivery.

- A delivery person will drop off clean diapers and pick up the soiled ones, usually on the same day. You can also arrange to leave your diapers in a special spot if you are not home during a delivery.

- A deodorized hamper is provided to store the soiled diapers. Some services allow you to keep the hamper, and others ask you to return it upon cancellation of the service.

- A vacation credit is standard for most diaper services. Simply contact your company one week in advance to let them know when you will be traveling. Your account should be credited for the time you are away.

- Most diaper companies require a minimum service period and need notification of at least one week before cancelling the service.

- Watch your baby's blankets or other personal items to make sure they don't drop in the diaper pail. Because of the large number of customers most diaper companies serve, it would be difficult to return personal items accidentally dropped in the diaper pail.

- A free diaper cover may be provided or rented by your diaper service. Diaper covers make it easier to use cloth diapers and come in various colors and sizes. Check with your diaper company for details.

- Diapers are the company's inventory, so they ask customers to return the same number of cloth diapers as they receive.

⮞ RESOURCES ⮞

■ **BABY DIAPER SERVICE** [Baby Pages]
800-562-2229
634-BABY Seattle
Hours: M-F   7:00 a.m. - 5:00 p.m.
        Sat.   9:00 a.m. - 1:00 p.m.
383-BABY Tacoma
Hours: M-F   1:00 p.m.-5:00 p.m.
                 for pick-up

Baby Diaper Service is the largest and one of the oldest diaper services in Washington. It serves customers throughout King, Pierce, Snohomish, Kitsap and Thurston counties. We were impressed with the customer service when inquiring about using the company. The representative, Vicky, was knowledgeable and offered an array of information. Baby Diaper Service offers a variety of sizes of diapers from preemie to toddler.

They also offer a diaper cover purchase program. To begin with, Baby Diaper Service recommends 80 newborn diapers at the low price of $13.35 a week. There is a four week minimum sign-up with the service and if you're a new customer you receive six weeks for the price of four. Similar promotions are available for longer sign-up periods. One other unique feature Baby Diaper Service provides is a day care diaper credit. If your day care charges you for diapers and you provide Baby Diaper Service with a receipt, they will give you a maximum of $15 per month towards any diaper charges.

Baby Diaper Service will deliver diapers before your baby is born. The first set of newborn diaper covers you purchase are offered at a special price of 3 for $10; these covers have space for the umbilical cord as part of their design. All of its diapers are pH balanced and 100% cotton. There is no setup fee for the service. A monthly newspaper entitled Northwest Baby and Child, published by Baby Diaper Service, is distributed at no charge throughout the greater Puget Sound Area and is delivered free to customers. Baby Diaper Service is also a member of the National Association of Diaper Services.

■ PURE AND NATURAL
545-1075

Pure and Natural's philosophy is to provide a quality diaper and excellent customer service. With its customer base, this service is able to offer special services unavailable through other diaper services. Pure and Natural offers a great variety of sizes from preemie to toddler plus training pants. The monthly service includes weekly pick-up and delivery, a diaper pail, hamper liners, deodorizers, and a free subscription to Seattle's Child. Diaper wraps are also available for purchase at a competitive price.

Specials are available for parents who sign up for at least one month. The most common promotion offers two weeks free for the first four weeks committed (with a 4-week minimum order). Another money-saving special they offer is a referral credit. Pure and Natural also has a total satisfaction promise which means if anything is not right, they will fix your customer concern. Pure and Natural delivers throughout the greater Seattle and Eastside area.

■ QUALITY DIAPER SERVICE
825-4171 South King County
226-7490 Seattle

Quality Diaper Service serves the South King County area and Enumclaw plateau. For all new customers it offers one diaper wrap, a set of pins, a diaper pail, hamper liners and deodorizers. Also, when you first sign up for the service you receive the fifth week free when paying for one month. Costs are competitive with other services. Eighty newborn diapers are about $52 a month.

CHILD CARE

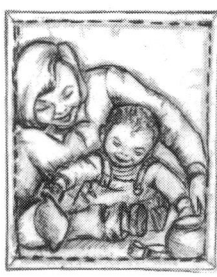

Whether you work full-time, part-time or stay at home with your child, quality child care is a necessity. Selecting the right type of care can be an overwhelming task. Although child care facilities must meet certain state and county guidelines, you should have your own list of preferences and expectations. Listen to your parental instincts when making your selection. Trust may be the single most important factor in making the final decision of who becomes your child's caregiver. Leaving your child is difficult anyway, but to do so with a child care arrangement that you are not 100 percent satisfied with is even more stressful.

To help you choose a caregiver, a number of agencies will provide names, phone numbers and information on care providers. We have chosen not to list specific child care facilities, since individual providers change frequently. Instead, this guide refers you to local child care agencies that will help you find the right caregiver for your specific needs.

To begin your child care search, it is important to examine the options available to you. Below is a brief description of the most common child care choices, including child care centers, licensed family child care and live-in or in-home child care.

❧

Although child care facilities must meet certain state and county guidelines, you should have your own list of preferences and expectations.

❧

CHILD CARE CENTERS

Child care centers are facilities licensed to care for more than 12 children. Centers that care for infants have an adult-to-child ratio of 1:4. (One adult must be available to care for every four infants under the age of 12 months.) For toddlers from 12-29 months, the ratio is 1:7. Ratios for children 30 months to 5 years are 1:10; 5 years and older, 1:15. These ratios are established to make sure your child will receive ample care and attention.

Besides following the adult-to-child ratio, child care centers are also expected to fulfill educational requirements and provide more than just a baby-sitting environment for children. Many child care centers will give you written reports on your child that include everything from the number of diaper changes to the achievements of special milestones, such as a first step. Child care centers must also follow specific fire, building, and zoning codes.

Some child care centers go beyond minimum requirements and seek to become accredited by the National Association for the Education of Young Children (NAEYC). This requires meeting nationally recognized high standards of quality and includes a site evaluation by a NAEYC accreditor.

A growing trend in recent years are on-site (or near-site) child-care centers that are provided by employers. Several local businesses and organizations offer this option in the Seattle area, including the City of Seattle and The Seattle Times. Hospitals and medical centers with child care centers for their employees include Fred Hutchinson, Group Health, Northwest, Providence, Swedish and Virginia Mason. The federal government has also been very supportive of this concept, with on-site centers at NOAA's Western Regional Center, EPA's regional headquarters, downtown Seattle, Federal Center South, GSA in Auburn, and several more on the way.

Specific arrangements with each on-site center and employer vary: employers may or may not subsidize care costs, some contract with child care companies to operate the centers while others hire their own employees, and some are overseen by a nonprofit board made up of parent-employees. Many allow children of non-employees to attend their center too, if space is available. While an on-site center is not necessarily less expensive than centers elsewhere, parents enjoy the convenience of having their children nearby and the opportunity to see them during the day. For working mothers of nursing infants, these centers provide an option to continue nursing during the workday.

According to Child Care Resources, the local child care referral agency, costs for full-time infant care at child care centers in King County range from $3,515 to $11,700 per year, with an average yearly cost of $7,224.

Some advantages of choosing a child care center may be:

- Convenient location for parents.
- Reliability of the center's caregivers.
- Written daily reports on your child's activities.
- The provider's educational background may include some early childhood education and/or previous child care experience.
- Planned activities (some centers schedule field trips).
- Programs are offered for every age, so your child can stay at the same center through the years.
- Licensing requirements are very strict, and there is constant supervision.

Disadvantages may include:

- Larger and less of a "homey" environment for infant care.
- Lack of "sick" care. Most centers have very strict sick care rules and will not accept ill children. (This can be an advantage too!)
- More caregivers—so your child may have less of an opportunity to bond with a provider.
- May cost more than licensed family day care.
- May be less flexible than in-home or licensed family child care providers. Check when they close for holidays; some operate on schedules similar to local school districts.
- Most child-care centers are businesses that cater to a large number of families, rather than a single provider who may serve only a dozen families or less.
- Most centers have policies that you must follow under all circumstances.
- Many centers have high staff turnover.

FAMILY CHILD CARE HOMES

Family child care refers to child care in the private home of a licensed individual. The number of children a single provider can care for depends on the age range of the children and the experience of the caregiver. A new licensee can care for six children, with no more than two under the age of two. With one year of experience, the caregiver can also choose to care for eight children, ages 2-11, or 10 children ages 5-11. With an assistant caregiver and one year of experience, the home can care for nine children, with up to four under age two.

To evaluate each licensed family child care provider, the licensing board visits each child care home before the initial licensing and is supposed to make annual inspections, too. Because of the large number of child care homes and the small number of licensors in King County, homes usually get visited once every two to three years. Licensors also visit homes whenever a complaint is made.

According to Child Care Resources, annual costs for family child care in King County range from $975 to $14,040 per year, with an average cost of $5,760 per year.

Some advantages of working with family child care homes are:

- The provider is licensed and therefore must follow certain guidelines provided by the state and county to retain licensing.
- A smaller and more family-like environment.
- More likely to have the same primary care provider, so your child can bond with one person.

- Can be less expensive.
- Social interaction with other children.
- May be more flexible. Some home care providers will watch your child after hours if you have special needs.

Disadvantages may include:

- Since you're often dealing with only one provider, if he or she becomes ill or takes a vacation you must work around that person's schedule.
- No educational requirements are needed to be a licensed family child care provider.
- Child care may be treated more casually because the provider is in her own home and not supervised by others.
- If the provider's own children are also being cared for, there is the possibility that her own child could be favored.
- The provider may not stay in business for the length of time your child needs care, i.e., may stop providing services if economics or family needs change.

ABOUT LICENSING

All child care centers and family child care homes in Washington state are licensed by the Department of Social and Health Services.

A child care license limits the number and ages of children in care. A license requires that all child care providers are checked for criminal and child abuse records. Before a license is issued, all child care centers and homes are checked for health and safety hazards.

If you have questions about the care your child is receiving at a center or home,

If you have concerns about a particular provider, you may wish to contact one of these resources:

LICENSING QUESTIONS OR COMPLAINTS
Department of Social and Health Services
King County: 721-4080 (centers)
               721-4160 (homes)
Snohomish County: 339-4780

REPORTING ABUSE OR NEGLECT
DSHS Child Protective Services
Seattle: 721-4115
South King County: 872-2665
East King County: 649-4110

talk to the teacher, director or home provider about your concerns or impressions.

If you think the children in care are at a risk of health and safety hazards and you have talked to the provider without any results, you can call the licensing authority and request an investigation of the care situation.

LIVE-IN OR IN-HOME CHILD CARE

There are several options for those who prefer to have their child care in their own home. Live-ins can be arranged through various nanny services or au pair organizations. An au pair is a foreign student who exchanges child-care services for living arrangements and/or a salary. You can also make an agreement with a private party or individual.

Although many nanny agencies have strict screening requirements, no government agency regulates care in your own home. Past employment references serve as the primary screening tool for nannies and other in-home providers. Annual salaries for a full-time nanny hired through an agency can range from $9,000-$22,000. Most agencies also charge a one-time placement fee.

The advantages of care in your own home may be:

- Convenience—someone will come to or live in your home.
- There is less travel and preparation time for parent.
- Your child is in a familiar environment.
- Many in-home providers may also do light housework, cooking and other household duties.
- In-home providers may be experienced and have some type of child education background.
- Providers are thoroughly screened by nanny placement services, and most services offer a guarantee.
- Some care givers will also provide sick-care.

Disadvantages may be:
- The cost.
- Lack of licensing and supervision.
- Household space requirements and loss of family privacy with a live-in.
- Reliance upon one individual for child care.
- Your child may not receive the same socialization skills compared to being in a group setting.

STEPS FOR CHOOSING CHILD CARE

The following checklist should help you select the best child care situation for your child. This is reprinted with permission from "Choosing Child Care," an information sheet provided by Child Care Resources.

- List things you feel are important for you and your child.
- Screen potential caregivers on the phone to see if they meet your basic requirements and make appointments with those you would like to visit.
- During your visits, use a checklist to evaluate programs. Visit more than once and at different times of day.

- Check references by talking to parents with children in the program and calling the child care licensor of the program.
- Take your child to visit the final choice(s).
- Trust your intuition and observations.
- Read the caregiver's written policies and procedures carefully.
- Consider substitute plans in case your child is ill or your child's care provider or the child care center is on vacation or closed.
- Work together with your caregiver to make the best child care experience for your child.

❧ RESOURCES ❧

REFERRAL AGENCIES

■ **CHILD CARE RESOURCE AND REFERRAL NETWORK**
258-4213
Hours: M-F   8:30 a.m.-1:30 p.m.
This referral line is operated by the Volunteers of America and provides referrals to child care homes and centers in Snohomish County. It is free for Snohomish County residents.

■ **CHILD CARE RESOURCES**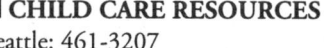
Seattle: 461-3207
1265 South Main St., Ste. 210
Seattle, WA 98144

Bellevue: 865-9350
15015 Main St., Ste. 206
Bellevue, WA 98007

S. King County: 852-3080
841 N. Central Ave., Ste. 126
Kent, WA 98032
Hours: M-Th   9:00 a.m.-3:00 p.m.,
                     6:30 p.m.-9:30 p.m.
        F   9:00 a.m.-1:00 p.m.
Telephone information and referral that connects parents seeking child care with licensed care providers is just one of the things Child Care Resources accomplishes. Through its computer data base it can link you with a provider near your work or home. It also offers the "Needs 'n Kids" program which lists providers who care for children who have various physical or developmental disabilities. Child Care Resources also provides employer programs, seminars, workshops and advocacy on child care-related topics. Operated as a nonprofit agency, Child Care

Resources serves the Seattle/King, East King and South King counties. Costs are determined on a sliding scale basis.

■ **DAYCARE FINDERS**
932-3677
Hours: 24-hour voice mail
A new business begun in 1995, Daycare Finders is run by a woman who previously owned a day care for 20 years. The company helps individual parents, as well as corporations seeking child care referrals for employees. For a $25 fee, Daycare Finders will provide a list of all licensed day care openings meeting a client's specific needs, such as age of child, location of child care center, special schedules, etc. They will provide lists for up to a three-month period for the $25 fee and only list those with openings that fit the client's requirements. The client is responsible for interviewing caregivers and making the final decision.

■ **KING COUNTY FAMILY CHILDCARE ASSOCIATION**
467-1552
Hours: M-F   9:00 a.m.-4:00 p.m.
This nonprofit organization will send you a list of licensed child-care homes in King County, ordered by zip code. The roster is free and is updated continuously.

■ **SEATTLE DEPARTMENT OF HOUSING AND HUMAN SERVICES**
386-1050
If you're eligible, you may have 25-90% of the cost of child care subsidized by the city. You must live within the Seattle city limits, be employed or in job training, and qualify based on income guidelines.

■ **WASHINGTON STATE CHILD CARE RESOURCE AND REFERRAL NETWORK**
800-446-1114
This is the number to call in Washington state if you live somewhere other than King or Snohomish County and need to find child care. The state line can put you in touch with your local child care resources agency.

OTHER RESOURCES

■ **OFFICE OF CHILD CARE POLICY**
State Department of Social and Health Services
P.O. Box 45710
Olympia, WA 98504-5710
You can order a free copy of "Choosing Child Care: A Consumer Guide for Parents" by sending a postcard to this address. The booklet was prepared by DSHS and the Seattle Department of Human Resources, and includes a checklist to complete as you visit potential child-care sites.

IN-HOME CHILD CARE AGENCIES

■ **ANNIE'S NANNIES**
784-8462
5018 Greenwood Ave. N.
Seattle, WA 98103
Hours: M-F   9:00 a.m. - 5:00 p.m.
In business since 1984, Annie's Nannies is the Puget Sound area's original nanny service. Annie Davis and her partner and daughter, Suzanne Royer McCone, personally interview with all families and nannies. Families rely on the partners' skills in matching just the right nannies

with parents and their children. The company's goal is to make sure that every family has the best nanny to share in the parenting of their children. Annie's Nannies' screening process includes a criminal background and driving record check in any state in which the nanny has lived. Also, all references are personally spoken to by the agency.

Salaries for nannies range from $1,200 to $1,800 per month for full-time live-out and $900 to $1,200 plus room and board for live-in, depending on the position and their experience. Part-time nannies make between $7 to $10 per hour. Annie's Nannies' placement fee is $1,600 with $150 of the fee as a deposit at the time they meet the family. The remainder is due after hiring the nanny. They give a one-year guarantee on all placements. This means that if the nanny does not work out for whatever reason, she/he will be replaced. Annie's Nannies is always available for a phone consultation as needed with the family or nanny for duration of employment. Most of their nannies are with families for many years.

■ CAREWORKS INNOVATIVE NANNY SOLUTIONS
325-7510 (24 hour voice mail)
Careworks is a nanny placement service dedicated to supporting families in finding child care solutions to suit their individual needs. CareWork's unique approach to matching nannies and families assures compatibility in the areas of parenting style, personality and values. The owner, Linda Stacey, started her business after seeking nannies for her own family and finding that the kind of service she had pictured wasn't being offered. Her focus on being service-oriented has been

well-received by her clients, since she was voted the Best Nanny Service for two years in a row by readers of Seattle's Child newsmagazine and given their Golden Bootie Award.

Careworks' first step in working with a family is an in-home interview to help define the family's parenting philosophy and to develop a clear picture of what a nanny's role can be. Both the family and prospective nannies are asked to complete two evaluations designed to assess compatibility in the areas of parenting, communication style and temperament. Defining these elements at the start is the key to establishing long-term successful relationships. Careworks also does a complete screening of all nanny applicants, including criminal and traffic checks, and requires CPR and first aid certification. They personally interview the references of applicants, and select only applicants who receive "glowing" recommendations. The cost for the initial application is $100 and includes this in-home interview. The placement fee is $1,200 which includes a one-year guarantee. Full-time nannies are paid $1,200-$1,800 monthly for live-out and $1,000-$1,400 for live-in.

Because Careworks recognizes that different families have different needs, and because they want to make nanny services available to more people, they also offer a free nanny share network for parents who want to share the services of a nanny and reduce their costs. Names of families interested in sharing are kept in a data base and matched by needs.

■ CARRIE CARE NANNY AND CHILDCARE SERVICE

844-2802

Hours: M-F   8:00 a.m. - 4:00 p.m.

This service provides both live-in and live-out placements. Their screening includes criminal and driving record checks, medical statement, and reference verification (both child care and character). They require two years of previous child care experience and current CPR and first aid and updated immunizations. This service is unique in that the owner, Carrie Dovenbarger, and Director Stephanie Hanson interview both the clients and potential nannies personally in their homes (versus their office) for better placement compatibility. Their initial application fee is $50, for which they will provide you with up to four nannies to interview. The placement fee is $650 for a three-month guarantee and $850 for a six-month guarantee for a part-time (24 hours/week or less) nanny or $1,050 for a three-month guarantee and $1,250 for a six-month guarantee for a full-time nanny. Nannies are paid between $7 and $10 per hour. This service has a strong ongoing support system: they provide temporary nannies to act as substitutes for vacationing nannies and have nanny workshops in order to enhance the nannies' childcare skills.

■ DREAMBOAT NANNIES

232-2553

Hours: M-F   8:00 a.m. - 6:00 p.m.

Dreamboat Nannies matches parents with live-in or live-out nannies. They require nanny applicants to provide between four and eight references, and besides verifying these, the agency also checks the criminal and traffic history and health of the nanny. Nannies also need to have CPR and first aid training. The $75 applica-

tion fee gets the process started and includes as many potential nanny interviews as needed to find a match. The placement fee is $950 and there is a nine-month guarantee. Nannies generally are paid from $6-$10/hour for live-out and usually not less than $800/month for live-in.

■ JUDI JULIN, R.N., NANNYBROKER INC.

624-1213 or 392-5681

25620 S.E. 157th Street

Issaquah, WA 98027

Hours: M-F   9:00 a.m.-9:00 p.m.

    Emergencies anytime

Nannybroker Inc. is owned by a registered nurse, Judi Julin, who has been interviewing nannies for 25 years and placing nannies for nearly nine. As the owner of her business, she strives to be as accessible as possible to her clients. Julin has also authored a book entitled "So You Want to Hire your Own Nanny."

Nannybroker Inc. offers live-in or live-out, permanent or part-time care. All applicants are fully screened and both personal and work references are thoroughly checked. You pay no up-front fees and only pay the agency once a child care provider is found. The fee for a permanent provider normally equals a monthly salary which runs about $1,300. For temporary help, the fee equals about $8-$10 daily and wages are between $8-$10 per hour. Overnight stays are also available with wages at $100 each 24-hour period and the agency fee approximately $15 per day. For permanent placement, a 90-day guarantee is offered through this service which means if your nanny does not work out, Nannybroker should replace him or her at no additional cost.

■ A NANNY FOR U

745-9882

24-Hour Pager: 969-1119

Rebecca Anderson-Vidmore, owner of A Nanny For U, brings five years of nanny experience to the nanny placement business. The philosophy of A Nanny For U is to provide a nurturing environment in which your child is both stimulated and secure. They also focus on providing on-going support and communication to their clients and nannies in order to sustain long-term placements.

Offering 90-day and one-year guarantees, with fees ranging from $700-$1,100, A Nanny For U is unique in that no upfront or application fee is paid until a nanny is placed with the family. Rebecca personally meets the families in their homes to ensure a long-lasting nanny-parent relationship. A Nanny For U does not limit the number of nanny candidates that a family may consider. Each nanny is carefully screened after completing the application and interviewing with A Nanny For U. Criminal and driving records are checked, as well as three childcare references. Upon being hired, nannies are sent to Kid Safety Plus, a class which thoroughly educates and certifies them in CPR, first aid, and overall child safety. Nanny salaries range from $8-$10 per hour for part-time, $1,200-$1,600 per month for full-time live-out, and $800-$1,400 for full-time live-in.

TEMPORARY AND SICK CHILD CARE

■ BEST SITTERS

682-2556

Best Sitters is one of the oldest temporary child care services. In business for more than 25 years, Best Sitters provides temporary child care in your home and at major hotels. There's a four-hour minimum and fees for one child begin at $33 (first four hours) and $6/hour after that. Rates vary depending on number of children, whether there is another adult on the premises, starting time for care, if child is ill, and if overnight care is needed. Babysitters must be at least 25 years old or have two or more years of nanny experience.

■ OPTIONS IN CHILDCARE

562-8905

13238 N.E. 20th (Northup Way)

Bellevue, WA 98005

Options' "Under the Weather Center" is the first licensed child care center authorized to care for mildly ill children. A professional registered nurse is on-site to screen and direct the care of the children in the center. Care is offered Monday-Friday, 6:00 a.m.-7:30 p.m.

Options also offers the "Fill the Gap Center" which provides back-up or open-door care for parents whose primary caregiver may be unavailable, or who otherwise need short-term care for their children. The center operates Monday-Friday 6:00 a.m.-1:00 a.m. and Saturdays 8:00 a.m.-8:00 p.m.

Care at Options is available for children from 11 months to 12 years old. Rates vary depending on age of child, number of hours, and whether sick child care is needed. In general, it costs about $6.15-$6.25/hour for temporary care. Costs for sick care are $45 for four hours, $60 for four to eight hours, and $11.50/hour for over eight hours.

■ **PEDIATRIC HOME CARE TEMPORARY CHILDCARE SERVICES**
747-7161
800-564-1906
13400 Northup Way, Ste. 42
Bellevue, WA 98005
Hours: M-F   7:00 a.m. -5:30 p.m.
         Sat.-Sun. 7:00 a.m. -3:00 p.m.
If your child is mildly ill or injured and cannot attend regular school or day care, PHC Temporary Childcare can help you secure appropriate child care; they can also provide this service if your child is well. Common illnesses or conditions appropriate to this program include, but are not limited to: chicken pox, ear infections, strep throat, tonsillitis, conjunctivitis (pinkeye), mumps, flu, mild injuries. You first must register with the service and complete a service agreement and preregistration form. If you are unable to preregister, you can get help the day you need service for a $5 fee. When you need the service, PHC's staff may help find the right provider for you. Prices for the service are $12 per hour for one child and $5 per day for each additional child with the total limit 3 children. The child care providers are nursing assistants who are experienced in sick childcare needs and developmentally appropriate craft activities. They are also certified in CPR. PHC Temporary Child Care has an on-call nurse available 24 hours a day.

Life Experiences...

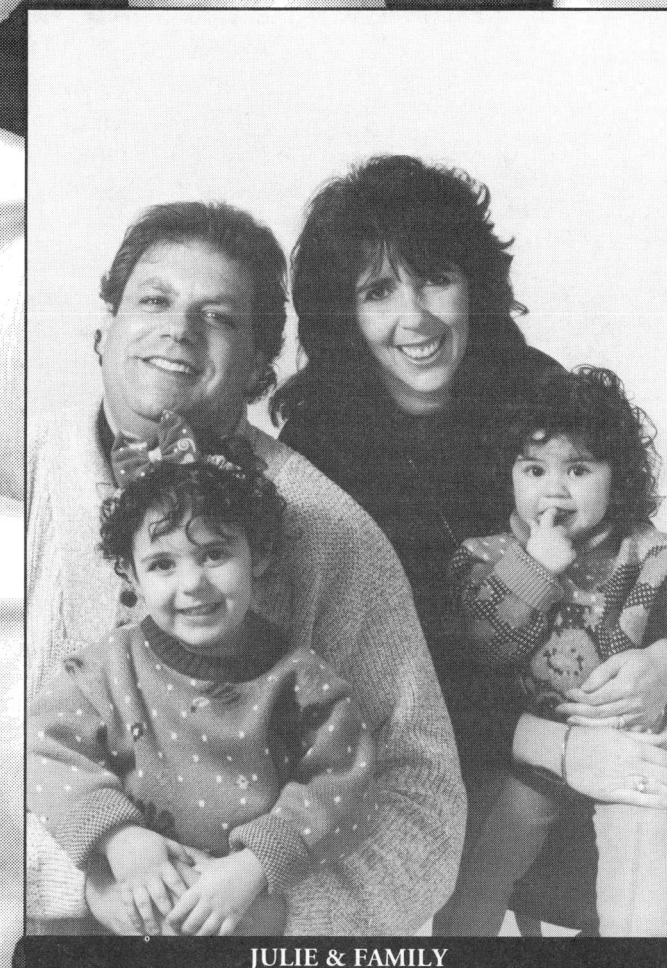

JULIE & FAMILY

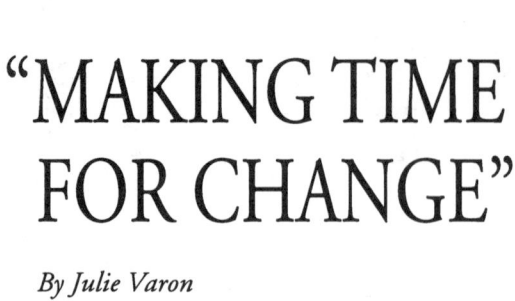

"MAKING TIME FOR CHANGE"

By Julie Varon

I always imagined that I could "have it all"...family, career, social life. I set the stage for this dream early on by having great success in sales. If I wasn't working, I was traveling, golfing, skiing and searching for that special some-one. However, finding the man I would spend the rest of my life with was a challenge. And then I met Ben. I think some of what I found so appealing about Ben was his love of children. This was apparent on our second date when he willingly came to a baby shower for a friend of mine, bearing a gift. I then discovered he had a entire photo album dedicated to his nephews and nieces, not to mention other friends' kids. I immediately knew he'd be a great dad!

We had a storybook engagement and wedding, knowing that the next chapter would be the addition of children. We were both in our mid-thirties and saw little reason to wait. Evidently our friends who knew us expected the same. One of our wedding gifts was an ovulation kit! Within the first year we were pregnant and very happy. We were ready for "domes-tic bliss"...or so we thought. Everyone always says how much having a baby will change your life. I guess I just thought that some additional hormone would kick in along with the baby, making it easy. Unfortunately, I can't say that I was right. The juggling act was about to begin.

I went back to work six weeks after having my first child, Sarah. The biggest obstacle was finding a comfortable, safe child care situation. With that in place I proceeded to resume my work schedule much as it has been before. It helped to know that there were many other working moms that were sharing my experience. The lunchroom discussions changed radically for me—from which cruise I had returned from to how few hours I slept the night before. The good news was that Ben far

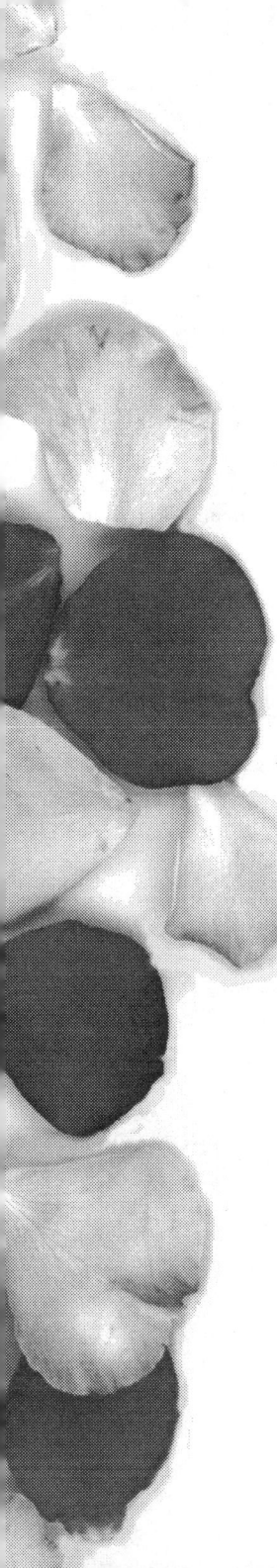

exceeded my expectations and was a fully involved father. I can't imagine it any other way. I understand that I should be (and am) thankful.

Just as we were starting to adjust to parenthood, we had the once-again-exciting news that I was pregnant. Sarah was 15 months old when we brought Rachel home. She greeted her little sister with hugs and kisses. Only now as they get older are we beginning to referee.

Now I was faced with a much bigger dilemma...two babies and an imminent move from Los Angeles to Seattle, to better our quality of life and be closer to our extended families. Although I had to give up the 14-year career that had given us financial security, I chose in favor of improving our family's position. As difficult as it was deciding to make the move, the aftermath of finding myself in a new city with a new baby was overwhelming. I discovered how much of me was invested in my job and how much of my own identity was tied to what I did. I wasn't sure that being "mom" was going to fulfill me, not to mention my pocketbook.

The obvious thing was to try and find part-time work. In fact that is what I am now doing. Wearing both hats has a whole new set of challenges. In the morning I could be working on a contract and in the afternoon I might be found running through sprinklers with the girls. I'm still working on getting to know "the new me." The thing that I constantly remind myself of is how precious the time I get to spend with the kids really is. It's more than just a cliché as to how fast the time goes. So maybe I don't exactly "have it all" yet, but what a fun ride it has been trying to achieve that goal. ❧

MATERNITY LEAVE

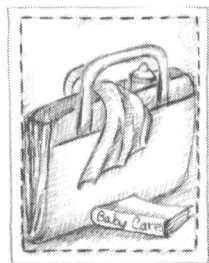

Planning ahead for your maternity leave is the key to making a smooth transition from leaving your job to enjoying your time at home with your new baby. The more informed you are about your rights in the workplace, the better you can maximize your options.

This section of the resource guide focuses on the laws that protect pregnant women and on the "gray" areas that surround maternity leave. This section is not intended to replace legal advice. It should also be noted that the laws change often in this area, so use the resources given to fully understand the most current information.

One resource we found very helpful is a book entitled *Everything a working mother needs to know** by Anne C. Weisberg and Carol A. Buckler. The book offers both a legal and logistical approach to maternity leave. It also offered great resources during maternity leave.

❧

The more informed you are about your rights in the workplace, the better you can maximize your options.

❧

THE FAMILY AND MEDICAL LEAVE ACT

In 1989, the State of Washington enacted a Family Leave Act. Four years later, President Clinton signed the Family and Medical Leave Act of 1993 (FMLA). The provisions in the Federal government's FMLA are more generous to employees in most cases than Washington State's, so employees will usually request an FMLA leave, although both laws must be followed. The FMLA requires employers with 50 or more employees to permit most personnel to take up to twelve weeks of unpaid family care leave. (The 50 employees is limited to worksites with 50 or more persons employed within 75 miles of the worksite.) This leave can be for the birth or adoption of a child, to care for a parent, spouse, or child, or personal leave if that individual has a serious health condition.

The Act also requires employers to guarantee reemployment in the same or equivalent position to workers who return from family leave. Employers are also required to pay for employees' existing health benefits while they are on leave. If the employee does not return to work at the end of the FMLA leave, the employer may collect the cost of the premium, so long as failure to return to work is not beyond the employee's control.

WHO IS ELIGIBLE FOR FAMILY LEAVE?

All employees with more than one year of service and at least 1,250 hours in the last twelve months with the employer are covered by this Act. Both spouses may take the full amount of the leave, as long as they do not work for the same company. The employer may limit the family leave for birth or adoption, not to exceed a total of twelve weeks between both spouses working at the same company.

Another provision in eligibility for the FMLA is the "Key Employee Exception." This means if you are a salaried employee among the highest paid 10% in a company and if restoration or taking the leave would lead to substantial and grievous economic harm to your employer, you may be refused the leave. This places a heavy burden on the employer to justify exempting an employee. If your employer does refuse your leave based on the "Key Employee Exception" it would be to your benefit to contact the U.S. Department of Labor, Wage and Hour Division to clarify this clause.

WHAT CAN THE LEAVE BE USED FOR?

This leave may be used to care for a newborn or adopted child, a seriously ill child, or a parent or spouse who suffers from a serious health condition. The act defines "child" as a biological, adopted, or foster child, a stepchild, a legal ward, or a dependent adult child.

HOW ARE THE TWELVE WEEKS DEFINED?

In accordance with the FMLA, you may take twelve unpaid work weeks in a 12-month period. Employers may require, or an employee may elect, to substitute paid vacation or any other accrued time off for a portion of an employee's available unpaid FMLA. An employee may only substitute accrued sick time for a portion of the unpaid family care leave if the reason for the leave would otherwise entitle the employee to use sick leave.

You may want to check with your employer and further discuss your company's maternity leave policy.

ARE YOU PAID DURING YOUR LEAVE?

The employer does not need to provide any salary unless the employee uses vacation time or other paid time off during the period of family leave.

During your leave, you can not be forced to sacrifice any seniority or benefits. When you return from the family care leave, you will have the same seniority and benefits as before your leave. Your employer also cannot consider your leave a break in service for purposes of a layoff, promotion, job assignment, employee benefits (including vacation) and for any seniority provision under a collective bargaining agreement. Your employer, however, does not need to pay into your pension or retirement plan during your leave. You must be allowed to make contributions to your retirement plan.

WHEN TO NOTIFY YOUR EMPLOYER

You should give your employer at least 30 days advance notice or as soon as possible when taking your leave for birth or adoption. Longer notice is always appreciated.

Contributing authors: Michael J. Killeen and Cliff Elliott from Davis Wright Tremaine.

PREGNANCY DISABILITY LEAVE REGULATION

For employees who work for companies that are not required to follow the FMLA, you are protected under the Washington law against discrimination and Washington's maternity disability regulations (WAC 162-30-020) which consider pregnancy discrimination to be sex discrimination. This is a violation of the state law. Companies with eight or more employees are subject to comply with this act.

In the "average" situation, a woman is disabled by pregnancy at least two to four weeks before her due date and four to six weeks after a vaginal birth. The period is a bit longer for recovery from a Cesarean birth. Your health care provider will determine when and if you are considered "disabled" by pregnancy and childbirth. Your provider holds the "answer" on how long you are physically disabled. *You are only entitled to the amount of leave your doctor certifies you to be disabled.*

If you are medically able to return to work, but choose not to, you are not covered by the Pregnancy Disability Leave Regulation.

Here is a summary of the state's maternity regulations.

- An employer may not refuse to hire you because you are pregnant.
- Your employer may not discharge or penalize you because you are pregnant.
- Your employer must give you a leave of absence for the period of time you are disabled because of pregnancy or childbirth.
- You must be allowed to return to the same or a similar job with the same pay.
- Your marital status does not matter.

In general, your employer's leave and benefit policies for pregnancy should be applied in the same way as leave for other temporary disabilities. There may be exceptions to the above based on an employer's business necessity.

QUESTIONS & ANSWERS
Your Maternity Leave

The following interview with the Microsoft Corporation Benefits Department answers commonly asked questions about maternity leave. The information below should not take the place of legal advice or information from your company's human resources professional.

Q: When should I notify my employer about my pregnancy?

A: At Microsoft, we encourage our employees to notify their manager regarding their estimated leave of absence dates as soon as possible. This enables the manager to arrange for contingent staffing and/or time to determine what duties will need to be temporarily reassigned.

Q: Although the law provides guidelines for maternity leave, is there room for negotiating a flexible or longer leave than what the law or current company policy stipulates?

A: It's important that the employee be familiar with her company's leave of absence policies. In some cases, employers may allow you to extend your leave of absence by using your floating holidays or accrued vacation. Additionally, based on the type of work you do, in rare instances some employers may be open to allowing you to take your leave of absence on an intermittent basis.

Q: What is the benefit of a short-term disability plan?

A. If your physician determines that you will not be able to work up until the time you deliver, short term disability plans allow the expectant mother time off prior to her delivery and maternity leave. Some short term disability plans provide benefits only after sick leave benefits are exhausted.

Q: If I do all my homework and present my employer with a reasonable request for maternity leave, could my leave still be refused?

A: Most employers are required to allow you to take leave of absence under the provisions and in accordance with the 1993 Federal Family and Medical Leave Act (FMLA). Further, in the State of Washington, the Pregnancy Discrimination Act protects individuals who work at a company with eight or more employees. Per this act, employers must provide disability leave for pregnant women for the length of time when a woman is actually disabled due to pregnancy and birth. Situations may vary based on the number of hours you work, how long you have been employed and other circumstances.

Q: Once my employer knows of my pregnancy, should I expect to be treated any differently and will my responsibilities change?

A: Based on the type of work that you do, your health care provider may indicate that some of your job duties may need to be modified until after you return from maternity leave. It is best to discuss this with your health care provider and your employer, so that your employer can determine the feasibility of your request for this temporary accommodation.

Q: After I've had my baby, should I call my employer? And what should I say?

A: Employers and co-workers are usually anxious to hear if you had a boy or girl, how you are feeling, and information about your new family. Additionally, if your employer has a health care plan that your newborn will be a part of, this is a good time to enroll them in the plan.

Q: Can a man take advantage of a parental leave?

A: New fathers are eligible for leave under the provisions and in accordance with the 1993 FMLA unless both spouses work at the same company. In this case, they may choose to share the allotted time allowed by the Act.

Q: What if my maternity leave is up and I decide I really don't want to return to work?

A: If at the end of your leave, you decide not to return to work, it is best to inform your employer right away so that they can work toward hiring someone to replace you. Also, under the FMLA of 1993 the employer may require you to pay for your health benefits that were paid for during your family leave.

Here is a checklist that may be helpful while planning your maternity leave.

- Consult your library and review the Family Medical Leave Act of 1993.
- Review Washington State's Pregnancy Disability Act.
- Write a letter to your employer regarding your pregnancy and anticipated leave.
- Visit your Human Resources department to ask and discuss the following items:
  - Will I receive any income from my employer during my leave?
  - Does my company provide short-term disability insurance?
  - Does my company allow the use of vacation and sick days during a maternity leave?
  - Will my current position, or a comparable one, be held open for me?
  - What expenses does my company medical plan cover, and what expenses should I expect to pay?
  - Is health plan coverage available for my new baby, and how soon must I enroll the baby?

Here is a sample maternity leave letter, which you may choose to copy or rewrite into your own words.

> *Dear Employer,*
>
> *I have recently discovered that I am expecting a baby. According to my doctor, my due date is (insert date). I would like to take approximately (insert number) weeks leave prior to my due date and (insert number) weeks of leave after my delivery.*
>
> *I fully intend to resume my work here at the end of my maternity leave and request that my current position, or a similar position, be made available to me at that time.*

❧ RESOURCES ❧

■ WASHINGTON STATE HUMAN RIGHTS COMMISSION
(360) 753-6770
711 S. Capitol
402 Evergreen Plaza Building
Olympia, WA 98504-2490
This department has the information on the pregnancy discrimination regulations. If you have questions or would like a complete copy of the regulations, this is the department to call.

■ U.S. DEPARTMENT OF LABOR WAGE-HOUR DISTRICT OFFICE
553-4482
1111 Third Ave., Ste. 755
Seattle, WA 98101-9795
This department's staff are the experts on the Federal FMLA. They can send you a complete copy of the Act. They also are a good agency to call if you feel you are being discriminated against.

Life Experiences...

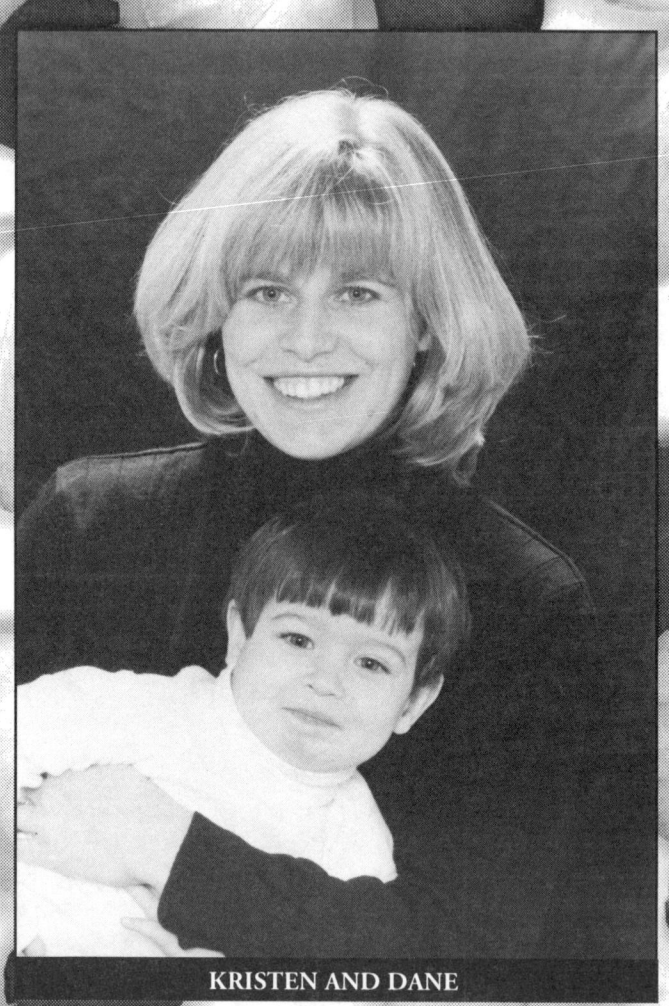

KRISTEN AND DANE

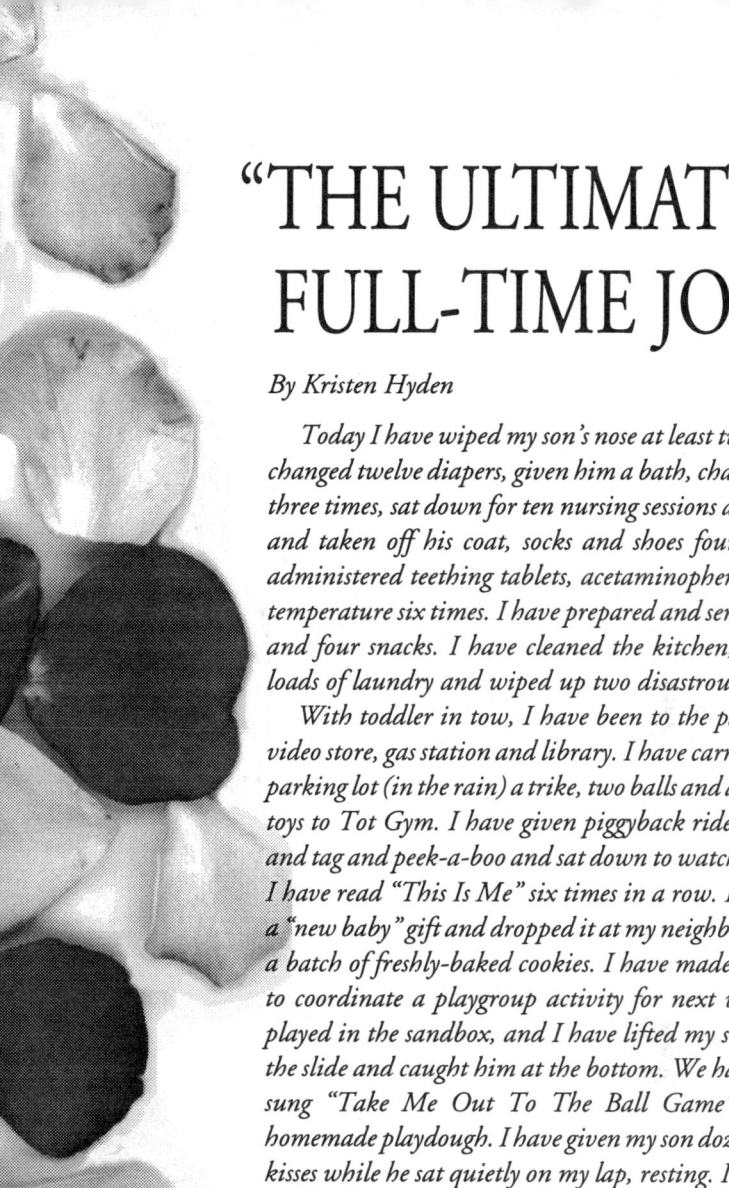

"THE ULTIMATE FULL-TIME JOB"

By Kristen Hyden

Today I have wiped my son's nose at least two dozen times, changed twelve diapers, given him a bath, changed his clothes three times, sat down for ten nursing sessions and have put on and taken off his coat, socks and shoes four times. I have administered teething tablets, acetaminophen and taken his temperature six times. I have prepared and served three meals and four snacks. I have cleaned the kitchen, finished three loads of laundry and wiped up two disastrous spills.

With toddler in tow, I have been to the park, post office, video store, gas station and library. I have carried through the parking lot (in the rain) a trike, two balls and a bag of assorted toys to Tot Gym. I have given piggyback rides, played soccer and tag and peek-a-boo and sat down to watch "Mr. Rogers." I have read "This Is Me" six times in a row. I have wrapped a "new baby" gift and dropped it at my neighbor's, along with a batch of freshly-baked cookies. I have made six phone calls to coordinate a playgroup activity for next week. We have played in the sandbox, and I have lifted my son to the top of the slide and caught him at the bottom. We have danced and sung "Take Me Out To The Ball Game" and sculpted homemade playdough. I have given my son dozens of hugs and kisses while he sat quietly on my lap, resting. I have soothed a bad spill, a bad dream at naptime and an upset stomach. I have coaxed, praised and cheered my son today, even though he has not slept through the night since he was born, and we have been up since five a.m.

Ironically, I receive no salary for these responsibilities. I work a 24-hour day but have no paid vacation, no job security and no potential for a raise or promotion. I am a stay-at-home mom: the ultimate full-time job.

That is not to say, however, that I do not receive any

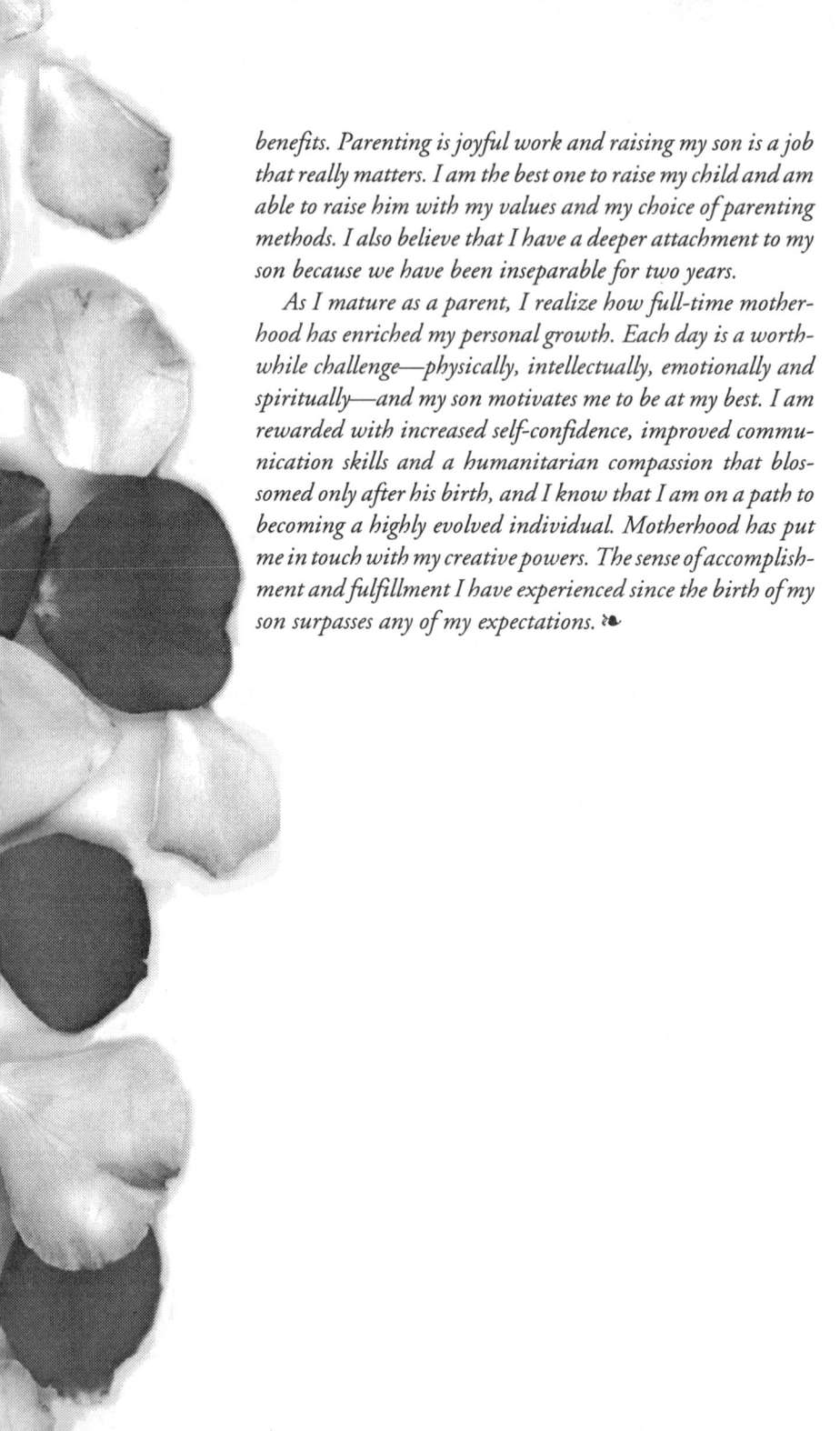

benefits. Parenting is joyful work and raising my son is a job that really matters. I am the best one to raise my child and am able to raise him with my values and my choice of parenting methods. I also believe that I have a deeper attachment to my son because we have been inseparable for two years.

As I mature as a parent, I realize how full-time motherhood has enriched my personal growth. Each day is a worthwhile challenge—physically, intellectually, emotionally and spiritually—and my son motivates me to be at my best. I am rewarded with increased self-confidence, improved communication skills and a humanitarian compassion that blossomed only after his birth, and I know that I am on a path to becoming a highly evolved individual. Motherhood has put me in touch with my creative powers. The sense of accomplishment and fulfillment I have experienced since the birth of my son surpasses any of my expectations. ❧

DIAPERS TO DORMITORIES

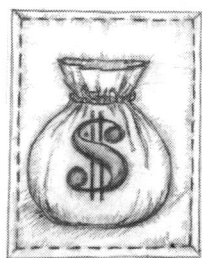

PARENTAL GUIDE TO MONEY MANAGEMENT

By Laura Harger Pajak, CFP

Preparing ahead financially for a baby is not unlike planning ahead for any financially-related event. Whether it's buying a new car or home or changing jobs, the idea is to be prepared.

When you buy a new car, the dealer explains all the costs involved with the purchase. Your friendly banker calculates the monthly payment, your insurance agent quotes insurance costs, and you can estimate maintenance and gasoline expenses with the service schedule and mileage figures.

Such specific information regarding the costs of having and raising a baby is not so readily available; first-time parents may have difficulty effectively planning ahead. Financial surprises only add stress to what can become an increasingly stressful environment.

The goal here is to provide information and resources that will assist you in financially planning for your child through every stage—from diapers to dormitories.

✿

Your first phase of planning can occur long before you even feel your baby's first kick.

✿

PREGNANCY

Your first phase of planning can occur long before you even feel your baby's first kick. Some financial considerations:

1. *Medical cost:* Evaluate your insurance coverage to determine the costs for which you are responsible. Pay close attention to deductibles, co-payments, costs above what your insurance company deems appropriate, and costs not covered by insurance.

2. *Maternity clothes:* This expense will vary depending on the mother-to-be's need for a professional wardrobe, as well as casual attire.

3. *Nursery:* Just the basics can add up fast in this category: a crib ($100-$250), bedding ($100-$150), and dresser/changer ($100-$300). The extras include diaper bag ($35), hamper ($15) and decorations (your basic mobile runs $40!).

4. *Loss of income:* Because most couples depend on two incomes these days, planning for the temporary or permanent loss of one income is vital. See if your employer offers any type of disability program. Planning for a decrease in income is tough any time, but especially so during a time of increased expenses. Keep in mind that even though you might want to work right up until labor begins, doctor's orders come first and disability often starts earlier than planned.

5. *Life/Disability Insurance:* Review your current life and disability insurance coverage. Your need for insurance increases with a new dependent. You might be able to increase your group coverage at work for little added cost. If that's not possible, you can purchase an individual policy. Information on individual policies can be obtained through your financial advisor or insurance agent. Either of these professionals should evaluate your current coverage. Make sure your advisor understands what you would want to happen in the event of disability or death.

6. *Will/Guardianship:* Have your attorney draw up a will that includes designation of guardianship. There are also software programs available very reasonably priced. At the very least, fill out standard forms available at most stationery stores ($2-$5). Don't leave it up to others to decide who would raise your children.

THE FIRST YEAR

With the arrival of your bundle of joy, a whole new set of expenses needs to find a way into your budget:

Monthly Expenses	
Formula (if applicable)	$50 - $65
Diapers (disposable)	$50 - $80
Diapers (cloth w/service)	$50
Baby food	$40
Clothes/Toys	$30 - $50
Day care (group/nanny)	$350 - $1,500
"Well baby" medical care	$35 - $100
Photography	$10 - $30
(film, processing & studio portrait)	
Increase in utility costs	$10 - $50
Baby clothes detergent	$5

One-time Expenses	
Infant car seat	$40 - $65
Regular car seat	$70 - $100
High chair	$50 - $100
Infant clothes	$100 - $150
Bottles	$2 each

Optional items include:	
Stroller	$60 - $300
Swing (manual)	$70 - $140
Breast pump	$15 - $250
Toys	$10 - $250
Playpen	$60

As you can see, there are many expenses involved with having a baby—long after the delivery room charges have been paid! Parents get into trouble trying to juggle the initial expenses without a game plan. This leads to frustration, added debt and debt payments.

Here are some tips for putting together a first-year plan:

❶ List all the one-time expenses you anticipate. Then make a timeline of when you will incur the expenses.

This will indicate whether you need to save ahead of time or if you can just absorb the expenses into your monthly budget. The key is to avoid surprises.

❷ Prior to your baby's birth, create a mock (soon to be real) budget that includes your decreased income figures, added monthly expenses, and monthly savings for the one-time expenses (see your timeline). Be realistic about your other expenses. Fudging your food budget from $500 to $200 to make the numbers work is not the answer! Evaluate your life-style and make realistic changes: quit the health club, reduce the frequency of weekend trips, sell the sports car, etc.

We've covered the pregnancy, your newborn's arrival, and the first twelve months. Now that you're over the initial hump, let's tackle the growing years.

THE GROWING YEARS

Anticipating expenses will keep you sane as your child grows, needing and wanting more and more.

One planning technique to help you stay ahead of the game is to list all the expenses you anticipate for the coming year (make it a New Year's resolution). For example, a trip to Disneyland, soccer

club, orthodontic expenses, Christmas or Chanukah gifts, two big birthday parties and camp add up to $4,000 for the year. The plan is to save $333 per month instead of trying to come up with one lump sum.

Keep these savings in an account other than your regular checking just to make sure it doesn't get spent! This technique will smooth out your monthly budget, eliminating large surprises.

COLLEGE PLANNING

Putting money toward your child's college education can be an overwhelming concept when there are so many other expenses to be dealt with in the interim.

First, decide what percentage of the college expense you want to pay. Will you pay 100 percent? 50 percent? Just supplement when needed? Do you have a preference for state or private schools?

After these questions are answered, you can more accurately determine what you will need to save on a regular basis to meet your goal. Amounts will vary depending on when you start saving and the return you get on your account.

College costs increase seven percent per year on average, so the savings calculation can get tricky. There are many investment vehicles you can use to fund your child's education savings. Here are a few and their advantages:

❶ Bank/credit union savings account - easy to open, low minimums (especially credit unions).

❷ U.S. savings bonds - interest is tax deferred until bond is cashed.

❸ Zero coupon bonds - you can buy them to mature in the year needed.

❹ Life insurance cash value - the cash accumulates tax deferred.

❺ Balanced or growth mutual fund - takes advantage of the higher returns in the stock market and dollar cost averaging.

Your financial advisor will help you pick the vehicle or combination of investment vehicles that best suits your personal needs.

Additional resources for college funding include grants, loans and scholarships. It is important to research all the available sources prior to your child's final year in high school. High school counselors should have all this information, or know where it can be found.

Also, let your relatives know that you have opened a college account. They might want to contribute instead of buying another toy.

❧ RESOURCES ❧

Resources to help you plan for your child's financial future

■ INSTITUTE OF CERTIFIED FINANCIAL PLANNERS
800-282-PLAN
Call for a free booklet, "Your Children's College Bill: How to Figure It...How to Pay for It."

■ MUTUAL FUND/FINANCIAL COMPANY BROCHURES
800-782-6620
Dreyfus Service Corp. of New York publishes "Guide to Investing for College."

800-544-6666
Fidelity Investments of Boston offers "College Savings Work Sheet."

800-525-2440
Founders Funds of Denver offers "The Gift of a Lifetime" about the Uniform Gift to Minor Act and Uniform Transfer to Minors Act.

800-403-KIDS
Stein-Rowe of Boston offers "Young Investor Parent's Guide."

800-638-5660
T. Rowe Price Associates of Baltimore has the "College Planning Kit."

■ QUICKEN SOFTWARE
800-781-5999
The makers of this very popular financial software have created an interactive CD-ROM version, "Parents Guide to Money: How to Raise Kids Without Going Broke." The purchase price is $29.95 plus $6.50 for shipping and handling.

QUESTIONS & ANSWERS
Financial Information

Q: *When does a child need a Social Security number?*

A: It is recommended to get your child's social security number shortly after birth. The federal government mandates that children over age 1 must have a social security number.

Q: *How do I get a Social Security number for my child?*

A: Parents can call 800-772-1213 and request form number SS-5 to be mailed to them.

Q: *What is the benefit of using a dependent care assistance plan offered by some employers?*

A: With this plan you pay for your child care with pre-tax dollars. You can use a maximum of $5,000 for joint ($2,500 single). There is no distinction for number of children.

Q: *How does the child care deduction on the tax return differ from an employer-sponsored dependent care assistance plan?*

A: The child care deduction is limited to $2,400 for one child and $4,800 for two or more children.

If you earn more than $16,000, it is usually more advantageous to use the dependent care plan. See your tax advisor and discuss which plan is best suited for your situation.

Q: *How much interest can a child earn before it is taxed at the parents' tax rate?*

A: Children under age 14 can have unearned income of $1,200 (1996) before it is taxed at the parents' highest marginal rate.

Q: *If I'm unmarried do I need to declare my partner as the father of my child and is he responsible financially?*

A: The State of Washington requires that parents establish paternity (fatherhood) at the time of your baby's birth. This requires that both parents financially support the baby. You can receive paternity information at the hospital you give birth at or contact your local OSE (Child Support Enforcement Office) at 800-526-8658.

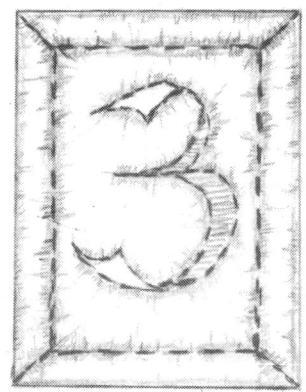

BABY
PRODUCTS

REFERENCE NUMBERS

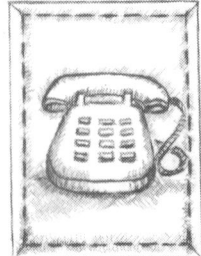

LOCAL BABY SPECIALTY STORES	
Baby Depot, Burlington Coat Factory	776-2221 or 575-3995
Bellini	451-0126
Children's World	451-0833
A Child's Room	643-7050
Go to Your Room	453-2990 or 528-0711
Kid's Club	524-2553 or 643-5437
Kym's Kiddy Corner	361-5974
Merry Go Round Baby News	454-1610
Once Upon A Child	774-8393

CUSTOMER SERVICE & CONSUMER INFO	
Aprica	201-883-9800
Century	800-837-4044
Chesebrough Ponds	800-243-5804
Combi	800-992-6624
Cosco	800-544-1108
Emmaljunga	800-848-3864
Evenflo	800-837-9201
Fisher Price	800-432-5437
Gerber	800-443-7237
Gerry	800-362-3200
Graco	800-345-4109
Johnson & Johnson	800-526-3967
Kolcraft	800-453-7673
Little Tikes	800-321-0183
Peg Perego	219-484-3093
Playskool	800-PLAYSKL

CAR SEAT PRODUCT RECALL NUMBERS	
Auto Safety Hotline	800-424-9393
National Highway and Traffic Safety Administration	202-366-2768

❧

Here are

some quick

references to

baby specialty

stores,

product

information

and car seat

recall

numbers.

❧

BABY PRODUCTS

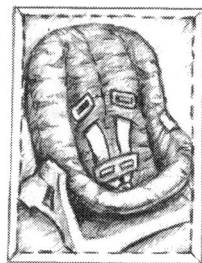

It can be difficult to choose baby products that meet your needs and budget. This section includes information on a variety of baby products, including their features and benefits. It is not meant to take the place of Consumer Reports or other scientific baby product reviews, but rather to give you a starting point on baby product purchases.

Products included in this chapter are: *strollers, car seats, cribs, swings, portable cribs, high chairs, and local specialty items.* Books and publications are also included. We hope this information will prove helpful as you evaluate your upcoming purchases. We do not endorse any one brand or product nor do we validate the safety of any product. Readers should make their own choices based on personal preference and on the safety of each item. With that in mind...read on!

PURCHASING DECISIONS

How do you find products that best meet your needs and your budget? Start by asking yourself the following questions:
- Are you looking for products that will last through more than one child, or is this it?
- Do you care about added convenience features, or do you want to purchase products for the lowest possible price?
- How informed are you about the baby products on the market?
- Does your partner have an opinion on the baby products you purchase?

BABY PRODUCT TIPS

Once you've answered these questions regarding your purchasing decision, consider the following general tips which can help you decide where to shop and what to look for.

DURABILITY AND CONVENIENCE

If you are looking for products that will last beyond one child, you may want to consider purchasing a higher quality product that offers durability and convenience. Consider a duo stroller, a high quality mattress or a crib that converts into a toddler's bed, and colors that will work as well for a boy as they do for a girl.

🐾

This section includes information on a variety of baby products, including their features and benefits.

🐾

PRICING

Although some department stores and discount stores offer low-priced baby products, you will probably not find available staff in these stores to assist and inform you about the individual items. You may be left to make your product decisions and choices alone. For those of you who know little about baby products this can prove to be a frustrating experience. However, once you know what you are looking for, you may want to shop around for the best price.

PRODUCT INFORMATION

We found baby product stores more responsive to parents' needs since they can provide a valuable source of information. The staff at most baby product stores is well-trained and available to assist you and answer your questions.

Several publications review baby products that will help you become more informed. The *Childwise Catalog*, written by Jack Gillis and Mary Ellen R. Fise, published by Harper & Row, is an excellent source of information on baby products. Another useful resource is Consumer Reports. This magazine periodically reviews baby products. They also have a book entitled *Consumer Reports Guide to Baby Products*, which is updated almost every two years. It evaluates the safety, convenience and durability of hundreds of baby products. It also includes buying advice, price guidelines for products and recall information. Becoming informed before you make a purchase may save you time and money, as well as aggravation.

OPINION

Check with your significant other before shopping. You may be surprised by your partner's opinions and besides, it is fun to shop for baby items together.

SOME GENERAL SUGGESTIONS

In case you don't have time to read the entire baby product chapter, here are some "biased" random opinions regarding products.

- Double check the buckle on your car seat. Make sure it is easy to get the baby in and out of the car seat without fumbling with the buckle.
- Buying a stroller that is lightweight and has the features you want, although it may be more expensive, it is well worth the purchase. For parents on the go, a stroller is a lifesaver.

- Consider a swing with a bassinet feature. The bassinet can be used when the infant is newborn and placed directly in the crib. This alleviates a separate bassinet purchase and the swing with this feature is only about thirty dollars more than the swing-only seat.
- If you don't have a walker, it is probably the one purchase you should skip. The American Academy of Pediatrics recommends that parents not use walkers for their children due to the high rate of walker-related injuries.

BOOKS

It seems that the one time in your life that you are continuously reading is during pregnancy. There are so many changes that take place both physically and emotionally; so many questions arise that you can never get enough to read. Here are books that are great to read during pregnancy and beyond.

■ *WHAT TO EXPECT WHEN YOU'RE EXPECTING*
Eisenberg, Murkoff, and Hathaway
Workman Publishing
This book has been one of the best selling pregnancy books for the past decade; it is easy to see why. *What to Expect When You're Expecting* is a very practical book that clearly and concisely responds to the fears, anxieties and hopes that mothers-and fathers-to-be may experience. It is organized by your stage of pregnancy, in a month-by-month format. This makes it easy to read and to relate to the book's content. It seems to have just about anything you are looking for on the topic of pregnancy.

■ *WHAT TO EXPECT THE FIRST YEAR*
Eisenberg, Murkoff and Hathaway
Workman Publishing
The follow-up book to *What to Expect When You're Expecting*, this parent's manual follows a comprehensive month-by-month format that clearly explains everything parents need to know. It includes information on baby's monthly growth and development, feeding, sleeping habits, infant illnesses, and safety. The infant first aid chapter is also very useful.

■ *DR. SPOCK'S BABY AND CHILD CARE*
Benjamin Spock, M.D.
E.P. Dutton, Pocket Books
This is America's oldest and most successful child care book with more than forty editions printed. Recently revised, this book is broken down by topic and is well-organized. Dr. Spock gives his advice on a wide array of topics, including the new role of fathers, children's fears of nuclear war, breastfeeding for working mothers, new discoveries about diseases, and child development and behavior management. The book covers information on children from birth to age eleven.

■ *A CHILD IS BORN, REVISED EDITION*
Lennart Nilsson
Delacorte Press
From the beginning of conception and for the nine months that follow, this book photographically documents life in the womb. It is a great book to read during pregnancy. To actually view each stage of fetal development is thrilling!

■ *YOUR BABY AND CHILD - FROM BIRTH TO AGE FIVE*
Penelope Leach
Random House
This book takes you through many stages of your child's development. Complete with useful illustrations, advice and an easy-to-read reference section, the book

outlines subjects from teething to discipline. This is a great book to have on the shelf during your child's first five years.

■ *A CHILDBIRTH KIT*
Marie Fellenstein Hale and Liz Chalmers
644-1401
Swanstone Press
Two local women have created a unique book to assist pregnant women (and their labor support persons) through the labor process. The book contains a range of natural childbirth techniques, such as using water, positions, massage, and music. It also includes a set of abstract and real life images in full color on separate cards, which are used as focal points during labor. The images are designed to communicate themes during childbirth, such as Opening, Energy, Floating, and Release, which help women channel their energy for an easier labor and delivery.

■ *THE BABY BOOK*
Dr. William Sears
Little Brown Press
Dr. William Sears and his wife Martha have gained national recognition for this book as many—especially Seattle health care providers—rave about Dr. Sears, his writing style and his medical advice. A father of seven children, his information is from the heart. The book is subtitled, *Everything You Need to Know about Baby from Birth to Age Two*, which is very appropriate.

LOCAL PUBLICATIONS

■ *A NEW ARRIVAL*
441-0191
A New Arrival Guide is published twice a year by Northwest Parent Publishing, Inc. This information-packed magazine is geared solely to new and expectant parents, and is available locally at children's stores, child care centers and almost any place children visit.

■ *NORTHWEST BABY AND CHILD*
232-0301 (Voice Mail)
Published by Baby Diaper Service, *Northwest Baby and Child* is a free publication that offers wonderful information regarding infancy and the toddler years. It is available at baby and maternity stores and at other infant related spots. The monthly calendar lists support groups, places to go with your child and much more.

■ *SEATTLE'S CHILD, EASTSIDE PARENT*
441-0191
Both publications are published by Northwest Parent Publishing, Inc. Run by two mothers, these publications are well known for their editorial content and excellent calendar. Their monthly publications, *Seattle's Child* and *Eastside Parent*, have a large circulation. Articles are geared to parents of children of all ages, rather than just infants or toddlers.

These publications are available at many locations throughout the area. Also look for the long list of local books this company publishes.

STROLLERS

Purchasing a stroller may be one of your more interesting baby product experiences. It is also one of your most important, as you will use a stroller for a longer period of time than almost any other baby product (depending on the brand). There are a variety of brands and styles of strollers on the market. You'll find everything from umbrella strollers to old-fashioned buggies to double strollers. This is one of the products that you may consider buying what you really want, if it is in your budget. Sometimes, for a little extra money, you receive more features and a stroller that will last (and that you want to last) for more than one child.

WHAT TO LOOK FOR

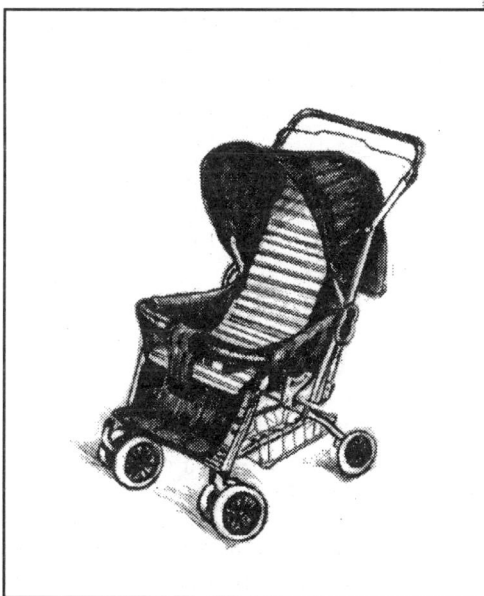

WHAT PARENTS LIKE
- ✓ FOLDS EASILY
- ✓ MANEUVERS EASILY
- ✓ RECLINES, SO INFANT MAY LAY DOWN
- ✓ HANDLE IS REVERSIBLE
- ✓ DURABLE

WHAT PARENTS DON'T LIKE
- ✓ HARD TO MANEUVER
- ✓ TOO LARGE AND HEAVY
- ✓ THE WHEELS STICK
- ✓ TOO BULKY
- ✓ DIFFICULT TO CLEAN

POINTS TO CONSIDER

- ■ Check out the storage availability that your stroller offers. Not all strollers come with baskets; those that do are preferred. The size of basket makes a difference— the larger the better.
- ■ Children are notorious for making a mess; strollers with removable, washable pads are a real plus.
- ■ Strollers which have an up-and-down adjustable handle come in handy, especially if one parent is much taller than the other. Also, check out a new product which

you can add to your stroller to make it adjustable to your height. Available at most baby stores, it costs about $15.

■ Since many parents want to take their newborns out for a stroll, finding a stroller which completely reclines makes this possible. Remember, babies don't sit up until four-plus months.

■ Umbrella strollers are very affordable and make an excellent investment, as you can continue to use them as your child grows older. They are also very convenient to use when traveling.

POPULAR BRANDS

JOGGING STROLLERS

Jogging strollers have grown in popularity during the past several years and are a favorite for locals. Light and easy to push up hills and on rugged terrain, jogging strollers offer one of the smoothest, lightest rides available.

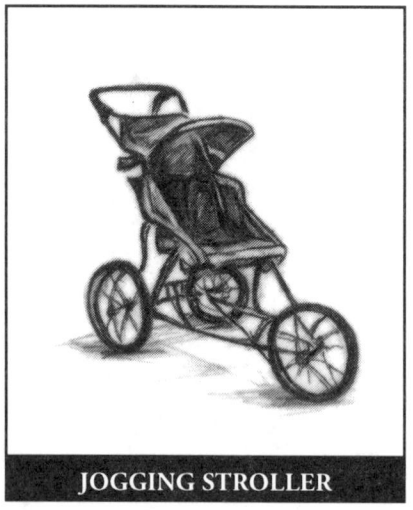

JOGGING STROLLER

Prices start at about $150 for a baby jogger and go up from there depending on special features or if you want a double jogger.

Jogging strollers are available primarily at bicycle stores and a few baby specialty stores. They are also available by mail order. We found jogging strollers at bicycle specialty stores and at the baby specialty stores. To order by mail you can call Racing Strollers, Inc. at 800-241-1848 for a free brochure.

GRACO STROLLERS

Graco is one of the most popular and affordable strollers available. Graco offers various styles, including the basic model that comes with both removable and non-removable padding to its top of the line stroller that features four sets of swivel wheels plus extra storage. Graco also manufactures double seat strollers. Their double seat stroller is very large with ample room to hold two children and is available with either non-removable or removable padding. Graco has spent the last year working on improving their strollers' wheels. This continuous improvement has resulted in a wheel that is dependable, durable, and handles with ease.

Graco offers two styles of umbrella strollers, one with a top shade, the other without. One of its most popular models is called the "Lite Rider." This model is in between an umbrella stroller and a "traditional" stroller. It offers wide wheels, a huge basket, a canopy with a rear window, and it is very light for ease of use. The only major features this model does not offer are an adjustable stroller handle and a handle which moves back and forth. Prices for Graco strollers start at $29 for an umbrella stroller to $79 for the basic

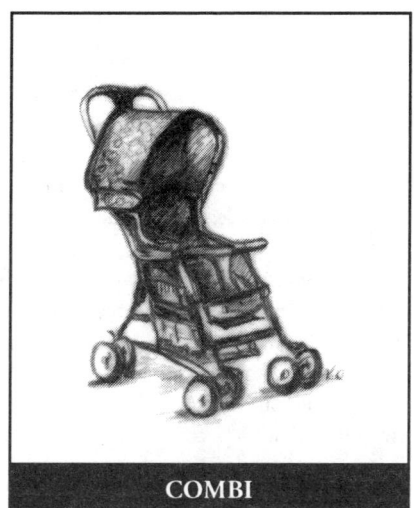

COMBI

wheel suspension, swivel lock system, one hand opening/folding, and compactness. Combi also offers a double stroller which weighs about 20 pounds. It offers the convenience of a double stroller without the weight. Their double stroller starts at about $300.

CENTURY STROLLERS

The two types of Century strollers you will most likely use with an infant are their convenience and carriage models. Their convenience strollers are lightweight with a seat that reclines, and have an extra large basket below for storage. They also have dual swivel wheels on the front, and brakes on the rear wheels. The convenience model comes in a variety of colors and styles and costs between $50 and $80. One of the newest stroller introductions into the market is the Century "4-in-1 System." It functions as a car seat and stroller. It can also be used as an infant carrier and toddler stroller. We found this product at baby specialty stores and in mail-order catalogs. It starts at $100. Ask the staff at baby specialty stores to show you how this product works. You might also check with other parents for their opinion on whether the convenience is worth the price.

Century's carriage strollers offer features such as: six-wheels, duo wheels in front and single wheels in the rear, reversible handles, rear brakes, large mesh storage baskets, removable pads, multiple seat positions, and a canopy. These strollers also have a window on the top of the canopy making it easy to see baby without physically moving to check on your child. You can expect to pay from $90 to $140 for a Century carriage stroller.

model. The double stroller starts at about $110. Graco strollers are available at baby specialty and major discount stores.

COMBI

Combi makes a stroller that is one of the lightest, most durable strollers made. Their umbrella-style stroller weighs as little as seven pounds and their carriage/stroller weighs from 16 to 21 pounds. This is an excellent feature for parents on the go. The lighter the stroller, the more often parents will use it. Combi strollers also offer features such as a canopy, large basket, reclining seat, and a removable guard. Combi's lowest priced stroller starts at about $159.

For parents wanting a little more stroller, Combi features a carriage/stroller which costs about $179. You can expect the features on the carriage/stroller to vary, but look for the following: a removable boot, reversible handle, reclining seat, removable basket, storage space, stylish design (the more stylish, the more you may pay), a one year warranty, special

EMMALJUNGA

Emmaljunga strollers were originally manufactured in Sweden. A very popular European brand, the Emmaljunga stroller offers such an old-fashioned high-quality feel that many parents save their stroller as an heirloom. The strollers are an investment with the least expensive model around $220. They also weigh about 27 pounds, but do fold very compactly. Other models are more expensive and fold less compactly, yet offer more stroller. Emmaljunga's most expensive and largest stroller is a "duo" stroller which holds two children face to face. This duo model retails around $450 and weighs close to 60 pounds. Emmaljunga strollers are sold primarily through baby specialty stores.

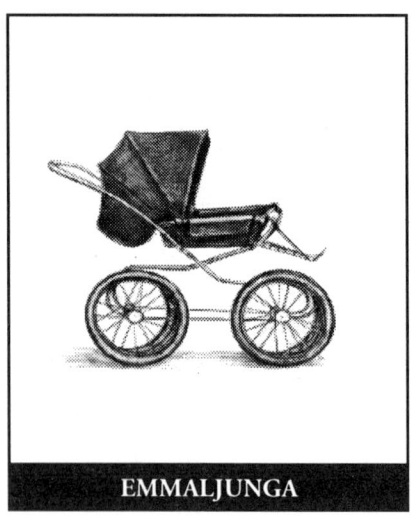

EMMALJUNGA

PEG PEREGO

The Peg Perego stroller is a "current" favorite of Consumer Reports. The Perego stroller comes from Italy and shows fine, quality Italian style. Lightweight, a Perego stroller weighs between nine and 13 pounds. All models are made with an aluminum chassis (frame) which guarantees sturdiness and practicality. Their carriages offer an old-fashioned feel, but without the bulk and weight. The Peg Perego Carriage System offers interchangeable parts: a chassis, a bassinet, a stroller seat with a cover for the baby's legs, and a hood. They also come with removable quilting, rear wheel brakes, a large basket, extra storage, shock absorbing suspension, a safety device that prevents accidental folding, and much more. One of the best features of this stroller is its removable bassinet. Yet, as your child grows, it becomes a portable well-made stroller. Perego's carriage line costs around $375.

For parents looking for a few less features, Perego offers a wide and versatile stroller line. (There are so many styles and brands it is impossible to list them all.) You'll find many of the same features of the carriage line such as: removable upholstery, reversible handle bar, swivel wheels, ample storage, removable front bar and more. Expect to pay between $200 to $250 for a Perego stroller. Peg Perego strollers are sold through baby specialty stores.

CAR SEATS

Since 1978, all 50 states and the District of Columbia have passed child restraint laws. Although state laws vary, most require a child to be restrained in a special child safety seat until he is four years old or 40 pounds in weight. This standard is the one accepted by the American Academy of Pediatrics (AAP).

According to the National Highway Traffic Safety Administration (NHTSA), proper use of child safety seats can cut the risk of death or serious injury by about 70%. But there are still an estimated 700 deaths and 60,000 to 70,000 injuries each year to children under five years of age due to automobile accidents.

WHAT TO LOOK FOR

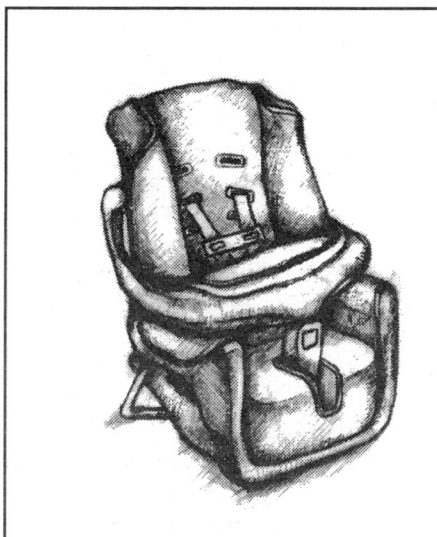

WHAT PARENTS LIKE
✓ STURDY AND SAFE
✓ EASY TO GET BABY IN AND OUT
✓ ALSO A CARRIER

WHAT PARENTS DON'T LIKE
✓ TOO HEAVY, BIG AND BULKY
✓ HARD TO BUCKLE AND UNBUCKLE
✓ HARD TO PUT IN THE CAR
✓ UNCOMFORTABLE FOR A NEWBORN

POINTS TO CONSIDER

■ Try out your infant car seat's handle. Many of the handles used to carry the car seat are extremely difficult to move from front-to-back or vice-versa.

■ The advantage of car seats with a detachable base is the seat is removable from the car without undoing the seat belt each time.

■ Car seats that are vinyl may be washed off but not removed and placed in the washing machine. Babies also sweat more often and seem hotter in vinyl car seats.

■ When shopping for your car seat, spend extra time to make sure the buckle meets your satisfaction. As one parent commented, "Nothing is more frustrating than trying to get a screaming child in the car seat and then having to fiddle with the buckle for five minutes before it finally secures the baby."

■ If you have a newer car that offers a built-in, rear-seat, fold-down restraint system, know this should never be used for infants.

■ To check on a car seat recall, know your seat's brand, model and date of manufacture and call the Auto Safety Hotline (800-424-9393).

■ The American Academy of Pediatrics offers a free information kit on car seats, including a shopping guide. This kit lists all products currently on the market with the type, approximate price and safety features. You can receive this by calling 800-433-9016. Ask for the "Family Shopping Guide to Car Seats."

■ If you can't afford a car seat, you may want to check with your hospital or community agency to see if any programs are available. Also Midas Muffler and the Easter Seals have special car seat programs.

Portions of this section were written by Pamela McCarthy, a free lance writer from Toledo, Ohio and the mother of two sons.

POPULAR CAR SEAT TYPES AND BRANDS

There are currently three categories of seats available:

1. Infant-only, for birth up to about 20 pounds or 27 inches tall
2. Convertible, for children from 7 pounds to 40 or 43 pounds
3. Booster, for children weighing 30 to 50 pounds

POPULAR BRANDS

Here are some car seat brands you may find on your shopping expedition:

■ Century
■ Cosco
■ Evenflo
■ Fisher Price

INFANT-ONLY SEATS

All infants must face the rear of the car until they reach 20 pounds or one year of age. The AAP recommends that infants be kept facing the rear as long as possible. Some infants reach 20 pounds well before they are a year old, but their necks and heads are still not strong enough to withstand the force of being thrown forward in a crash.

It is not always necessary to have an infant-only car seat to start out with, but they are clearly more convenient to use and there is no question about proper fit as with some convertible seats. Parents of premature infants and low-birth-weight infants, however, should use an infant-only seat at birth.

If your vehicle is equipped with a passenger side air bag, do not use a rear-facing car seat in the front passenger seat. The air bag could throw the car seat up and into the headrest or between the seats upon inflation. A convertible seat that faces forward or a booster seat can be used in these passenger seats, but the car's seat should be moved back to the farthest position. For safety's sake, however, children are always better off in the back seats. The middle of the back seat is actually the safest position.

CONVERTIBLE SEATS

Convertible seats are the most commonly purchased type of car seat as they can be used for a longer period of time. If you are buying one to use with an infant, Consumer Reports recommends one with a five-point harness rather than those with a T-shield or car-shield.

A five-point harness secures the child's pelvis and shoulders and goes across the chest as a secondary point of contact. It will also have a crotch strap to hold down the pelvis or a lap strap. A T-shield can reach a very small infant's head; for proper fit, the shield should only be chest-high.

If an infant's head flops forward, tilt the seat slightly by wedging a towel where the base sits on the car's seat. Towels or blankets can be used as bolsters to support a small child in a large seat.

Children should remain in convertible seats until they have reached the upper weight and height limits (40-43 pounds and 40 inches) or until they have completely outgrown the seats. Their ears should not be higher than the top of the safety seat. When a child reaches this height, he should be moved into a booster or properly-fitted seat belt to prevent whiplash.

OPTIONS FOR OLDER CHILDREN

Children should never put a shoulder belt behind their bodies or under their arms. If the shoulder portion is behind the child's body, the latching mechanism will not engage during a sudden stop and the child can slip out of the lap portion of the belt. Putting the shoulder belt under the arm can lead to internal injuries.

If your child sits too low in the seat and cannot see out of the window, use a booster designed for a lap/shoulder belt. As long as the child's ears are not higher than the top of the car's seat he can use a booster.

POPULAR BRANDS

CENTURY

Century offers a wide variety of car seats from infant to toddler sizes. The infant car seats are the "570" and "590" models. The "570" is a basic model without a canopy, but it does have a handle. The "590" model has a canopy and detachable base. Century's infant car seats run from $50 to $70. Century's convertible car seats begin with the 1000 Series. Their least expensive model costs about $50 and has a five-point harness with no shield. The top of the line model runs about $100, but offers a wide variety of luxury features including a pillow, shield and extra padding. Century also offers a car seat named "Smart Move," designed to let infants ride in a more reclined position, at a 47 degree angle rather than current infant car seats' more upright angle. The car seat is designed to meet the needs of both infants and toddlers. It costs around $119 to $139.

Century also offers an infant car seat/stroller combination named the "4-in-1 System." It can be used as a car seat, an infant/car seat stroller, a carrier, and a toddler's stroller. This product runs around $150. We found it at baby specialty stores and in a mail order catalog named One Step Ahead.

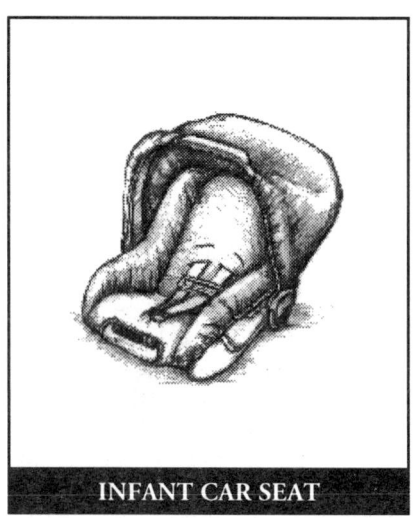

INFANT CAR SEAT

EVENFLO CAR SEATS

Evenflo is a large manufacturer of a variety of juvenile products. In their car seat selection alone, they offer more than 15 styles. Their infant car seat offers cloth padding, a handle and canopy. Prices begin at $50. The same model car seat is also available with an auto base bottom, which means the base always stays buckled in the car, eliminating the need to use the seat belt every time. With this added feature, the name for the car seat is the "On My Way." It costs about 10 to 15% more than the "Joyride." The "On My Way" also has rear storage available in the base for items such as diapers, pacifiers and other necessities. Many of the Evenflo infant seats also have a unique handle style which is curved making it easy to carry baby.

Evenflo makes three styles of convertible car seats: the five-point harness, the T-shield and the overhead shield. The five-point harness offers the advantage of having a buckle that attaches to the harness rather than the base of the car seat, making it easily accessible. The five-point harness car seats run from $60 to $120 depending on the features you choose. In reviewing Evenflo's car seats, we found only one T-shield model which buckles at the base of the car seat costing about $60. Evenflo sells a large selection of car seats with overhead shields. A large plastic shield is pulled down in front of your child's body. You buckle the child in through the base of the car seat. The overhead shield model costs between $80 and $120.

SPECIAL SEAT BELT ADJUSTERS FOR OLDER CHILDREN

Once a child *weighs more than 50 pounds*, he or she reaches the stage where a car or booster seat is no longer needed. Products are available which fit over the shoulder belt portion of a seat belt to make the seat belt fit better. We spoke with the manufacturer of a product called Safe Kid. Although a seat belt adjuster cannot assure safety for your child, here are some benefits:

- It keeps the shoulder belt from pulling across the child's neck.
- Special designs ensure the proper placement of shoulder and lap belt.
- It may reduce internal injuries if properly placed and there is a car accident.

Safe Kid retails for about $6-$9 and is available at baby specialty stores and major discount stores.

PORTABLE CRIBS

Portable cribs have become a popular item with parents, especially those who do a lot of travelling. They are the preferred choice over their older counterpart, the playpen, because they are easier to set up, and fold up into a small bundle.

WHAT TO LOOK FOR

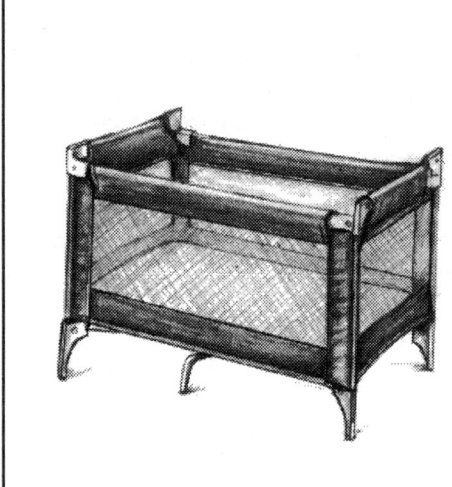

WHAT PARENTS LIKE
✓ PORTABLE
✓ EASY TO SET UP
✓ ADJUSTS TO A
   BASSINET
✓ STURDY

WHAT PARENTS DON'T LIKE
✓ DIFFICULT TO PUT
   TOGETHER
✓ TOO HEAVY
✓ MATTRESS IS TOO
   THIN

POINTS TO CONSIDER

■ There are no separate Consumer Product Safety Commission (CPSC) standards for portable cribs. Most of the new models, however, meet voluntary safety standards set by the manufacturer.

■ The most important thing to consider when shopping is that a portable crib should be portable! They should set up quickly (within a few minutes) and fold up into a convenient carrying size. The best ones come with a travel/carry bag.

■ They can be used either as a temporary bed or play area for babies up to 30 pounds or under 34 inches in height. When used as a playpen, the play area is slightly smaller than in a conventional playpen.

■ They are also rectangular like a crib, instead of square.

■ Portable cribs should not be used in place of a regular crib for everyday use.

POPULAR BRANDS

Companies manufacturing portable cribs include:

- Evenflo
- Fisher-Price
- Gerry
- Graco

Most have a plastic or metal frame with woven fabric and mesh sides. Gerry does make a wooden fold-away crib on wheels that is narrow enough to fit through a doorway. It is not as convenient to store as the mesh/fabric models. Most brands have two mesh sides and two fabric sides, but Graco has a model with four mesh sides. There are flaps that can be left down or rolled up. The total mesh models afford easy viewing from all sides.

EVENFLO

The Evenflo portable crib ("Happy Cabana") is easy to put together and is affordable, retailing at around $100. This model has two large wheels and two legs, making it easy to maneuver. A canopy with a roll-down flap makes it great for outdoor use. Just one side has a mesh panel, with a roll-down flap, and the top rail is padded. Evenflo notes that the "Happy Cabana" folds and sets up in just one minute. And, along with the convenient features, Evenflo's "Happy Cabana" is also very cute.

FISHER-PRICE

Fisher-Price has redesigned its portable crib. Formerly, the "3-in-1 Portable Crib" was difficult to put together. The new model is a bassinet, portable crib and playpen. Its newest design is assembled similarly to the Graco models. The Fisher-Price portable crib comes in one style and one color making it easy to make a product decision. It costs about $110.

GRACO

The Graco "Pack 'n Play" is one of the easiest portable cribs to use. Once you put it together once, the second and third assembly is simple. Basically, you pull one lever and pull the sides up and the crib is assembled. The "Pack 'n Play" also offers added features such as bug netting, a thick quilted cover and toy bag. The Graco "Pack 'n Play" comes in bright colors and costs from $70 to $140.

HIGH CHAIRS

High chairs are an essential for your baby once he or she is ready to eat solid foods and can sit up easily. This usually occurs during the fourth or fifth month. Parents have a wide selection of types of high chairs—from the basic to the sophisticated.

The basic high chairs are plastic with vinyl seats. They may require one or two hands to put the baby in the high chair. Most models today offer the one hand option which makes it much simpler for the busy parent. You can also purchase a "no frills" wooden high chair for your child. Although these chairs look beautiful, they may be more difficult to clean and they also take up a little more room because they don't fold. There are also high chairs available that will "grow" or adjust to your child. Many of the large

WHAT TO LOOK FOR

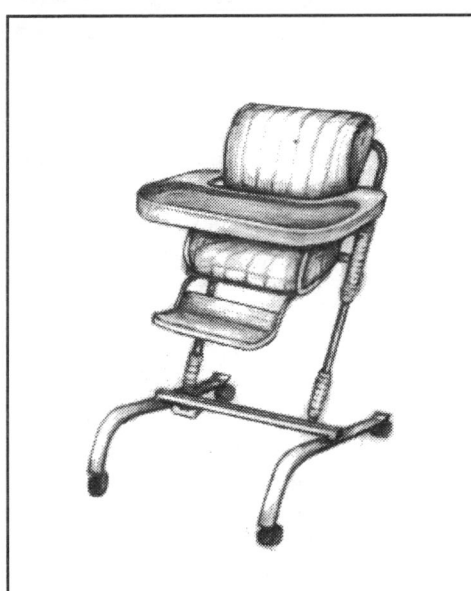

WHAT PARENTS LIKE
✔ LARGE TRAY
✔ EASY TO CLEAN
✔ ONLY NEEDS ONE HAND
✔ STURDY
✔ APPEARANCE
✔ ADJUSTABLE
✔ WHEELS

WHAT PARENTS DON'T LIKE
✔ HARD TO CLEAN
✔ TRAY STICKS
✔ SEATBELT STRAP IS DIFFICULT TO USE

baby product manufacturers offer this option. The advantage of these high chairs is they may be used as a high chair, youth chair and also a play chair. They may be placed in several positions, extending the life of the high chair. The adjustable models also come with the convenience features of large tray, non-splash sides and one hand adjustments. Some also come with wheels! You'll pay more for this type of high chair, but it will also last longer too.

The final type of high chair is a portable high chair. Portable high chairs may either be strapped onto one of your chairs or placed directly on the table (it hangs on your table). If you travel or visit friends and family, the portable high chair is great.

One safety feature that is a must on any high chair purchase is the waist belt to secure your infant. According to CSPC, injuries from children falling out of high chairs is one of the leading causes of injuries. Make sure every single time you put your child in the high chair that you buckle him in.

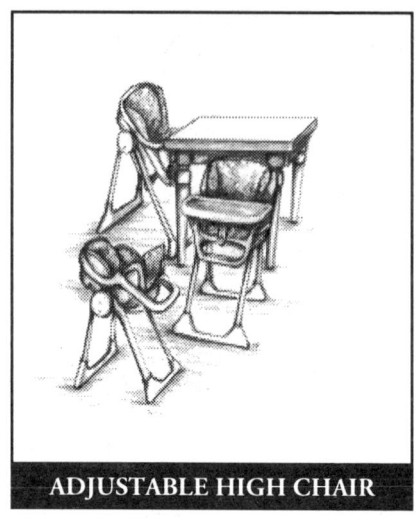

ADJUSTABLE HIGH CHAIR

POPULAR BRANDS

EVENFLO

Evenflo's basic high chairs offer high sides, a one-hand tray latch and a tray which swings down to the side for storage. It also has a three-position foot rest. Evenflo's newest model is an adjustable high chair. This model, costing around $80, adjusts to fit different heights. Evenflo high chairs start from $35.

FISHER-PRICE HIGH CHAIRS

Fisher-Price offers two styles of high chairs: a deluxe model and adjustable height model. The deluxe Fisher-Price high chair has been around for many years and each year minor modifications are made. It has a wide tray and one-hand entry. The deluxe high chair costs about $80. It comes in one color and style. Fisher-Price also has an adjustable high chair with six different positions. This model, however, does not have wheels. It costs between $65 to $75.

PEG PEREGO

Peg Perego was one of the first manufacturers that offered the adjustable high chair. Each model also comes with wheels making it convenient to move around. The Peg Perego high chair comes in one color, white, and is easy to clean. It costs about $120 to $150.

GRACO HIGH CHAIRS

Graco offers a wide variety of basic high chairs. Almost all of its models fold and have the one hand entry-and-release feature. Graco high chairs range from $40 to $60. Graco also makes a portable high chair which sits directly on the dining room table and costs around $27.

SWINGS

An infant swing is a product that isn't absolutely necessary to have, but many parents swear by them. It can be used to stimulate a baby's senses, rock a tired baby to sleep or soothe a colicky baby when nothing else can.

Early swings were crank operated and vinyl covered. Most have been changed over the years to make them more convenient, accessible and comfortable for the infant. Most newer models are battery operated, although crank models are still available. They are quieter and will run considerably longer. Some models claim to run up to 150 hours

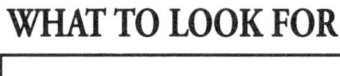

WHAT TO LOOK FOR

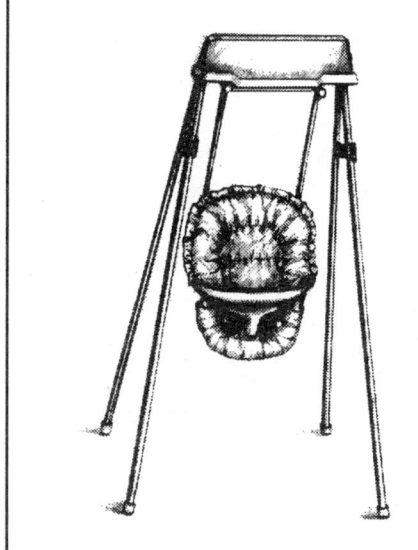

WHAT PARENTS LIKE
✓ AUTOMATIC
✓ THE BABY LOVES IT!
✓ QUIET
✓ SEAT RECLINES
✓ PORTABLE

WHAT PARENTS DON'T LIKE
✓ DOESN'T SWING LONG ENOUGH
✓ DIFFICULT TO PUT BABY IN AND OUT
✓ TOO LOUD
✓ NOT STURDY

on a single set of batteries. Other features that you'll find on many newer models involve the seat itself. Many can be removed from the swing to be used as a separate baby seat. The trays now swing away to make it much easier to take the infant in and out. Also available on many models is a cloth cover on the seat that can be removed and laundered. It keeps the baby more comfortable, especially when asleep.

One thing to keep in mind is that not all infants like swings. Before purchasing one it might be wise to borrow one to try first to see how your baby reacts to the swing.

POINTS TO CONSIDER

- If space is limited, look for a swing with detachable legs for easier portability and storage.
- Parents mentioned that they liked swings that detach from the frame and can also be used as a carrier.
- Some swings are vinyl; others have removable, washable covers. Parents again commented that they preferred the cloth removable covers over vinyl. They are easier to clean and parents felt their babies looked more comfortable.

POPULAR BRANDS

GRACO

At most discount and baby department stores, you'll find Graco swings, as they offer a wide selection of this product. Their low end swings have vinyl seats and parents start them manually. This basic style of Graco swing costs about $30 to $40. It is a little more difficult to find, as many of the stores we visited offer the cloth seat more dominantly. A cloth seat swing has the advantage of washability and it is softer and does not stick to the baby. It costs only about 10% more than the vinyl manual swing. Graco also offers automatic, battery operated swings. This style of Graco swing only comes with cloth seats and it costs around $50 to $70. One of the most practical swing styles Graco offers is their "Three-in-One Swing." This style offers a cradle which is a lifesaver during the early weeks and a swing which can also be used as a baby carrier. If parents choose this model, they can use the cradle as a bassinet and eliminate the need for one additional purchase. The cradle also fits easily into a crib. If you are thinking about purchasing or borrowing an older model of this type of style, specifically models #1830 or #1801, don't! These models were recalled. Call Graco for recall information. The new styles have been redesigned and at the time of print did not have any safety problems. Graco's newest battery operated swing has an open frame which makes it easy to access. It costs about $90 and also includes a reclining, adjustable seat with thick padding.

CENTURY

The new Century swings are only available as battery operated. Their battery-powered motor runs on two "D" batteries for up to 100 hours. All of the Century swings patterns coordinate with other Century products' patterns such as their walkers, strollers and car seats. For the fashion-concerned parent, this is an advantage. Each Century swing model also comes with a machine-washable pad, and detachable links and toys which gives your baby something to look and play with. All of their models offer at least a two-position posture seat which reclines for your baby's naps. Their most expensive model offers a four-position carrying angle and rocking base. These swings range from $75 to $100.

CRIBS

There are many decisions and purchases for new parents to make. One that seems to involve the most time and money is the crib. Everyone has a different idea about how they want their nursery to look. This is evident by the wide range of colors and styles available. The crib decision is usually one based on looks. There are, however, safety features to be considered. Most were mandated by the CPSC in 1973. Major manufacturers also follow voluntary standards as developed by the Juvenile Products

WHAT TO LOOK FOR

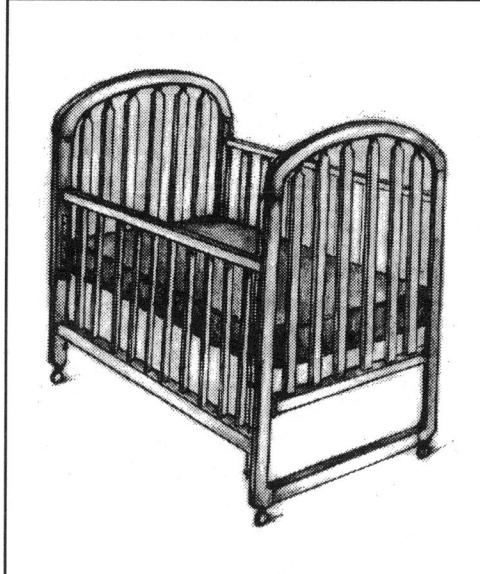

WHAT PARENTS LIKE
✓ APPEARANCE
✓ STURDY
✓ THE MATTRESS
   ADJUSTS
✓ SIDES GO UP AND
   DOWN EASILY
✓ THE PRICE WAS
   RIGHT

WHAT PARENTS
DON'T LIKE
✓ SIDE RAILS STICK
✓ HARD TO CHANGE
   THE SHEETS
✓ NOISY

Manufacturers Association (JPMA). Products that meet these standards usually carry a JPMA certification sticker, but a crib without a sticker doesn't necessarily mean that it does not meet the safety standards. What all this means, basically, is that if you purchase a new crib, you can safely base your choice on convenience, price and looks. The rest has been taken care of for you.

According to Consumer Reports, the 1973 CPSC regulations were prompted by some grim statistics. Crib accidents were accounting for 150 to 200 deaths each year and some 50,000 injuries. The majority of these were caused by slats that were too far apart. The child's body would fit through, but the head wouldn't, causing strangulation death. The federal government came up with the following requirements that are still in effect today:

- Crib slats must be no further apart than 2-3/8."
- A lowered dropside must be at least 9" above the mattress support at its highest setting. The raised dropside must be at least 26" above the support at its lowest position.
- A dropside must take at least two separate actions to activate. If it is too easy to drop, an older baby could activate it.
- The mattress must fit snugly. You should be able to fit no more than two fingers between the crib interior side and the mattress.

Voluntary standards cover aspects such as corner posts and mattress supports. Corner posts should be either practically flush with the top of the end panels or very tall, such as on a four poster bed. If they are not completely flush, they should be nor more than 1/16" above it. Mattress supports should be firmly secured to the brackets at the end panels. Also, the end panels should extend lower than the mattress support at its lowest position. This prevents accidents caused by a child becoming trapped between the end panel and the support.

There are a few features of convenience that you may consider when making your choice of a crib. Wheels make a crib easier to move. Round, ball casters move better, especially on carpet, than narrow, disk-shaped wheels. The dropside release mechanisms vary from model to model and some are easier to work than others. Try them out at the store when shopping. Keep in mind that you may be holding an infant when putting the side down. A mechanism that can be worked with one hand is preferable.

Cribs are available with either one or two drop-sides. A one dropside model is less expensive and if your crib is going to sit against a wall it may be a better choice. The extra money isn't worth it if you aren't going to use both sides. Ease of assembly is also a consideration. Some cribs require only a screwdriver to put together while others are more complicated. Some stores offer the option of having the crib assembled at your home when it is delivered. There is an extra fee for this service, but it may be worth it.

The major crib manufacturers are Child Craft, Bassett, Simmons, Welsh, Cosco, Evenflo and Bellini. To help you choose a crib, you can write to the CSPC for their free brochures called "Tips for your Baby's Safety" and "Nursery Equipment Buyer's Guide." Their address is U.S. Consumer Product Safety Commission, Nursery Equipment Buyer's Guide, Washington, DC, 20207. Specify which brochures you want and send along a self-addressed stamped business size envelope.

Crib mattresses need to be purchased separately and there are a few things to look for. Mattresses are either foam or inner-spring. It is just a matter of preference which you choose. Inner-spring models may keep their shape better, although a high-density foam can be just as good. There are many variations of inner-spring models which contain anywhere from 60 to 360 coils. A large number of coils doesn't guarantee firmness. You will want to purchase as firm a mattress as you can afford and the only way to measure firmness is by giving it a "squeeze" test.

Squeeze the mattress in the center and around the edges to test firmness. Vent holes in the sides are also good to have. They help keep the mattress fresher and reduce pressure on the seams. There are new mattresses on the market that are firmer on one side than the other. The softer side is for infants up to 20 pounds. The other side is firmer and more durable for older infants and toddlers. Whichever mattress you choose should fit snugly in your crib.

Even with the current safety regulations, Consumer Reports magazine reports that more infants die each year in accidents involving cribs than any other child product. General consensus is that most of these involve older model cribs that were manufactured before 1978. If you are purchasing a used crib or using a family hand-me-down, you'll need a tape measure to check to see if it meets the CPSC requirements. Also check to see that there are not cutouts or decorative items attached to the head or footboards. These can pose a choking or strangulation hazard. All bolts and screws should be present and fit tightly. Another thing to check for, especially on cribs manufactured before 1970, is that they may be coated with paint that contains lead. If the used crib you are considering does not meet the current safety requirements, don't use it. Special Note: If your infant is in child care and is using a crib there, check the crib to see if it meets the safety standards.

There are a few things to remember so that you use your crib safely. First, position it away from windows, heating elements, lamps, wall decorations, cords, and climbable furniture. When your baby is alone in the crib, keep the dropside up

and locked. Hanging toys and mobiles should be out of the baby's reach and as soon as the child can pull itself up on hands and knees, remove any toy that goes across the top of the crib. Don't leave pillows, stuffed animals, or large toys in the crib. A tiny infant could smother in them, and an older child can use them as steps to climb out. Also, as soon as your child can stand in the crib, you should remove the bumper pads. They can also be used as steps to climb out. A rule of thumb to use is that when your child either reaches a height of 26" or can climb out of his or her crib, it's time to make the move to a regular bed.

When considering bedding, be aware of a warning issued by the CPSC in 1994 which is against soft bedding because they found it could cause asphyxiation in small infants. The warning is based on research done at Washington University in St. Louis. They have found that soft bedding may be responsible for up to 25% of infant deaths from SIDS. The infant can become wrapped in the bedding which leads to re-breathing of exhaled air that can eventually lead to death from carbon monoxide poisoning. To avoid this the CPSC recommends:

- Putting the baby to sleep on his or her back on a flat, firm mattress without any plush, fuzzy bedding.
- Don't use soft, fluffy products such as pillows, sheepskins or toys under the infant as he or she sleeps.

To check on a particular model for recall information, write to or call the CPSC at 800-638-2772. Many manufacturers also have consumer information hotlines which are listed in the Reference Numbers section in this chapter.

LOCAL PRODUCTS

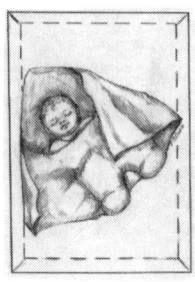

Locally, there are many companies that offer baby products. Most companies were started by creative parents seeking to fill a personal need. Many of these products are specific for our way of life. If you know of other products that should be highlighted in future revisions, please take the time to send us the information.

■ **BIRTH AND BEYOND**
324-4831
2610 E. Madison St.
Seattle, WA 98112
Birth and Beyond is owned by mother Lyndsey Starkey. It is a unique store that carries many local products, as well as just about anything else you would need during pregnancy. Books, nursing clothing, tapes, breast pumps, slings, and music are just a few of the items we found. Besides offering products, Birth and Beyond also offers childbirth classes, a resource lending library and just a great place to hang out. During my visit to this bright store, I was surprised at how many people knew each other and how open the environment was. Birth and Beyond must be a definite stop for you to find local items or just about anything else you would want for pregnancy and baby.

■ **DREAMLAND RECORDS**
639-4944
Dreamland Records, a division of Sound Storm Music, is a locally-owned family business with an award-winning lullaby tape. The tape, "Blanket Bay Lullabies," was awarded the National Parenting Publications' highest honor, the Gold Award. The tape includes five traditional lullabies and five original compositions written by members of the extended family of Kevin and Kelly Kunz. Local singer Jennifer Lind sings the songs, with harmony provided by family members. Two songs, "Blanket Bay" and "Barges" make this even more of a family project, as they are songs that have been sung to their families' children for about 50 years. "Blanket

Bay Lullabies" is available in local stores and can be purchased for $9.95 by phone at the number above.

■ MARIE MEARS, MURAL PAINTER

365-4754

Marie has an impressive background in scenic art—she's worked at most of the theaters in the area. After having a baby recently, she's begun sharing her artistic talents in a new way by painting murals and other room decor in homes. Her consultation is free and she'll provide an estimate after meeting with the client, based on a rate of $20 per hour, which includes materials. You can see an example of her work at Birth & Beyond, where she's painted a mural.

■ NANNY AND WEBSTER

800-392-4975

10838 Main St.

Bellevue, WA 98004

Hours: M-F 8:00 a.m.-5:00 p.m.

Nanny and Webster features baby blankets with a message: "bringing warmth and comfort to children and the people who care for them." Profits from the sale of the blankets are donated to children's charities.

The Nanny and Webster blanket is crafted to the highest-quality specifications. All blankets are 100% cotton with a two-piece flannel design. The 36" x 42" blanket comes in five different patterns and retails for $24. A quilted flannel blanket with satin trim sells for $30.

■ STITCHES IN TIME

768-2658

7749 16th S.W.

Seattle, WA 98106

Stitches in Time manufactures the Rosado Sling, a product developed by Julianne Rosado to ease her daughter's colic. Because she personally used the sling many hours a day, she came up with a design that allows much more freedom of movement for parents. Julianne believes that babies take to the sling because of the closeness, security and comfort they provide. The sling is available in a variety of fabrics and is machine washable and dryable. It has wide fabric which gives you added support and privacy while nursing. It is easy to use as it has a one hand adjustment. Depending on the fabric, the sling costs around $40 and is available via mail order (checks or cash only) or at local retail locations which can be found by calling the number above. The company's other products include nursing tops, diapers and hats.

■ TEDDY TOES [*Baby Pages*]

284-3404

800-51TEDDY

3213 W. Wheeler St., Ste. 254

Seattle, WA 98199

Teddy Toes is manufactured by Sisters 3 of Seattle. The product is an innovative blanket which your baby can wear. An advantage for Seattle natives is that Teddy Toes won't absorb more than one percent of its weight in water and it insulates even when it is wet. The material is colorfast and both machine washable and dryable. Teddy Toes comes in a variety of wonderful colors. The product costs around $45. One of the beauties of Teddy Toes is that it can be worn up to 18 months or 30 pounds, saving you money on a coat purchase. Sisters 3 also recently began offering a new product, called Tiny Toes. It's smaller than the original product and is primarily used for a receiving blanket. It's available in a cotton interlock fabric (pastels, primary prints, pastel prints) for $25. It's also offered in a certified organic, undyed, no-bleach cotton thermal, which comes with a hat and costs $33.95. Teddy and Tiny Toes can be purchased in Seattle at Nordstrom stores, Group Health Take Care Stores, and at baby and children's stores, as well as directly from Sisters 3.

■ THE UNCOMMON WALL
615-7528

Barbara Rich creates "whimsical and sophisticated" hand painted murals, furniture, and personalized items like keepsake boxes. Call her for a free consultation. She'll bring her portfolio and idea book to help you visualize the possibilities. She charges based on the time spent, not the project size.

TOP 10 GIFTS TO GIVE AND RECEIVE

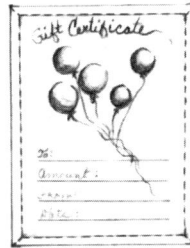

As there are many products to purchase with a new baby, there are also some great items to consider buying as a gift or simply to pamper yourself. Most of these gifts may not seem like a necessity, but we found them extremely helpful. Also, the recommendations are biased as they are products we or parents we know really appreciated. Take a look:

🔊

...there are also some great items to consider buying as a gift or simply to pamper yourself.

🔊

❶ The Diaper Genie. After a discussion with my husband about the smell of diapers in our house, we found a solution: a Diaper Genie. This is one of my favorite products, as it is virtually impossible to smell diapers in the house—even the "worst" ones! It may be a little tricky to figure out the first time. But, once you do, you'll use it with every diaper change. It retails at about $25 and is available at baby and discount stores.

❷ An exersaucer. Exersaucers or stationary walkers are a great invention for babies (from about the time a baby can sit up until walking) and parents as it provides exercise for the baby, but holds the child in one place. It runs about $50. Since this is a short-term product, check local resale stores for the latest deals.

❸ A locking clip. Retailing at only $2, this is probably the most useful and inexpensive item you can purchase. A locking clip is to be used with your car seat to hold the seatbelt in place. It keeps your baby and the car seat secure. You can find a metal locking clip in the plastic bag attached to the back of almost all new car seats. It should be used at all times. We found this item at discount stores and local baby stores.

❹ A front pack. For some the front pack can be a blessing, as holding the baby close soothes and calms even the crankiest child. For others, the front packs don't quite do the trick. You can purchase a front pack only, a front pack that allows the baby to be in different positions or a sling. In most cases, you may only use this item for a few months. Packs may cost from $20 to $70 depending on the brand.

❺ A gift certificate for a cleaning service. What all new parents need is time and order. Surprise yourself or a friend with a cleaning gift certificate.

❻ A back pack. This is a great product for parents on the go, as it gives your child a view of the world and parents an easy way to carry their child. Check into the different styles and manufacturers as price and quality really does vary.

❼ A night of baby-sitting. Offer your time and your care. It is probably the least expensive and most appreciated gift you could give to tired new parents.

❽ A great nightgown. Between nursing, sleepless nights, and wanting your old body back, a button-down night shirt or pajamas makes you feel like a new mother.

❾ Computer software. To help the new parent get and stay organized, consider some of the many software programs avail-

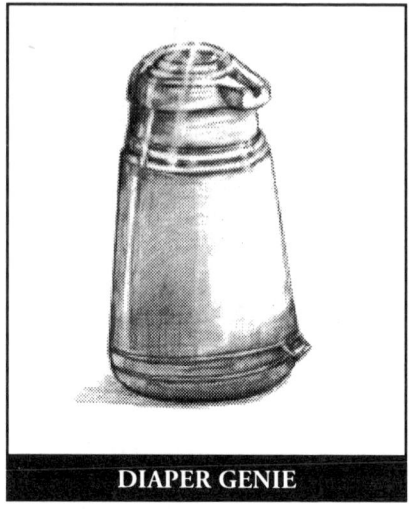

DIAPER GENIE

able. Two of our favorites are "A Womb with a View" (pregnancy software) and "Simply Kids" (an organization software program from Parents Magazine.) Both programs cost about $30.

❿ The Teddy Toes blanket. This product is a lifesaver for babies, as it functions as a coat and a blanket all-in-one. This makes a great gift. Stop by the baby specialty stores for a better look.

Other items to consider: A lullaby tape, sure to soothe a newborn baby to sleep; a baby book, to record all the essentials; film and a photo album, something new parents need; and just about anything with Winnie the Pooh or Peter Rabbit, as these characters are the current "hot" gift items. Remember, anything that comes from the heart makes a wonderful gift.

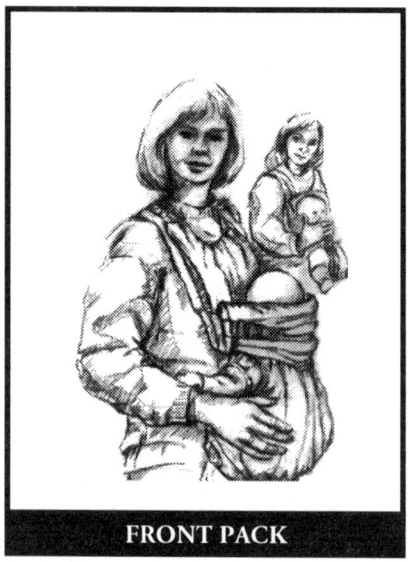

FRONT PACK

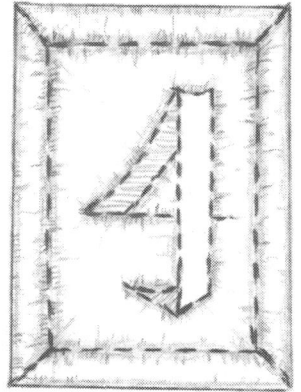

ESSENTIALS
FOR
YOUR
BABY

QUESTIONS & ANSWERS
An Interview with a Local Pediatrician

All physicians are not alike, and your challenge is to find one who relates well to both you and your child. Today, many parents choose either a family physician or a pediatrician to care for their baby. A family physician must graduate from four years of medical school and then serve three years of residency training. Family physicians who have successfully passed an oral and written examination given by the American Board of Family Practice are known as "Board Certified" and the initials "ABFP" will follow their name and title.

To become a pediatrician, one must graduate from a four-year medical school and then serve three additional years of residency training in pediatrics. Pediatricians who pass the written examination given by the American Board of Pediatrics are issued a special certificate. These doctors will have the initials "FAAP" following their names.

Every physician is committed to helping parents raise healthy children; however, individual doctors take different approaches so you may want to interview several doctors before selecting the one who best meets your needs. A physician should be selected before your baby is born. This will allow the provider the opportunity of giving your newborn its very first examination. The information below was obtained through an interview with Dr. Bernard J. Alberda, M.D., FAAP, of North Seattle Pediatrics.

Q: How do I choose a physician?

A: There are several good sources to check with. I think it's important to ask friends and family who have built a relationship with a physician. If you are new to the area, check with professionals who work with physicians. Your health care provider probably has some suggestions. Or check with different hospital nursing staff in the maternity or pediatric units. It all comes down to your preferences. For example, some families prefer a close location, while others will drive across town for office visits.

Q: What type of relationship should I expect to establish with my child's doctor?

A: Expect a good professional relationship with your child's physician, but over time that often becomes a close friendship—the physician almost becomes a member of the family.

Q: May I call the physician during non-office hours?

A: That's a good point to discuss with the physician on your first get-acquainted visit. There are a variety of ways to communicate with the physician during non-office hours, so it's important to clarify this point early on. You should try to take care of your non-emergency questions during regular office visits.

Q: *Are there times when an appointment is not necessary and I can call for additional advice over the telephone?*

A: Absolutely. One of the primary purposes of your pediatrician is to be an information center for new parents. There are many times when children are sick but do not require an office visit. A phone call can help your doctor identify what the problem is and suggest solutions over the phone.

Q: *What happens during the doctor's first visit with a newborn?*

A: This is a time to celebrate and enjoy the birth of a child. Often the doctor will check the newborn in the parents' room with the mother, father and siblings present. The newborn will be checked from head to toe and all of the normal newborn characteristics will be shared with the parents. This is a good time for parents to ask any questions they may have. Some doctors may spend a lot of time talking about what to expect in the coming years, but most tend to focus on what's going on right now; all of the normal, wonderful things that are going on with this newborn. I think it's important for parents to know that they have a normal, healthy baby.

Q: *What else should I expect during this first visit?*

A: A first office visit appointment will be arranged and information about how to reach the physician in the meantime will be shared.

Q: *Once we leave the hospital, what are some of the things I may notice with my infant?*

A: This bundle of joy is a lot of work! Mothers are often very tired and the child can be very demanding. You may also notice this is a very smart little person who knows how to get attention by complaining when there's not really a big problem. Parents need to appreciate and understand how smart their baby really is. It's important for parents to establish a relationship and a message with their baby, even early on, that parents are in charge.

Q: *What are some issues I should discuss with the doctor and/or nursing staff before leaving the hospital?*

A: Before you leave the hospital it's really important that you understand how to care for yourself and your newborn baby, and know where to get additional support for the questions you will have once you get home. You should have additional help at home when you return so that you can spend time resting and getting to know your newborn.

IMMUNIZATIONS

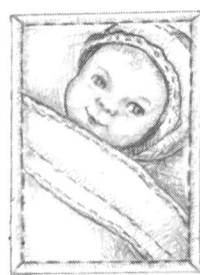

All normal and healthy children should be immunized against diseases which may be crippling or fatal. Benefits of immunization are partial or complete protection against the consequences of disease, which range from trivial and inconvenient symptoms to paralysis and death. No vaccine is completely effective or completely safe. Minor reactions to vaccines are frequent; severe reactions are extremely rare. It is more likely a child will have severe health problems from serious illnesses than to have significant problems from the vaccine against the illnesses. Minor illnesses, even those with some fever, are not sufficient reason to postpone vaccination. Vaccines should not be given if an individual is hypersensitive to a vaccine component or has altered immune response. "Important Information Statements" have been prepared by the Communicable Disease Center for each vaccine to inform parents of the benefits and risks of the vaccines. Be sure to ask your provider if you have any questions about immunizations. Below is information about the different diseases for which your child may be immunized.

❧

The American Academy of Pediatrics recommends that all normal, healthy children in the United States receive immunizations.

❧

DPT IMMUNIZATION:
DIPHTHERIA, PERTUSSIS, TETANUS (DTP, DTAP)

Diphtheria occurs primarily in children. The throat infection produces a toxin which damages the heart, kidneys and nerves, and may cause death.

Pertussis (whooping cough) is most severe in young infants. The illness produces protracted coughing, and may cause lung damage, seizures, brain damage and death.

Tetanus (lockjaw) is caused by a toxin produced by a wound infection. The toxin causes severe, painful muscle spasms, breathing problems and death.

OPV IMMUNIZATION:
ORAL POLIO VACCINE (OPV)

Polio is a viral infection of the nervous system which may produce extensive paralysis and death. Polio vaccination has been very successful; wild polio virus is no longer causing disease in the Western Hemisphere. Expect a modification in polio immunization practices to include inactivated polio vaccine (IPV) for the first two immunization doses for infants.

MMR IMMUNIZATION:
MEASLES, MUMPS, RUBELLA (MMR)

Red measles or "rubeola" is the most serious common childhood illness. The illness lasts ten days, with a high fever and generalized rash. Complications are pneumonia and encephalitis, which can produce deafness, blindness, and retardation. The mumps virus causes painful swelling of the salivary glands. It may cause inflammation of the pancreas. Fortunately, complications are rare.

Rubella, also called "German measles" or "three-day measles," is usually a mild illness with fever and rash. Infection in a pregnant woman can result in disastrous defects in the fetus.

HIB IMMUNIZATION:
HEMOPHILUS INFLUENZA TYPE B (HIB)

Invasive hemophilus influenza type B disease is one of the most serious bacterial infections in the young child. This bacterium causes meningitis, which has a high rate of residual neurological effects, and serious infections of the throat, lungs, bones and joints. This vaccine has dramatically reduced infections with this organism.

HBV IMMUNIZATION:
HEPATITIS TYPE B (HEP-B)

Hepatitis B can cause a serious liver infection which may produce chronic liver damage, liver cancer and death. An infected person passes the virus in blood and body fluids.

VARIVAX IMMUNIZATION:
CHICKEN POX (VARICELLA)

Chicken pox is a highly contagious, common childhood illness with fever and a blistery rash as the primary symptoms. Although the complication rate of this disease is low, it causes significant economic problems with disruption of child care and school attendance. Talk with your pediatrician about the pros and cons of this vaccine.

IMMUNIZATION SCHEDULE

The age at which the recommended immunizations may be given is indicated in the table below. Your child's schedule may vary, depending on the recommendations of your health care provider.

Immunization Schedule	
Birth	Hep-B
2 months	DTP, OPV, Hib, Hep-B
4 months	DTP, OPV, Hib
6 months	DTP, OPV, Hib, Hep-B
12-18 months	DTP, MMR, Hib, Varivax
4-6 years	DTP, OPV, MMR

Recommended childhood immunization schedule for birth to age 6, approved in January 1996 by the Advisory Committee on Immunization Practices (ACIP), the American Academy of Pediatrics (AAP), and the American Academy of Family Physicians (AAFP).

❧ RESOURCES ❧

■ KID CARE HOTLINE
800-756-KIDS
Call this toll-free line for information and referrals for pediatrician, dental, and immunization services.

■ SEATTLE-KING COUNTY DEPARTMENT OF PUBLIC HEALTH
296-4949
Call the department's hotline for recorded health-related information and for the hours and locations of public health centers. The health centers listed below have walk-in clinics during the hours noted, although it's best to call first to confirm those hours and find out about lunch-hour closures. The charge is $10 per immunization but no one is turned away if unable to pay. DSHS medical cards are also accepted.

■ COLUMBIA PUBLIC HEALTH CENTER
296-4650
4400 37th S.
Seattle, WA 98118
Hours: M-W   8:00 a.m.- 5:30 p.m.
              Th   8:00 a.m.-7:30 p.m.
              F   8:00 a.m.-4:30 p.m.

■ DOWNTOWN PUBLIC HEALTH CENTER
296-4755
2124 4th Ave.
Seattle, WA 98121
Hours: M-Th   7:00 a.m.-Noon,
                     1:00 p.m.-5:00 p.m.
              F   8:00 a.m.-Noon,
                     1:00 p.m.-4:00 p.m.

■ **EASTGATE PUBLIC HEALTH CENTER**
296-9722
14350 S.E. Eastgate Way
Bellevue, WA 98007
Hours: M-F   8:00 a.m.-4:30 p.m.

■ **NORTH DISTRICT PUBLIC HEALTH CENTER**
296-4990
10501 Meridian Ave. N.
Seattle, WA 98133
Hours: M,W,Th,F 8:00 a.m.-4:00 p.m.
       T   8:00 a.m.-4:00 p.m.,
              5:00 p.m.-7:00 p.m.

■ **NORTHSHORE PUBLIC HEALTH CENTER**
296-9787
10808 N.E. 145th St.
Bothell, WA 98011
Hours: M-F   10:00 a.m.-11:30 a.m.
           & 1:00 p.m.-4:00 p.m.

■ **SOUTH PUBLIC HEALTH CENTERS**
833-8400 (296-8400 from Seattle)
20 Auburn Ave.
Auburn, WA 98002
Hours: M,W,Th,F 8:00 a.m.-11:30 a.m.
              1:00 p.m.-4:00 p.m.
              (arrive by 3:30 p.m.)
       T   8:00 a.m.-3:30 p.m.,
              4:00 p.m.-6:00 p.m.

296-8410
33431 13th Pl. S.
Federal Way, WA 98003
Hours: M-F   8:00 a.m.-11:00 a.m.,
              1:00 p.m.-3:30 p.m.

■ **SOUTHEAST PUBLIC HEALTH CENTER**
296-4700
3001 N.E. 4th
Renton, WA 98056
Hours M-F   8:00 a.m.-5:00 p.m.
              (arrive by 4:15 p.m.)

■ **SOUTHWEST PUBLIC HEALTH CENTER**
296-4620
10821 8th Ave. S.W.
Seattle, WA 98146
Hours: M   8:00 a.m.-7:00 p.m.
       T-F   8:00 a.m.-4:30 p.m.

■ **SNOHOMISH COUNTY PUBLIC HEALTH DISTRICT**
339-5220
3020 Rucker Ave., Ste. 108
Everett, WA 98201
Hours: M,T,Th,F 8:00 a.m.-4:30 p.m.
       W   8:00 a.m.-6:30 p.m.

775-3522
19709-C Scriber Lake
Lynnwood, WA 98036
Hours: M-F   8:00 a.m.-4:30 p.m.
Low fees are charged for immunizations, and DSHS medical cards are also accepted for payment. Both sites offer walk-in services during their open hours.

■ COMMUNITY HEALTH CENTERS OF KING COUNTY
735-0166
105 A St. S.W.
Auburn, WA 98001
Hours: M,T,Th,F 9:00 a.m.-5:00 p.m.
      W   Noon-8:00 p.m.

486-0658
10414 Beardslee Blvd.
Bothell, WA 98011
Hours: M,T,Th,F 9:00 a.m.-5:00 p.m.
      W   Noon-8:00 p.m.

882-1697
16315 N.E. 87th, Ste. 36
Redmond, WA 98052
Hours: M,T,W,F 9:00 a.m.-5:00 p.m.
      Th   Noon-8:00 p.m.

852-2866
403 E. Meeker
Kent, WA 98031
Hours: M,T   8:30 a.m.-8:00 p.m.
      W,Th,F 8:30 a.m.-5:00 p.m.

226-5536
149 Park N.
Renton, WA 98055
Hours: M,T,Th,F 9:00 a.m.-5:00 p.m.
      W   Noon-8:00 p.m.

874-7634
33431 13th Pl. S.
Federal Way, WA 98003
Hours: M   9:00 a.m.-8:00 p.m.
      Th-F   9:00 a.m.-5:00 p.m.
Immunizations are given during well-child checkups.

■ COMMUNITY HEALTH CENTERS OF SNOHOMISH COUNTY
775-2589
21727 7th W., Ste. 107
Edmonds, WA 98026
Hours: M-F   8:30 a.m.-5:00 p.m.

258-4595
2722 Colby Ave., Ste. 318
Everett, WA 98201
Hours: M-F   8:30 a.m.-5:00 p.m.
The Community Health Centers accept DSHS medical cards and charge low fees on a sliding scale. A well-child visit will be scheduled to coincide with immunizations. Call to make an appointment.

■ NATIONAL VACCINE INFORMATION CENTER
800-909-SHOT
This is a nonprofit center that was founded by parents whose children responded negatively to immunizations. They will send information regarding these issues.

JAUNDICE: COMMON IN NEWBORNS

Jaundice is the yellow or yellow-orange discoloration seen in baby's skin and whites of the eyes due to the elevation of bilirubin in the blood.

Bilirubin is a product of the breakdown of red blood cells. As new red blood cells are being formed, old ones continue to break down. Before birth, the mother's liver processed the baby's bilirubin via the placenta. After birth, the baby's liver has to take over the job—it can take up to two weeks for the baby's liver to function at full capacity. During this time, extra bilirubin accumulates in the baby's system and jaundice appears. Approximately 80 percent of all newborns show some signs of jaundice during this period.

Certain factors can cause this process to be exaggerated, such as prematurity, bruising from the delivery and certain mother/baby blood incompatibilities. Babies also have a higher percentage of red blood cells than adults and they break down faster.

Approximately five to fifteen percent of babies will require treatment for elevated bilirubin. Phototherapy, a non-invasive procedure that can be performed in your own home, is the treatment of choice.

There are three simple tests you can do at home to determine if your baby has jaundice. Hold your baby in front of a window in the daylight. Look at your baby's skin color. Press down slightly on the skin and release.

- Is the skin yellow/orange?
- Does the yellow/orange color extend to the chest area? To the abdomen?
- Are the whites of the eyes yellow?

If you answered "yes" to any of these questions, notify baby's physician. The physician may ask you to take your baby to the lab for a simple blood test to determine the level of bilirubin (jaundice) in your baby's system.

Life Experiences ...

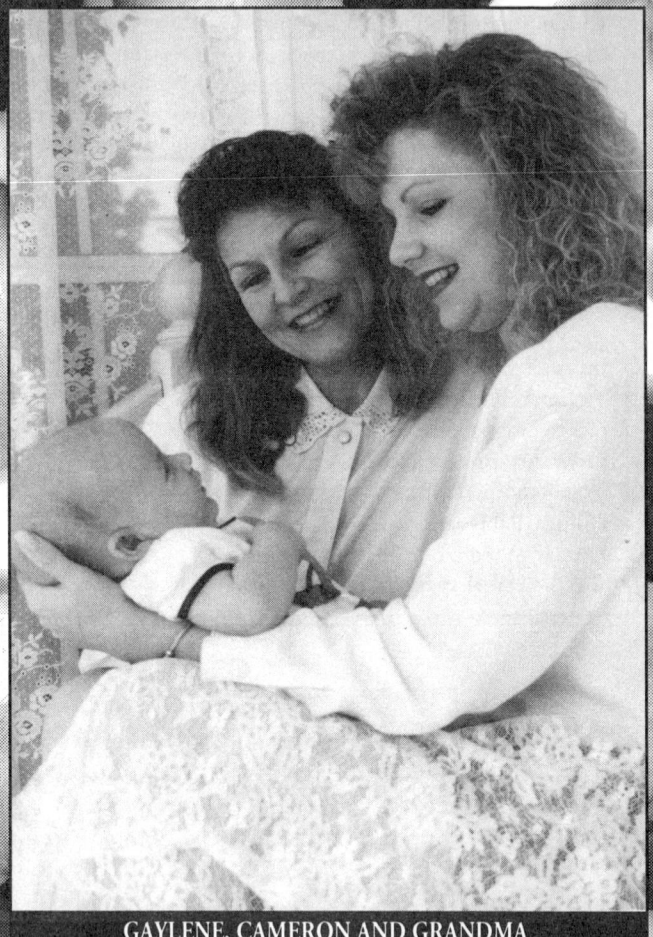

GAYLENE, CAMERON AND GRANDMA

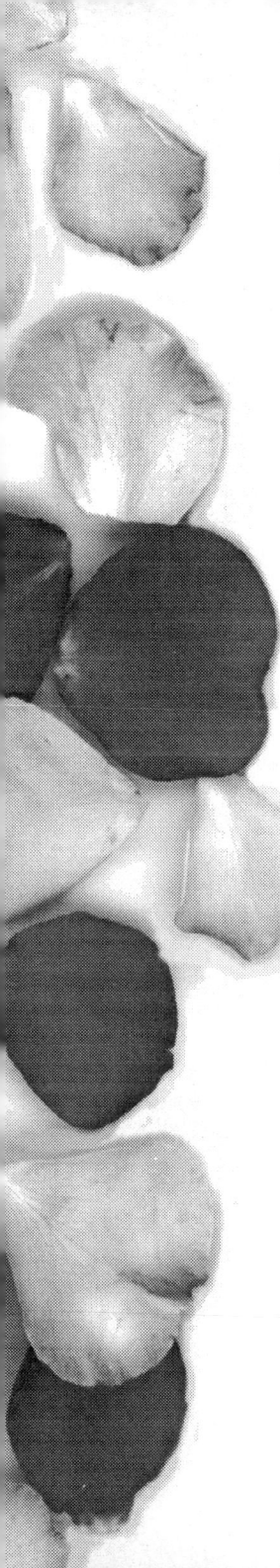

"A LETTER TO MY MOTHER"

By Gaylene Tompkins

It's 9:45 p.m. I've just put my son down for the third time this hour. As he begins to cry again, I fight my urge to pick him up and comfort him, and walk to the kitchen for a bowl of cereal before I fall into bed. I stare blankly at the flakes as they tumble into the bowl and pause to listen for his signal—do I pour the milk or head back down the hall for another round?

Silence. At last. My exhausted mind begins to wander and I think of you; of how many nights you must have spent the same way I have spent this one—comforting your child the way only a mother can.

I wonder if I'll remember the way his tiny hand wraps around my smallest finger and holds on like he'll never let go. I wonder if I'll remember how overwhelmed I felt those first weeks—how I yearned for someone to tell me I was a good mom and how, as if somehow he knew the incredible joy it would bring me, he picked the moment when I was the most exhausted to smile for the first time. I wonder if you remember these things about me. In my heart, I know that you do.

I could never have imagined the incredible love a mother feels for her child. But now I know. Now I know how much you love me. Of all the things you have taught me, the one that stands out is this: the most important job you'll ever have is raising a child. Of all the things you have given me, the most important is your love. Because I grew up feeling loved, knowing you were there for me no matter what, I was free to become the person I am today—strong and independent, able to think on my own, comfortable with who I am and able to love others because I love myself.

So thank you, Mom, for all those nights you picked me up and held me one more time. I couldn't tell you then, but I'll tell you now—you did a good job. You're the best mother I could have ever hoped for. I love you. ❧

SUPPORT GROUPS

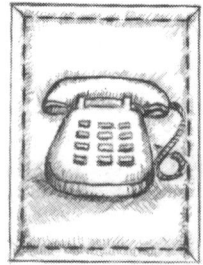

This section includes some of the many support groups in the greater Seattle area. A support group serves a dual purpose: companionship and information. It is also wonderful for your child!

See the special-concern resources section for more support group information on children with special needs.

Participating in a support group is a great idea, especially for first-time parents, who often have so many questions and concerns. The arrival of a baby can unleash many new emotions and demands. Sometimes just being with other new parents helps to remind you that you aren't alone in your new role. It is also fun to share your child's accomplishments and gain other parents' insights and clues to success.

■ FATHERS SUPPORT GROUP
721-5542
Southeast Youth & Family Services
3722 S. Hudson St.
Seattle, WA 98118
Fathers in Action presents this support group for dads on the second and fourth Wednesday of each month, from 6:00-7:30 p.m. Open forum discussions will explore the personal experiences of fathers.

■ F.E.M.A.L.E.
485-0822, Regional Coordinator
702-9044, Redmond Chapter
Meeting dates: M-W 9:30-11:30 a.m. playgroups (Redmond)
Thurs. 7:00-9:00 p.m. (bi-weekly meetings for moms)
Formerly Employed Mothers at the Leading Edge (F.E.M.A.L.E.), is a national organization for women who have chosen to take a break from their full-time career to stay at home with their children. Local chapters meet twice or more a month in the evening, without children. Most chapters also have play groups and family functions. The groups provide a place where Moms can find intimacy and support from other moms. Call Meg Nafziger, Regional Coordinator, at 485-0822 for information.

■ **MOMS & MOPPETS**
Eastside Foursquare Church
N.E. 145th & 100th N.E.
Bothell, WA 98011
Meeting dates: Tues. 9:00-11:30 a.m.
Moms & Moppets offers weekly get-togethers for mothers and their children from newborn through age 5. Meetings include teachings on parenting, health, crafts, and decorating. Refreshments and small group discussions are also offered.

■ **MOM'S GROUP**
St. John's Episcopal Church
827-3077
105 State St.
Kirkland, WA 98033
Meeting dates: Tues. 9:30-11:00 a.m.
This free group for mothers meets weekly for discussions, parties, special programs, and other activities. Child care is available for children through kindergarten age.

■ **MOTHERS & OTHERS**
226-6600
St. Madeleine Sophie Catholic Church
4400 130th Pl. S.E.
Bellevue, WA 98006
Meeting dates: Mon. 9:30-11:30 a.m.
This support group is for mothers, fathers, nannies, grandparents, and anyone else who nurtures children. Child care is available for babies and toddlers, and play activities for preschoolers.

■ **NEW MOM SUPPORT GROUP**
386-3606
Swedish Medical Center
747 Broadway
Seattle, WA 98114
The New Mom Support Group meets weekly at Swedish and provides a forum for discussion on a variety of topics. It covers the first three months of motherhood and costs $60 for the three-month session.

■ **PROGRAM FOR EARLY**
  PARENT SUPPORT (PEPS)
547-8570
4649 Sunnyside Ave. N.
Seattle, WA 98103
Hours: M-F   8:00 a.m.-4:30 p.m.
PEPS services include facilitating community-based parent support groups for parents with children birth to three, publishing and distributing a new parent resource list, and staffing a resource and referral line. The Neighborhood PEPS groups meet at members' homes for six months on a weekly basis, and provide education and support for parents whose children are age birth to four months when the group starts. The Neighborhood Program costs $50. A free Outreach Program provides ongoing weekly groups at community centers for parents with children birth to three years old. Facilitators of groups are volunteers from the community who are trained by PEPS. The goal of PEPS is to support all families through mutual support and shared information, building on their strengths as parents. The programs are offered to all families regardless of income (scholarships are available for the Neighborhood Program). PEPS also offers special programs for teen parents and for mothers in treatment for substance abuse.

■ **SEATTLE-KING COUNTY DEPARTMENT OF PUBLIC HEALTH MOTHER-INFANT GROUPS**
296-4765
North Seattle Public Health Center
10501 Meridian Ave. N., Rm. H-200
Seattle, WA 98133
These groups meet once a week for six weeks, and discussion topics include coping with crying, illness care, safety, growth and development, and nutrition and feeding. No preregistration is required and classes are free (donations accepted). Classes are held on Wednesday or Thursday afternoons. Call for session dates.

■ **SUPPORT GROUP FOR GAY AND LESBIAN PARENTS**
527-6068
This group is sponsored by the Adoption Resource Center of Children's Home Society and meets on a monthly basis to discuss the unique issues faced by adoptive gay and lesbian parents. Prospective adopters are welcome. The group is limited to gays and lesbians. Call for meeting times and locations.

■ **YOU AND YOUR NEW BABY**
688-5259
Overlake Hospital offers this five-week support class for new parents on an ongoing basis. Topics covered include infant feeding, sleep patterns, fussy babies, new parent adjustments, and more. Classes are held once a week at Overlake Hospital in Bellevue and at Issaquah Medical Center in Issaquah, and cost $40/person. Call for specific dates, times, and locations.

FAMILY SUPPORT CENTERS

Family Support Centers operate in many communities in the metro Seattle area. These centers provide resources, education, referrals, support groups, and more. Types of programs offered include parent-child activity time, WIC and maternity health support services, new parents support groups, an "evening out" (free drop-off care for your kids), and single parent and teen parent groups. The centers are operated by nonprofit organizations, often with financial support from local counties, cities, and communities. Most are open weekdays and some evenings; call for specific hours and a current list of programs.

SEATTLE

■ **NORTH SEATTLE FAMILY CENTER**
364-7930
13540 Lake City Way N.E., Ste. 5
Seattle, WA 98125

■ **SOUTHWEST FAMILY CENTER**
763-7929
5950 Delridge Way S.W.
Seattle, WA 98106

■ **SOUTHEAST SEATTLE FAMILY CENTER**
723-1301
7301 Beacon Ave. S.
Seattle, WA 98108

METRO AREA

■ AUBURN FAMILY RESOURCE CENTER
854-0700
4338 Auburn Way N.
Auburn, WA 98002

■ LYNNWOOD FAMILY SUPPORT CENTER
670-8984
6309 196th St. S.W.
Lynnwood, WA 98036

■ REDMOND FAMILY SUPPORT CENTER
869-6699
16315 N.E. 87th
Redmond, WA 98052

■ SHORELINE FAMILY SUPPORT CENTER
362-7282
17018 15th N.E.
Shoreline, WA 98155

PARENT EDUCATION COOPERATIVES

Community colleges and vocational schools throughout the area offer parent education programs that include a cooperative preschool component. These programs serve several purposes including parent education, opportunities for children to learn and socialize with other young children, and a built-in support group for parents. Programs vary but generally they include some on-campus time with other parents and a preschool/playschool for the children that meets 1-3 times a week, usually at neighborhood locations. Classes have an assigned teacher and parents rotate as helpers in the classroom. There are some fees for these programs, but usually they cost much less than a regular preschool. Some of the schools offer programs for parents with young babies (prewalkers). Many of the co-ops offer an open house in the spring, in preparation for fall enrollment, and classes do fill up quickly. For more information call the school nearest you:

Bellevue	641-2366
Green River	464-6133
Highline	878-3710
North Seattle	527-3783
Seattle Central	587-6900
Shoreline	546-4593
South Seattle	764-5321
Lake Washington	828-5600
Renton	235-2352
Edmonds	640-1665
Everett	388-9300

OTHER RESOURCES

■ CHILDREN'S HOSPITAL RESOURCE CENTER
526-2201 (center/education information)
526-2500 (resource line)
4800 Sand Point Way N.E.
Seattle, WA 98105
Hours: Resource center hours:
     M-F   8:00 a.m.-4:00 p.m.
     Resource line:
     Daily   7:00 a.m.-midnight
Children's Hospital offers the most comprehensive child health, safety, and parenting resource service in Washington State. On the fifth floor of the hospital you'll find the Parent Resource Center. It's filled with racks of free brochures related to parenting, including information on feeding, immunizations, community resources, and special needs programs, as well as safety and health issues. There is also a lending library.

Children's also operates a resource line, staffed by pediatric registered nurses. You can call and get information on child health and parenting, as well as referrals for physicians and community resources. A leader in community education, Children's offers classes in parenting, child development, safety, baby-sitting and more. Classes are offered at various times and are affordable. They also publish a quarterly newsletter, "Good Growing," and conduct a variety of community outreach activities.

■ CHILDBIRTH AND PARENTING RESOURCES
781-0858
This is an advocacy association of consumers and professionals which campaigns for improvement in all aspects of maternity care by promoting birth and parenting options, offering resources and referrals and providing support and encouragement to parents and the community.

■ COMMUNITY INFORMATION LINE
461-3200
Hours: M-F   9:00 a.m.-5:00 p.m.
Operated by the Crisis Clinic's Resource Center, this phone line provides information and referral to over 2,000 social services agencies in the area. The center maintains a current data base of agencies and also publishes an annual directory called "Where to Turn PLUS" which includes detailed information on agencies: a service description, eligibility requirements, fees and branch locations.

■ LULL-A-BABY
(900) 255-BABY
Parents and caregivers needing help consoling a distressed, crying baby can get

assistance by calling Lull-a-Baby, a 900 number with an informational taped message by Anne McElhinney, Infant Behavior Specialist. She describes techniques that she also teaches in a class at Children's Hospital. The call costs $1.80/minute (average 7 min./call).

■ MED-INFO AT NORTHWEST HOSPITAL
633-4636
Northwest Hospital provides their 24-hour MED-INFO line as a free community service. When you call, you'll talk to a registered nurse who can answer medical questions and refer you to additional resources as necessary.

■ PARENT RESOURCE LINE
259-2973
This phone line is operated by the Child Care Resource and Referral of Volunteers of America in Snohomish County. Besides providing phone referrals to agencies, parent support groups, and classes, a parent resource guide is published quarterly which lists information on programs for parents. This publication is published by Lifenet in conjunction with the Volunteers of America.

■ PARENTS ANONYMOUS
233-0139 (Family Help Line)
or 800-932-HOPE (outside Seattle)
Parents can call the help line 24 hours a day to get assistance in dealing with crisis situations and to locate local resources. They'll also send written material on positive parenting. Parents Anonymous offers free self-help support groups throughout the community, including free child care.

ONLINE SUPPORT

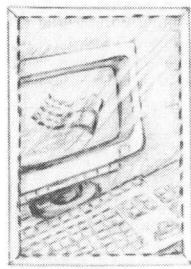

With just a computer, modem and phone line, parents can access a world of support and information. From checking an online version of a parenting book to chatting with other parents, the virtual community can be a wonderful resource. Here are some ways to get online. Note that the online world is rapidly growing; the resources were current when this book was published.

◼ LOCAL LIBRARY SYSTEMS

King County Library: 382-2116
Seattle Public Library: 386-4140

One of the least expensive ways of getting online is through the Seattle Public Library and King County Library systems. Both offer a local phone number which users dial using a communications software program. Once online, you can search for library resources and place holds on books, tapes, videos and more, which will be sent to the library you specify for pick-up. Both also offer some access to the Internet and listings of community resources and events. Using this method costs only a local phone call.

◼ ONLINE SERVICES

America Online: 800-827-6364
CompuServe: 800-848-8199
Microsoft Network: 800-386-5550
Prodigy: 800-776-3449

America Online, CompuServe, Microsoft Network, and Prodigy connect people throughout the country and beyond. You'll need to install their software and sign up as a member. It's easy to get free software and a free trial period, after which the monthly cost is about $5-$10, which covers the first 3-5 hours, and $2.50-$3 per additional hour.

These services offer bulletin boards for exchanging messages and "chat rooms" for real-time communications via the keyboard. They also offer e-mail, software files to download, and resource information on many different subjects.

Each provides one or more areas specifically for parents. America Online has "Parent Soup" with message boards, experts, chat areas, reviews, and much more.

Prodigy has message boards on parenting and adoption, as well as a parenting page on their Internet site. Microsoft Network offers both "Home and Family" and "People and Communities" areas, with message boards, chat rooms, and resources. CompuServe, well-known for its business-related features, has recently begun to offer a parenting forum.

All of these services also provide a way for users to access the Internet, which offers many places where parents can share and receive information. Here we've highlighted some of these sites.

■ INTERNET/WWW

Parents can access the Internet and its graphically-rich World Wide Web (WWW) through commercial online services like those mentioned above, or through a direct Internet provider. Check newsmagazines like Puget Sound Computer User for local Internet providers. With a direct provider, you'll also need Web browser software such as Netscape Navigator; many of the companies include this for free. The cost of accessing the Internet this way is somewhat less, generally averaging $1 per hour or less (usually with a minimum charge of $15). Here are some sites of interest to parents.

Family Planet:
http://family.starwave.com
Family Planet is a site created by Bellevue's Starwave Corporation. It offers daily news on family-related topics, experts discussing family issues, reviews, the *Parent's Resource Almanac* book online, and monthly calendars of family events from cities around the country.

Family.com: http://family.com
Family.com is part of Disney Online, and includes lots of local information from

parenting newspapers throughout the U.S., as well as feature articles and resources for parents.

Parent Soup:
http://www.parentsoup.com
This web site is the Internet version of AOL's parenting area, with much of the same information. There are bulletin boards and chat areas here too.

Resolution Business Press:
http://www.halcyon.com/ResPress/
This is the home page for the publisher of the book *Internet for Parents*. The 700+ Internet resources from the book are listed right here online, so instead of typing in a site's address, you can just click on it from this page.

Baby Web:http://www.netaxs.com/~iris/infoweb/baby.html
Contains baby-related resources.

Family Internet:
http://www.familyinternet.com
Includes a baby care section.

Family Web:
http://www.familyweb.com
Includes a pregnancy section.

Moms-at-home:
http://iquest.com/~jsm/moms/
An online support area for moms at home.

La Leche League International:
http://www.prairienet.org/llli/
Home page for this breastfeeding support organization.

National Parenting Center:
http://www.tnpc.com
Offers a variety of parenting resources.

Parents Place: http://parentsplace.com
Includes online news, resources, and areas to communicate with other parents.

PUBLICATIONS OFFERING SUPPORT

■ *AT-HOME DAD* NEWSLETTER
508-685-7931
Peter Baylies
61 Brightwood Ave.
North Andover, MA 01845
This quarterly newsletter promoting the home-based father publishes a list of local coordinators who help fathers meet, get parenting advice, and plan activities. A subscription costs $12 per year. There are listings for other sources of information such as books, online services, and magazines as they are developing rapidly. Examples include a new magazine called *Modern Dad* and an America Online chat group called "Stay-At-Home/Primary Care Dads Chat."

■ A *NEW ARRIVAL, SEATTLE'S CHILD, EASTSIDE PARENT*
441-0191
These three publications are published by Northwest Parent Publishing, Inc. Run by two mothers, these newsmagazines are well-known for their editorial content. *A New Arrival* is published twice a year and is geared solely to new and expectant parents. Free copies are available at maternity and baby stores as well as local libraries. The monthly publications, *Seattle's Child* and *Eastside Parent*, have a large circulation and are available free of charge at children's stores, child care centers, libraries, and almost any place children visit. Articles are for parents of children of all ages, rather than just infants and toddlers. The paper includes an extensive listing of activities for families, as well as classes and support groups for parents.

■ *NORTHWEST BABY & CHILD*
232-0301
Published by Baby Diaper Service, *Northwest Baby & Child* is a free monthly publication that offers wonderful information regarding infancy and the toddler years. A regular monthly column offers advice on breastfeeding; there are also many articles on health and safety and environmental issues. It is available at baby and maternity stores, toy stores, and other children-related spots and delivered to Baby Diaper Service customers in five counties. The paper also includes a monthly calendar of support groups and other happenings for parents and children.

Life Experiences...

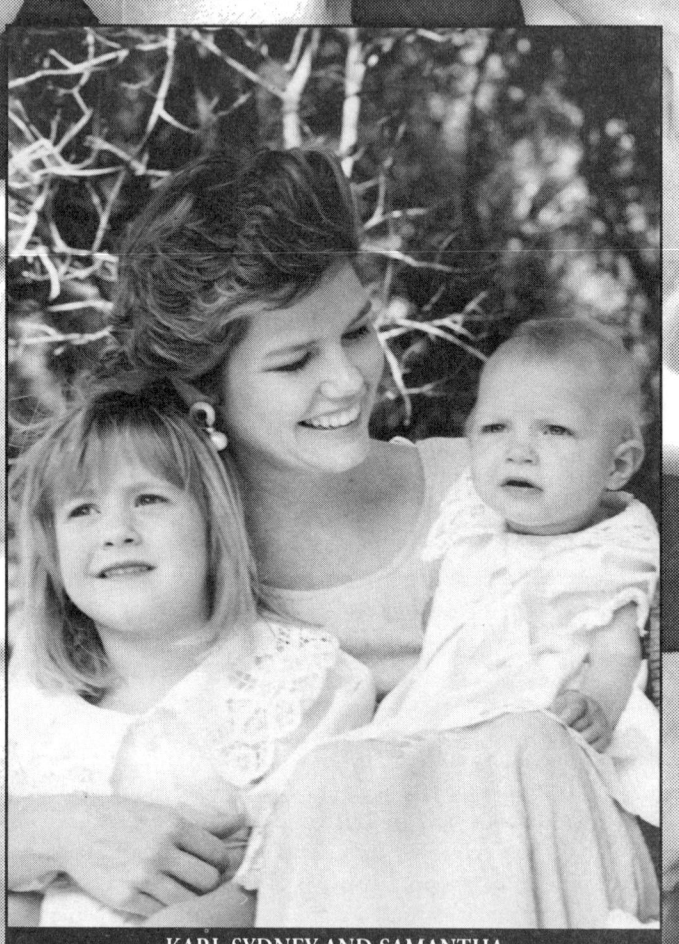

KARI, SYDNEY AND SAMANTHA

"UNCERTAINTY"

By Kari E. Hazen

The other day, my friend Joy shared her news with me—"Guess what? I'm pregnant!" After a year of trying, she and her husband had finally conceived. She was not only pregnant, but also subtly added, "Oh, and by the way, we're having twins." My heart sang for her, my soul chuckled. I kept thinking, "I wonder if she knows what she's getting herself into?" I knew instantly that she didn't. She couldn't. I also knew there was no way to prepare her. Not until you have entered this sacred sorority of motherhood can you begin to understand this rollercoaster ride of raising children.

A week later, I called to set up lunch. It took eight days for her to return my call. During that time, I fretted and worried. I wondered about her pregnancy. Was she all right? How were the babies? Did complications occur? I almost dreaded talking with her. Finally she left a message that she and the babies were fine. She had spent the last eight days plagued with morning sickness. Once I received her call I felt a huge sigh of relief.

That experience made me stop and reflect about the last five years of my parenting journey. It also made me realize all the uncertainties that come with the title of "mother." It begins at pregnancy and, so my mother tells me, never ends. With each new experience comes a question, a thought, or a concern. Am I doing this right? Why is my child doing what she's doing? How could I be a better parent? And, oh no, is she all right? I intensely recall celebrating each of my daughters' first birthdays. Along with the cake, ice cream and party favors, we also quietly celebrated that the "SIDS" critical period passed. With each new year, came a new set of questions. Being a concerned parent, I immersed myself in books, articles, and parenting conversations trying to understand my child better. I found there were as many opinions as there were parents. And, each "expert" has their own way of parenting. It's enough to make you feel slightly confused in a place which is already perplexing enough.

And then something happened with the birth of my second child. I stopped and learned to let go and relax a little bit. I began to trust. I didn't worry about doing everything the "right" way. I also quit caring about what others thought. I accepted the fact that having children and raising a family was not going to be a controlled or perfect experience. Letting go allowed me the freedom to enjoy my children and cherish the time I have with them.

There are still days that I stop and wonder about my children's futures. I really don't know if I can conceptualize my world without them. And there are mornings when my five-year-old looks up at me with her big blue eyes and says, "I love you, Mommy, more than anything in the whole world. Let's just stay home and play," that makes me question why I'm going to work. But, I simply do the best that I can. And that's all I can do. That's all any parent can do. I know that I give my children all the love, hope and dreams that exist in me. I hope by giving them the confidence they need, they will be able to survive happily in this uncertain world. And, like my friend Joy, they will get through every day with all the triumphs and snags life brings. ❧

BIRTH ANNOUNCEMENTS

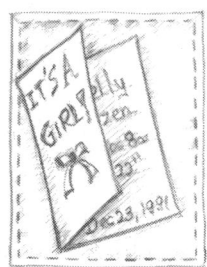

When considering birth announcements, spend some time thinking about and researching your options. Once the baby arrives it will be more difficult to find the time and energy to shop and make decisions. While this section may not include all of the stores that carry birth announcements, it gives you a good place to start. Happy shopping!

■ **ALL WRAPPED UP**
447-CARD
201 Pine St.
Seattle, WA 98101
Hours: M-Sat. 8:00 a.m.-6:00 p.m.
Sun. 10:00 a.m.-5:00 p.m.
All Wrapped Up carries a large selection of announcements, from pre-packaged to ones you can custom-order from several catalogs. They also can print on the many decorative card stocks that they carry in-house.

■ **DRUG EMPORIUM**
Drug Emporium is the place to go if you want pre-packaged announcements at a bargain price. Although the selection varies, there are always at least a few different designs to choose from and all are sold at 40% off the retail price. Brands carried include American Greetings and Marcel Schurman. The 40% off applies to all products in those two lines including wrapping paper, ribbons, bows, greeting cards, invitations, thank you cards, stickers, and package decor. Drug Emporium also has a good selection of baby accessories like packaged toys, rattles, bottles, teethers, and more, all at discounted prices.

■ **HALLMARK SHOPS**
Hallmark Shops are located in malls and in neighborhood shopping areas and offer a great selection of pre-packaged announcements. They have catalogs if you want to order custom announcements. Most stores also have an in-house service that customizes and prints your announcement on a laser printer.

■ LICENSED TO CRAWL
524-6352
21729 S.E. May Valley Rd.
Issaquah, WA 98027
Here's a unique idea for a birth announcement—a Washington Crawler's License. Postcard size and in full color, these announcements look a lot like a driver's license except they also include the parents' names. The order form comes with detailed instructions on how to get a good picture of your baby, which you send along with all the vital statistics and your check (starting at $30 for 25 "licenses"). Call and get a free sample and order form.

■ THE PAPER TREE
451-8035
Bellevue Square
Bellevue, WA 98004
Hours: M-Sat.   9:30 a.m.-9:30 p.m.
        Sun.   10:00 a.m.-6:00 p.m.
The Paper Tree is a popular place to shop for birth announcements. In addition to pre-packaged selections, there are more than 20 books of custom announcements that you can choose from. You'll also find plenty of shower invitations, thank you cards, photo albums and frames, and baby books.

■ PAPYRUS
771-5830
Alderwood Mall
3000 184th St. S.W., Ste. 562
Lynnwood, WA 98036
Hours: M-Sat.   9:30 a.m.-9:30 p.m.
        Sun.   11:00 a.m.-6:00 p.m.

464-1505
1210 4th Ave.
Seattle, WA 98101
Hours: M-F   9:00 a.m.-6:00 p.m.
        Sat.   10:00 a.m.-5:00 p.m.

451-4802
Bellevue Square
Bellevue, WA 98004
Hours: M-Sat.   9:30 a.m.-9:30 p.m.
        Sun.   11:00 a.m.-6:00 p.m.

363-8055
Northgate Mall
Seattle, WA 98125
Hours: M-Sat.   9:30 a.m.-9:30 p.m.
        Sun.   11:00 a.m.-6:00 p.m.
Papyrus carries both pre-packaged and custom order birth announcements. They also have a nice selection of scrapbooks, photo albums, brag books, mothers' journals, and grandparents' journals.

■ PHOTO TIDINGS
(503) 484-0896
Design your own birth announcement with a photograph of your new arrival. These unique cards are 5" x 7" and can be ordered with or without customization.

■ REAL CARD COMPANY
325-1854
2814 E. Madison
Seattle, WA 98112
Hours: M-Sat.   10:00 a.m.-5:00 p.m.
At Real Card Company you can select announcements from a wide variety of catalogs but the real emphasis here is on in-house custom designing. Designers make unique creations using any of a number of different processes: printing, calligraphy, letterpressing, and engraving, to come up with the final result. You can go in while you're expecting and select what you want, then call in the vital statistics when your baby is born. The announcements will usually be ready within a couple of weeks. Call for an appointment to ensure undivided attention, as the store can be busy.

■ SAB-TEC STATIONERS

523-2106
4710 University Village Pl. N.E.
Seattle, WA 98105
Hours: M-Sat. 9:30 a.m.-6:00 p.m.
Sun. 10:00 a.m.-6:00 p.m.

Sab-Tec has an excellent selection of birth announcements. They offer pre-packaged sets and you can also order by catalog. In-house, they have a nice assortment of blank cards with colorful borders and matching envelopes. They'll do pen and ink calligraphy on these and the result is very attractive. You pay by the card for in-house work, so you can get just as many as you need.

■ STORK EXPRESS

649-5490
Announce your baby's arrival with a personalized lawn sign. The seven-foot-tall stork has a blue or pink vest and displays your baby's first name and date of birth. Cost is $10 per day with a three day minimum, or $60 for a week. Delivery is free to Bellevue, Redmond, and Issaquah addresses, with a small delivery charge outside of these areas.

■ "THE STORK GAZETTE"

633-3988
"The Stork Gazette" is a personalized newsletter that shares the details of your baby's birth. You provide the information, including photographs, and they'll do the rest. Cost is $50 for the first 50 copies, and $10 per 25 for additional copies. The newsletter is printed on both sides of a sheet of high quality cardstock.

■ BABY PICTURES

462-9116
If you'd like to show your child what she looked like before she was born or find out for certain if your baby will be a boy or girl, Baby Pictures can help. For $50 they'll make a 15-minute prenatal ultrasound video, as well as still pictures from the ultrasound. The videos are done by a licensed (RT, RDMS, RVT) ultrasound technician in her home in Bellevue.

MAIL ORDER ANNOUNCEMENTS

A number of companies offer customized baby announcements by mail—here are a few. Call their toll-free numbers below to request a free catalog (some even provide free samples). Several will address and mail the cards for you within a day of receiving your baby's birth data if you pre-order and provide them with a mailing list.

Contemporary Statements	800-578-4711
Heart Thoughts	800-524-BABY
H&F Announcements	800-964-4002
MugShots	800-553-1412
The Personal Touch	800-453-3882
Photo-Flash	800-366-1363
Pride and Joy	800-657-6404

MEMENTOS FOR BABY

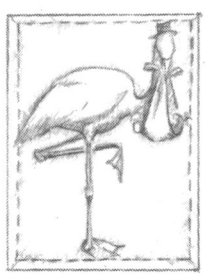

There are a few special mementos available to celebrate and remember your baby's birth. Some companies are fairly well-known in this area and others are individuals who provide some very special memories.

■ **BASKETCASES GIFT BASKET SERVICE**
338-3436 or 800-290-9330
Basketcases makes a "Baby's Time Capsule" gift basket. For $70, you get a huge gift basket of baby goodies like powder, lotion, and bath supplies, and the "time capsule." This is a large container that you can fill with such memories as baby's first photo, a photo of baby's first home, a newspaper from baby's birth day, a letter from baby's grandparents, your predictions for your baby's future, and any other mementos to help mark the day your baby was born (the receipt from the pizza you had delivered that night, maybe?).

■ **CREATIVE MEMORIES**
800-468-9335
You can design and create your own baby photo album with the photo safe supplies Creative Memories provides. Creative Memories' staff presents classes which help you organize and tell a story with your pictures. There is a small fee for the classes and you're encouraged to purchase supplies through Creative Memories.

■ **JACKSON'S BRONZED BABY SHOES**
322-4151
Several finishes are available to preserve your baby's shoes: bronze, gold, antique pewter, silver, clear, and chinakote (pink, blue, ivory, and pearl). All work is unconditionally guaranteed for life. They offer an assortment of mountings, include por-

trait sets, desk sets, even book ends. Prices range from $40 to $85. Call to receive a price list and full-color brochure that shows the many options available.

■ **JAN'S CUSTOM KNITS**
800-JAN-KNIT
You can order personalized baby blankets from Jan's. Two crib sizes are available, 28" x 28" for $39.95 and 30" x 40" for $59.95. There are 40 different designs available, and you can specify what you want embroidered on the acrylic blanket such as name, birthdate, time, weight, and more. Designs are available in Hebrew, Spanish, Japanese, and other languages upon request.

■ **KEEPSAKES, INC.**
800-447-0654
31200 LaBaya Dr., Ste. 304
Westlake Village, CA 91362
A beautiful ceramic bootie is available through Baby Keepsakes. Delicately hand-painted, your keepsake bootie includes your baby's name, height, weight, and date and time of birth. The provider's name or any ten-word saying can also be included at the bottom of the bootie. You may order over the phone with VISA or MasterCard, through the mail or by fax. The total cost, including first-class shipping and handling, is approximately $42.

■ **MY STORYBOOKS OF THE NW**
800-704-BABY
S. 428 Truax, P.O. Box 865
Tekoa, WA 99033
My Storybooks offers a very different kind of baby book: "My Baby Book" is a personalized keepsake book, told from your baby's point of view. The 8-1/2" x 11" hardcover book features beautiful color illustrations and your baby's name throughout the story. All your baby's vital statistics are included, and there are special pages for you to add all of baby's firsts and favorites, along with favorite photos. You can even order a Spanish language or single-parent version. Besides the baby book, My Storybooks offers more than a dozen other books that can be personalized with your child's name. Prices are very reasonable, $12.95 for the baby book and $10.95 for most of the other hardcover books.

■ **PRECIOUS PRINTS**
255-0736
12214 S.E. 96th Pl.
Renton, WA 98056
This is a really cute memento! A poem called "Baby's First Impression" is professionally printed and framed in glass. You get to personalize it yourself with your baby's foot prints. Complete instructions explain how to get a good stamp of baby's foot and how to apply it to the picture. The stamped foot prints are connected by a pink or blue ribbon. Order direct for $20 from Elizabeth at the number above. Elizabeth will also add baby's name and birthdate to make it even more special.

■ **SAFEWAY STORES PHOTO DEPARTMENT**

Safeway's photo company, Benco Inc., offers a line of photo mementos called Memory Lane Gifts. You can have a photo put on a mug, T-shirt, watch, button or magnet, porcelain china plate, plastic bank, keychain, and even a photo puzzle can be made. Photo sculptures are another interesting memento—they're freestanding, lifelike sculptures made from a print that's bonded to acrylic. Sizes range from 3" x 4" (ornament) up to 11" x 14". Ask your local Safeway store for current prices and other products available.

■ **SENTIMENTAL KEEPSAKE CO.**
575-0747

Sentimental Keepsake Co. is the regional outlet for the Senti-metal Company, the first national company for bronzing baby shoes. They will schedule an in-home appointment with you so they can see the shoes and explain the many different finishes and mountings available. Finishes include bronze, pewter, silver, gold, and a porcelain-like material. The cost for an heirloom quality job will run $100-$200 and all work is guaranteed.

SPECIAL PHOTOS

A number of photographers offer baby portrait clubs, special photos or black and white hand-tinted photography which make beautiful mementos. Here are a few:

- Nancy Clark
  324-5846
- Martine Fabrizio
  776-3178
- Joy Fischer
  822-1731

- Barry Hartman
  861-0600
- Debra Lacopolla
  634-3706
- Craig Larson
  885-5553

- Nancy Medwell
  285-1649
- Merrill Photography
  328-5234
- Michael Ziegler
  767-4547

Life Experiences...

MARY & PAUL

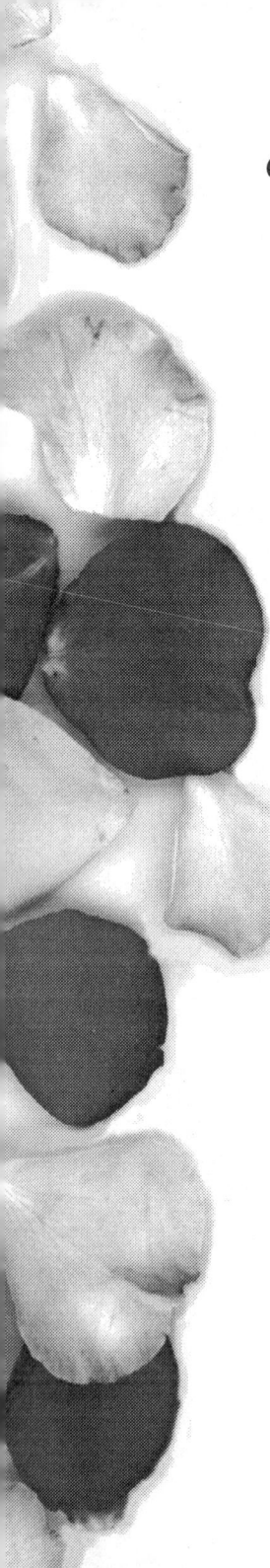

"YOU CAN WORK AND BREASTFEED"

By Mary E. Kessler

With a little planning and support, you don't need to give up breastfeeding when you go back to work. I was able to exclusively breastfeed my son, Paul, until he was almost a year old while working full time. Whether you rely on breast milk alone, or supplement with formula, I believe you and your child can reap the many benefits that breastfeeding provide.

One of the biggest benefits breastfeeding provides is to help you preserve the close relationship you enjoyed with your baby while on maternity leave. Noted pediatrician T. Berry Brazelton states, "I think breastfeeding is of extra importance to a working mother in maintaining the attachment between her and her baby."

My experience was that continuing to breastfeed reduced my guilt of leaving my child when returning to work. Even though I couldn't be with him all day, I knew he was getting optimal nutrition and protection against illness. Sitting down to nurse in the evening helped me to unwind and reconnect with my son. I was fortunate to find child care near my office, so was able to nurse at lunch time—a delightful break which also afforded an opportunity to tune into my child's daily activities. And, when I was unable to go to his child care center, I booked a locked conference room and pumped for 20 minutes which helped me maintain my milk supply.

I also got more rest! With no formula to mix or bottle to warm, I could nurse Paul during the night while I was half asleep and catch another 40 winks during his morning feeding, snuggled in bed.

One question people ask me often is how I was able to continue to breastfeed without worrying about juggling work and pumping. My answer is I didn't concern myself with caring about what people thought, nor did I tell very many

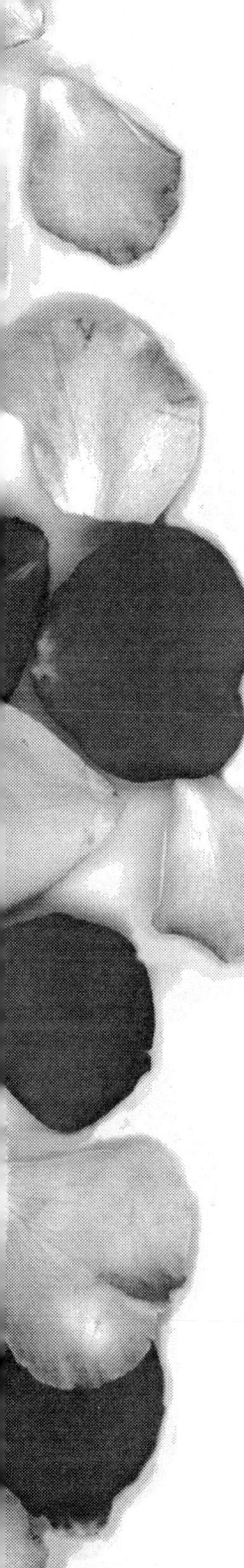

people what I was doing. As a regional vice president of a bank, I found myself in a traditional environment and yet I found a way to balance my personal needs with my work expectations.

I also found that a good support team was essential. At home, my husband, Michael, cooked and cleaned up many meals giving me time to nurse the baby. My child care provider was knowledgeable about breastfeeding and did not sabotage my efforts. I also arranged for a long enough maternity leave that allowed me to establish my milk supply and energy level. I also found that easing back into work with a flexible schedule allowed additional nursing time. And, finally, I found that I really needed to rest as much as possible to maintain my milk supply.

Most importantly, I found it was important for me to keep my priorities straight. Nursing a baby is one of life's greatest joys and it lasts for just a few short months—for me making the commitment to breastfeeding was worth every minute of the extra effort it took.

Mary's Tips for Fast, Easy and Effective Pumping:

To maintain your milk supply and provide milk for baby, pumping the breasts is important. Keep your pumping equipment at work. Here are a few hints I found were helpful:

■ Rent a top-quality electric pump. Some insurance companies will reimburse part of the cost. With a double hookup, you may be able to pump 6-8 ounces of milk during a typical coffee break.

■ Find a private space at work so you can relax (an office with a door that locks, a conference room, seldom-used restrooms).

■ Two piece suits work best for pumping and covering up an occasional "leak."

■ Assist your "let-down" reflex with your baby's picture or an item of clothing.

■ A Playmate cooler with reusable ice works well for private storage of milk and pump components that require daily cleaning, as well as a snack and drink for mom.

■ Sterilize the plastic parts of the pump in the dishwasher every night to save time.

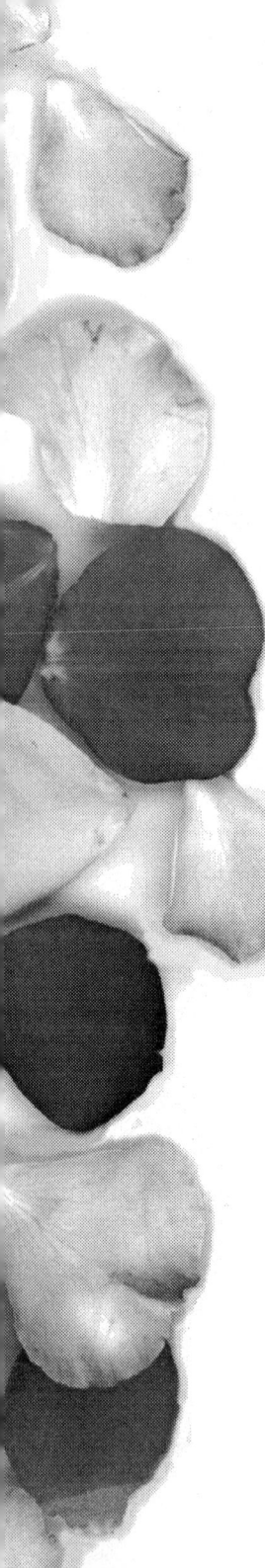

To help you stay organized, here is a list I found helpful each morning:

Work Checklist
- *Cooler*
- *Ice*
- *Pump kit (assembled to save time during pumping breaks)*
- *Empty bottles to store milk*
- *Snack and drink for mom*
- *Briefcase, purse, etc.*

Child Care Checklist
- *Breast milk pumped the previous day*
- *Baby food, juice for an older infant*
- *Baby's "lovey" and/or pacifier*
- *Mom's lunch (if nursing at lunchtime)*
- *Mom's "bib" for protecting work clothes from spit-up (made from an old towel)*
- *Weekly: diapers, wipes, clothes, etc.*

After Work Checklist
- *Refrigerate and label pumped milk*
- *Sterilize pump kit and used bottles in dishwasher*
- *Refreeze ice*
- *Pack cooler for tomorrow!*

BREASTFEEDING

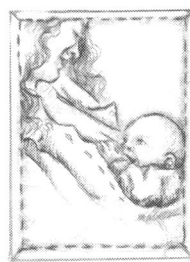

It seems one of the first questions people ask you once you become pregnant is: "Are you going to nurse your baby?" Your answer may depend on several factors that include:

- How much you know about breastfeeding
- Your and the father's feelings towards breastfeeding
- When and if you will go back to work
- Whether you have breastfed before

Regardless of where you are in the decision-making process, you will probably have many questions. Fortunately, there are more resources for you than ever before. In addition to a variety of nursing books available, there are many local resources including breastfeeding classes at many area hospitals (see childbirth education listings in chapter one); La Leche meetings, and private lactation consultants.

If you are thinking about breastfeeding, you probably have heard about the health benefits it provides your baby. There is no human-made substitute for breast milk. It is the best first food for your baby and provides the most balanced nutrition. Breast milk contains sugar (lactose), digestible proteins and fats plus minerals, vitamins, antibodies, and enzymes which help build up your child's immune system. Studies are continually showing other health benefits, such as breastfed babies have half the ear infections as bottle-fed babies.

Babies aren't the only ones who benefit from breastfeeding. Mothers benefit too! Breast milk is convenient—always available and at the perfect temperature. Nursing also represents an intimate relationship between mother and child. It is unique and individual. It can't be bottled and sold in the supermarket. It can't be duplicated and reconstituted and mixed with water. It is the one thing a mother can give to her child that is only hers. And, breast milk is free! It can save a family money when a mother chooses to nurse rather than purchase formula. Plus, moms who breastfeed may also find that their extra pregnancy weight comes off more quickly.

As the health and nutritional information surrounding breastfeeding is endless, so may the emotions you may be feeling. For some women, again, there is very little to consider. The intimacy and the maternal image that breastfeeding provides is enough to make their decision easy. For others, the thought of a baby on

❧

There is no human-made substitute for breast milk. It is the best first food for your baby and provides the most balanced nutrition.

❧

their breast does not stir the same "sweet images." Dealing with the sexuality and the modesty issues is something that can cause a woman to question her desire to nurse.

Once the baby is born, the answers to these questions will probably become clearer. The emotional issues tend to disappear and the maternal instinct may really kick in. Your physician and the local breastfeeding organizations will encourage you to at least start to breastfeed your baby...and that's good advice. By nursing for at least two to three weeks, you can see for yourself how you feel about it. The hospital staff or lactation specialists may provide excellent support to help make breastfeeding a special and positive experience.

After choosing to breastfeed, mothers become so happy with the experience that they often don't want to give it up! And, the good news is more working women are nursing than ever before and more employers are working with employees to make arrangements to include it in their daily routine.

DIFFICULTIES

If you have difficulties with breastfeeding or questions regarding your milk supply, contact your pediatrician and one of the many organizations listed in this chapter. Also, make sure your baby is urinating frequently and producing a stool after each feeding. If breastfeeding is very difficult or you have any questions at all, don't hesitate to pick up the phone and ask for help. You and your baby are the only ones who can determine your breastfeeding relationship.

BREAST PUMPS

Whether returning to work full time or planning for an occasional night out, most breastfeeding mothers need to express their milk at some time. Milk can be expressed manually or by using a breast pump. There are many kinds of pumps available, and choosing the right one for you may be confusing.

Manual pumps are widely available at drug and grocery stores for $15 to $30. These pumps are hand-operated and may work well for occasional use.

Battery operated and small electric pumps are available at many baby product stores and some drug stores. They are reasonably priced from about $35 to $100. These pumps create a continuous suction which is released in a rhythmic pattern by pressing a button or bar. If you use this type of pump, be careful not to let the pressure build for too long as this can cause sore nipples. The motors are small and they often do not stand up to long-term use. Some may not be sufficient for maintaining a good supply of milk with routine use.

If you choose to express on a regular basis, a quality electric pump is probably the way to go. This type of electric pump has an automatic suck-release action that closely matches the sucking of a nursing baby. Electric pumps may be rented or purchased from private lactation specialists, some hospitals, and retail outlets. Rentals range in price from about $35 to $65 per month, depending on the length of the rental period. You will need to purchase a pump accessory kit to use with these machines. There are single and double kits available; the double kit allows you to pump both breasts simultaneously which is a great time saver for busy women. These pumps also help you maintain a better milk supply. The cost of the kits range from $28 for a single kit to $39-$49 for a double. You can also call Medela at 800-TELL-YOU or Ameda/Egnell at 800-323-8750 (these are the two most well-known breast pump companies) for a breast pump rental station nearest you.

LACTATION CONSULTANTS

Lactation consultants are specially trained in breastfeeding education, management and support. Their goal is to help you breastfeed successfully, and to help you work through any problem. Most lactation consultants are International Board Certified Lactation Consultants (IBCLC), which means they have met the necessary qualifications set by the International Board of Lactation Consultant Examiners and meet continuing education requirements. Some area hospitals have lactation consultants on staff, and there are several private lactation consultants in the greater Seattle area. Fees for private lactation consultants vary yet usually start at $30 to $45 per hour depending on the services you need. Some lactation consultants also sell and rent electric pumps and related supplies.

REIMBURSEMENT

Some insurance companies may reimburse for lactation consultants or breastfeeding supplies or breast pump rentals; so be sure to check with your provider. You may also check with WIC for reduced or free breastfeeding pump rentals and supplies.

RECOMMENDED READING

Eiger, Marvin and Olds, Sally Wendkos. *The Complete Book Of Breastfeeding.* New York, NY: Workman Publishing Co., 1986.

Gotsch, *Breastfeeding Pure and Simple.* IL; La Leche League, 1994.

Grams, Marilyn, MD. *Breastfeeding Success For Working Mothers.* Sheridan, WY: Achievement Press, 1985.

Huggins, Kathleen. *The Nursing Mother's Companion.* Harvard's Common Press, rev. 1995.

La Leche League. *The Womanly Art Of Breastfeeding.* New York, NY: New American Library, 1991.

D. Mason and D. Ingersol, *Breastfeeding and the Working Mother.* St. Martin's Press, 1986.

Renfrew, Fisher, and Arms, *Bestfeeding: Getting Breastfeeding Right For You.* Berkeley, CA: Celestial Arts, 1995.

Sears, *William. The Baby Book.* Little Brown and Co., Boston, 1993.

& RESOURCES &

■ BIRTH AND BEYOND
324-4831
2610 E. Madison St.
Seattle, WA 98112
Birth and Beyond offers breastfeeding accessories, books and a supportive environment for the nursing mother.

■ BREASTFEEDING NATIONAL NETWORK (BNN)
800-TELL-YOU
P.O. Box 660
McHenry, Illinois 60051
They offer a 24-hour, 7-day-a-week service with information on where you can rent a Medela electric breast pump in your community and information on breastfeeding specialists.

■ CEAS BREASTFEEDING SERVICES
789-0883
10021 Holman Rd. N.W.
Seattle, WA 98177
The breastfeeding counselors at the Childbirth Education Association of Seattle are registered nurses and childbirth educators who have had special training as lactation specialists. They offer help for nursing mothers and their babies in the early days after birth and during the following months of breastfeeding. CEAS offers free telephone counseling on weekdays 9 a.m. to 3 p.m. and on weekends from 9 a.m. to noon (usually). To reach a counselor on the weekends, after hours, or on holidays you can use a telepager at 615-8078. If you need more than telephone counseling, a specialist can provide you an individual consultation for about $55. CEAS also offers two classes

on breastfeeding. The main office has the information.

■ DECENT EXPOSURE
800-524-4949
2202 N.E. 115th
Seattle, WA 98125
Decent Exposure offers a bra that is designed by two sisters who were unable to find comfortable fitting bras during their pregnancies. They offer an "Un-bra" which can fit women in every size from 28AAA to 58H. The bra that they offer can be lifted up or down for nursing. This Seattle company also offers nursing pads, underpants and other items. The Un-bra costs between $21 and $41 depending on the size and material you choose. Shipping is included.

■ FAMILY RESOURCES OF BOTHELL
485-3295
21029 W. Richmond Rd.
Bothell, WA 98021
Family Resources offers a complete line of breastfeeding supplies, including pumps to rent (Medela) and pumps to own (even a rent-to-own plan). Accessories include pillows, pads, baby slings, and more. There's a large assortment of nursing bras, gowns, and other clothing. Owner P.J. Jacobsen (former owner of two highly-popular local children's stores in the '80s—Babakies and Kinderkies) is a board certified lactation consultant and offers her services at a very economical rate.

■ **LA LECHE LEAGUE INTERNATIONAL**
522-1336
La Leche League is a nonprofit organization founded in 1957. It is the world's largest resource for breastfeeding and related information. The above local number will connect you with a recording which will supply you with a list of leaders in your area whom you may call with your nursing questions. The League strongly believes in nursing and they will do all they can to support you towards this goal. They also have monthly meetings with various topics. The leaders can provide you with this information. They will also mail you a free catalog featuring books and products related to breastfeeding.

■ **MILK DIAPERS**
800-929-0218
P.O. Box 961
Camas, WA 98607
Milk Diapers is a locally owned company that offers washable nursing pads. The nursing pads are available at local retail outlets or by mail order. The company also sells nursing sleepwear.

■ **MOTHERWEAR**
800-950-2500
P.O. Box 114BIC
Northampton, MA 01061
Motherwear publishes a free and complete catalog for the nursing mother. This includes nursing bras from size 32B to 46G, nursing shirts, dresses, and nighties. They also have breast pumps and pads, as well as 100% cotton diapers and diaper covers. The catalog also includes books and tapes.

■ **NORTHWEST MEDICAL SUPPLY**
368-1196
1530 N. 115th St. #112
Seattle, WA 98103
Hours: M-F   9:00 a.m.-6:30 p.m.
          Sat.   9:00 a.m.-1:00 p.m.
Northwest Medical Supply, located on the Northwest Hospital campus, is a Medela breast pump rental station. The certified lactation educators on staff provide support for breastfeeding mothers as well as home-to-work transition training. Northwest Medical Supply has satellite stations in both King and Snohomish counties which offer a full line of breastfeeding supplies. They offer on-call pump delivery and a 24-hour breastfeeding answer line.

■ **PEDIATRIC HOME HEALTH CARE**
747-7161
13400 Northup Way #42
Bellevue, WA 98005
An affiliate of Children's Hospital and Medical Center, PHC provides in-home breastfeeding support as well as temporary child care and newborn care.

■ **PEDIATRIC SERVICES OF AMERICA**
King and Snohomish County:
467-5559
South King and Pierce County:
922-9086
In-home breastfeeding assistance and intervention is offered, and electric breast pumps are also available.

■ **THE TAKE CARE STORE—** `Baby Pages`
   GROUP HEALTH
Central
326-3496
306 15th Ave. E.
Seattle, WA 98112
Hours: M-F   9:30 a.m.-5:30 p.m.
        Sat.   10:00 a.m.-3:00 p.m.

Northgate
527-7878
9800 4th Ave. N.E.
Seattle, WA 98115
Hours: M-F   9:30 a.m.-1:30 p.m.,
                    2:30 p.m.-5:30 p.m.
        Sat.   9:00 a.m.-2:00 p.m.

Redmond
883-5052
2700 152nd Ave. N.E.
Redmond, WA 98052
Hours: M-Th   9:30 a.m.-6:00 p.m.
        F   9:30 a.m.-5:30 p.m.
        Sat.   10:00 a.m.-3:00 p.m.
The Take Care Stores offer breastfeeding rooms in both the Central and Redmond locations so you can have a free trial of a breast pump and find the one that works best. Medela portable breast pumps are available for purchase and there's also a hospital style breast pump that can be rented by the day or month. Both pumps have the single or double pumping option depending on the parts that you purchase or receive from your hospital. The stores offer a full supply of accessories like pads and pillows, and are well-known for their excellent selection of educational books on a wide variety of health topics. Although located at Group Health, you don't have to be a co-op member to shop at the stores, and all three are open on Saturdays to make shopping even more convenient.

■ **WOMEN, INFANTS, AND**
   CHILDREN (WIC)
800-841-1410
Serving Seattle-King County
This 800 number will give you the nearest WIC office in your area. WIC is for pregnant or lactating women and their children under five years of age who are assessed to be at nutritional risk. The group offers prenatal nutrition counseling and vouchers for specific nutritious foods.

Also, check the stores chapter for information on where to find nursing clothing.

FEEDING BABY

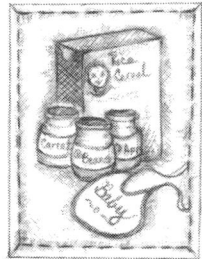

FORMULA

Scientifically, baby formulas are meant to imitate mother's milk as much as possible. For women who cannot breastfeed, or for those who choose not to nurse, formula is a safe and appropriate choice. It is recommended that cow's milk not be used until a child is one year of age because of the high amount of sodium and protein it contains, possible milk allergies, and its lack of other vital nutrients for infants.

There are several brands and types of formula on the market. Discuss with your baby's pediatrician the different choices available and ask for a recommendation.

If you have decided to bottle-feed your infant, you should know which formulas are the most balanced nutritionally. There is no formula that is identical in composition to breast milk; however, some are closer than others.

CHOICES

Commercial formulas are manufactured and ready for purchase in three different forms. They are listed here with the most expensive first, and the least expensive last.

❶ Ready to use single-serving bottles with sterilized nipples.
❷ Ready to pour from a can into your own clean or sterilized bottle.
❸ Ready to mix from a powder or concentrate that may be diluted with water and then poured into your own clean or sterilized bottle.

BABY FOOD

When should a parent introduce solids to their baby? The "typical" introduction period is when your baby is four to six months old. However, discuss with your pediatrician any questions you may have regarding solids and what is best for your child.

When you're ready to introduce baby food, there are two avenues you may choose to pursue. One is to purchase commercial baby food from the grocery store and the other is to make the food yourself. The choice is an individual one.

❧

For women who cannot breastfeed, or for those who choose not to nurse, formula is a safe and appropriate choice.

❧

BOTTLE FEEDING SAFETY

- Always check the expiration date on the formula.
- Follow the manufacturer's directions when preparing formula.
- Do not use leftover formula; leftover portions from a previous feeding may cause infection.
- Do not heat formula in a microwave oven—the formula may heat unevenly and burn the baby's mouth or throat.
- Do not use formula that has been frozen or shows white specks or streaks.
- Keep the bottles and nipples clean, and wash your hands before preparing formula.
- Follow manufacturer's guidelines for the refrigerator life for formula.
- Refrigerate unused portion or prepared amount of formula until feeding.

COMMERCIAL BABY FOOD

There are many advantages to purchasing commercial baby food, especially during your child's infancy. The texture is the perfect consistency for babies during this first early stage. You can also purchase single-ingredient foods, which make it easy to detect any food allergies your baby may have. The convenience of commercial baby food is undeniable. It saves you time and energy, while not necessarily compromising quality. Be sure to read labels so that you can avoid ingredients such as added sugars, salt, modified food starch, MSG, preservatives and artificial colors and flavors. It is possible to buy commercial baby food that consists of only the food and water.

Most full-service grocery stores carry major brand-name baby foods that offer a wide variety of single foods and food combinations. The most common brand names are Gerber and Beechnut. Most grocery stores also carry organic baby foods, such as Earth's Best and Beechnut Special Harvest.

HOMEMADE BABY FOOD

Taste some store-bought baby food and ask yourself, "Is this what I want for my child?" If taking food from a jar is not exactly your idea of a delicious, nutritious, satisfying meal, then read on...

For less then $15, you can purchase a baby-food grinder from most stores that carry baby products, including some grocery stores and pharmacies. Other than this, you need not invest more than a little time in order to offer your baby homemade baby food. Simply grind up the fresh vegetables, fruits, grains, and meats you already have at home. For less than half an hour per week, you can have homemade baby food.

If organic is what you want, you may want to shop at either the health food store or the natural food coop. Some grocery stores also sell organic foods. The easiest way to prepare baby food is to make it in quantity, then freeze it in double ziploc bags.

HOMEMADE BABY FOOD SUGGESTIONS

VEGETABLES:
(CARROTS, SQUASH, BROCCOLI, POTATOES, PEAS, CORN, ETC.)

❶ Steam or microwave your vegetable until soft.

❷ Let cool.

❸ Cut into slices that will fit into the grinder.

❹ Grind the vegetable.

❺ Spoon into plastic bags.

❻ Seal tightly and place in freezer.

❼ Remove from the freezer one hour before serving.

FRUITS:
(BANANA, APPLE, PEAR, PEACH, PLUM, ETC.)

Why give your child a banana in a jar when you can give her a fresh one? Banana has got to be the easiest food to prepare and one that most babies love. Take a fork and mash a ripe banana or, if this is still too chunky, put it through the grinder. Most fruits can be prepared quickly this way. Ripe pears were always a favorite of my girls. After you grind the fruit, if there is juice left over, mix it with a little water and your child has fresh juice to drink; or you can mix the juice with dry cereal instead of using water or breast milk/formula.

When on the go, instead of grabbing a few jars of baby food, go to your freezer and grab some bags of homemade food. Remember, it is best to stick with one new food a week in case of allergies and for the purpose of identifying which food may be causing the problem. But, once foods are well introduced, you can start mixing.

FOODS TO AVOID

Certain foods are best avoided until your baby is one year old because they are either highly allergenic, contain too much fat, or are difficult for a baby to digest. Avoid:

- wheat - until 6 months
- citrus fruits and juices - until 1 year
- egg whites - until 1 year
- honey - until 1 year
- raw vegetables - until 1 year
- peanut butter - until 1 year
- pudding and fruit desserts - avoid at all ages since they contain excess sugars and empty calories.

ORGANIC BABY FOOD

Many parents prefer to feed their baby certified organic baby food in order to avoid food treated with synthetic pesticides and fertilizers. Federal standards for production, processing and certification of organic foods, and independent certification that you will see noted on organic baby foods, such as Earth's Best, let consumers know the food is truly synthetic pesticide- and fertilizer-free. You can also make your own baby food with organic produce found at health food stores and farmer's markets.

ORGANIC FOOD

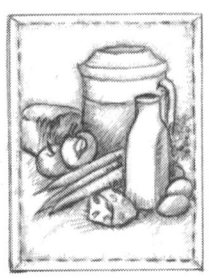

Buying organic food is more convenient than ever for Seattle families. Besides the many local suppliers of certified organic foods listed here, many of the major supermarkets also carry organic sections.

■ ALFALFA'S MARKET
525-3941
5440 Sand Point Way N.E.
Seattle, WA 98105
Hours: M-Sat. 7:30 a.m.-9:30 p.m.
Hours: Sun.   7:30 a.m.-9:00 p.m.
This is a full-service grocery store which has an in-store deli, a large organic produce section, and baked goods from a number of community suppliers. They have bulk grains and spices, organic juices and milk, goat's milk, and they carry Earth's Best baby food.

■ ALL OF WASHINGTON'S BEST
800-840-SAFE or 869-2984
Redmond, WA 98052
Hours: M-F   8:00 a.m.-7:00 p.m.
           Sat.   9:00 a.m.-2:00 p.m.
This local organic foods business is unique because all foods are shipped fresh to your door. They specialize in organic produce, as well as organically-grown seafood, meats and eggs. They emphasize no hormones, antibiotics, appetite stimulants or synthetic additives in feed. Known as the "Safe Food Grocers By Mail," all products are shipped with a 100% satisfaction guarantee. Call for a complete price list.

■ CENTRAL CO-OP
329-1545
1835 12th Ave.
Seattle, WA 98122
Hours: M-Sun. 9:00 a.m.-9:00 p.m.
Central Co-op carries Earth's Best baby food, Healthy Times teething biscuits and cookies, grains, organic juices, and lots of organic produce. They accept membership from any co-op; if you're not a

member you pay a 15% surcharge for purchases over $5. To become a member you pay an initial fee of $5 then $2 each month you shop until you've paid $60.

■ **MANNA MILLS**
775-3479
21705 66th W.
Mountlake Terrace, WA 98043
Hours: M-F   9:30 a.m.-8:00 p.m.
       Sat.   10:00 a.m.-6:00 p.m.
This store is a little hard to find. Take the 220th St. S.W. exit from I-5 and proceed west. Turn right at 66th W. and you'll see the store on your right a few blocks down. Inside you'll find organic juices, cookies, crackers, and a big selection of whole grains in bulk containers. Prices are very good on bulk items and, since they are a mill, flours are fresh as they are ground right on the premises.

■ **PUGET CONSUMERS CO-OP**
828-4621   *Baby Pages*
10718 N.E. 68th
Kirkland, WA 98034
Hours: Daily   8:00 a.m.-10:00 p.m.

525-1450
6504 20th Ave. N.E.
Seattle, WA 98115
Hours: Daily   9:00 a.m.-9:00 p.m.

789-7144
6522 Fremont Ave. N.
Seattle, WA 98103
Hours: M-Sat.   9:00 a.m.-9:00 p.m.
       Sun.   10:00 a.m.-7:00 p.m.

723-2720
5041 Wilson Ave. S.
Seattle, WA 98118
Hours: Daily   8:00 a.m.-10:00 p.m.

526-7661
6514 40th Ave. N.E.
Seattle, WA 98115
Hours: Daily   8:00 a.m.-10:00 p.m.

937-8481
2749 California Ave. S.W.
Seattle, WA 98116
Hours: Daily   8:00 a.m.-10:00 p.m.

632-6811
716 N. 34th
Seattle, WA 98103
Hours: Daily   8:00 a.m.-11:00 p.m.
PCC is the largest natural foods co-op in the country, owned by over 40,000 members. Many of their full-service grocery stores have an in-store deli and they feature baked goods from a number of different suppliers throughout the community. They have a large organic produce section, bulk grains and spices, organic juices, organic milk, butter and cheeses, goat's milk, and also carry Earth's Best baby food. The co-op has a large selection of free literature, and sells popular books on healthy eating and living. They also offer a variety of cooking and nutrition classes that address parents' and children's eating needs. To join you'll pay $8, then make regular payments towards a $60 lifetime membership that is fully refundable if you resign your membership.

■ **RAINBOW GROCERY**
329-8440
417 15th E.
Seattle, WA 98112
Hours: Daily   9:00 a.m.-9:00 p.m.
At Rainbow Grocery you'll find Earth's Best baby food, organic juice and produce, goat's milk, crackers and rice cakes.

INFANT CPR & FIRST AID

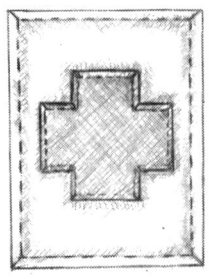

When we initially questioned parents on topics of interest for this resource guide, one of the top answers was infant CPR and first aid. Infant CPR and first aid teaches you how to respond if your baby begins to choke or stops breathing. The training also includes other injury prevention techniques. Every parent should learn CPR and first aid. It could save your baby's life.

Listed below are the local agencies that provide infant CPR and first aid classes. Prices are reasonable and schedules are varied to help accommodate even the busiest person's schedule. Many of the private companies will come to your home or workplace for a reasonable fee. Also, see the baby safety section of this book for further reading.

■ AMERICAN RED CROSS

323-2345
1900 25th Ave. S.
Seattle, WA 98144
Hours: M-F   9:00 a.m.-4:30 p.m.

252-4103
2530 Lombard Ave.
Everett, WA 98201
Hours: M-F   8:30 a.m.-4:30 p.m.
The American Red Cross has been teaching courses for more than 80 years. Their courses are standardized nationwide and are kept up-to-date with the latest information available. They offer a 9-hour class on Community First Aid and Safety, which teaches first aid and adult and infant/child CPR. The class costs $61. They also teach a 5-hour infant/child CPR class which covers CPR for infants and children and care for breathing emergencies. This class costs $26. Classes are held days, evenings, and Saturdays at many sites throughout the community.

■ **FIRST STEP FIRST AID/CPR**
328-1377
P.O. Box 22997
Seattle, WA 98122
Taught by a professional firefighter, the First Step program is certified by the Department of Labor and Industries and provides a full 8-hour infant/child/adult CPR and first aid course for $35. A 3-hour CPR class is offered for $15. Recertification classes are also available. Slides and videos are used to supplement the basic curriculum and the focus is on providing a flexible and low-stress environment for learning. Classes are held on a regular basis throughout the community and groups can also arrange to have a First Step course provided at their site. Discount rates are available for groups.

■ **HEART START**
235-7106
Heart Start offers first aid and CPR classes scheduled regularly at a location in Bellevue. Groups may also request a course at their own site. The cost for individuals is $39 for a full 8-hour infant/child/adult First Aid and CPR session or $15 for CPR only. Group rates are slightly less, averaging $25 (full course) and $11 (CPR only) per person. Discounts are available for new clients.

■ **HOLISTIC CHILDBIRTH EDUCATION & YOGA CENTER**
547-9882
4649 Sunnyside Ave. N., Rm. 300
Seattle, WA 98103
The center offers separate infant CPR (for ages birth to 1 year) and child CPR (ages 1 to 8) workshops. You can bring your infant to the infant CPR class. The cost is $25 per person or $35 per couple for a 2-1/2 hour session.

■ **LIFE TECH**
485-2529
This company provides a 6-hour CPR/first aid course for $30 per person and a group CPR class for $125 (up to 20 people per group). They also do private classes for $75/class. Sessions are held at sites in Kirkland, Bothell, and others.

■ **MEDIC FIRST AID**
747-5252
A national program, Medic First Aid is taught by EMTs both on-site and at group locations. The rate for a group of 10-12 is $350, and includes a full 8-hour first aid and CPR session.

■ **MEDIC II**
Seattle Fire Department
684-7274
This division of the Seattle Fire Department provides information on CPR and choking prevention, fire safety in the home and work place, and talks for preschoolers. Free CPR classes are offered at community locations, including fire stations.

■ **WASHINGTON CPR PROVIDERS**
800-933-5950
Infant/child/adult CPR and first aid classes are offered on-site in north Seattle and Kent or at specific group sites. Minimum group size is 10 and the classes cost $15 for a 4-hour CPR session or $30 for an 8-hour first aid/CPR session. Trainers are professionals who conduct these courses on a full-time basis.

OTHER SOURCES

Many hospitals, family support centers, YMCAs, and other community groups offer CPR and first aid classes too.

CHILD SAFETY

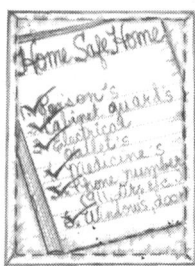

Accidents continue to be the leading cause of death among American children. However, most accidents can be prevented. As a parent, be aware of the kinds of situations that make accidents likely to happen. Get down on the floor and see the world from your child's point of view. This will open your eyes to the potential disasters waiting to happen.

- Teach safety at an early age.
- Check every room of the house and eliminate hazards.
- Be aware of the increasing abilities of your child.
- Never leave a child in a home alone.
- Be prepared in the event an accident does occur.
- Learn infant CPR and first aid!

Children get into everything. From the moment they begin to scoot across the floor, everything within reach is fair game. Take your time reviewing your environment and begin child-proofing before you bring your baby home from the hospital.

⧫

Children get into everything. From the moment they begin to scoot across the floor, everything within reach is fair game.

⧫

Stairs: Keep a gate at both the top and bottom; if the posts are more than four inches apart you should consider plexiglass or netting.

Electrical outlets: Keep them all covered...even the ones that are up high; children are great climbers.

Cupboards: Put safety latches on all cupboards that contain unsafe items. Especially beware in the kitchen and the bathroom.

Cleaning supplies: They should all be kept in a locked cupboard, preferably one that is up high.

Poisons: Always keep a bottle of syrup of ipecac on hand. It is available without a prescription and should be used to induce vomiting upon the advice of the Poison Center (526-2121).

Medications: Keep them in a locked tool box or fishing tackle box, then place the box out of reach of the child.

Water: 200 children have died by drowning in 5-gallon buckets of water since 1984. Never leave an infant or young child alone in the bathtub. Babies can drown in less than 2 inches of water! Keep infants away from buckets of water and use toilet latches to avoid accidents.

Pools: Pools should be fenced all the way around, and the doors leading out to the pool should be locked. Never leave a baby or young child out by a pool unattended...not even to answer the phone.

Toys: Any toy can be unsafe if it is misused or given at an inappropriate age level. Keep your older children's toys away from infants.

Auto Safety: An adult's arms are not safe! Use an approved infant carrier or child's seat from birth to 4 years or 40 pounds. (Also use your seat belt.) Auto deaths account for the largest group of fatal injuries among American children. The possibility of death or injury is reduced 80% when a child is in a safety seat.

Hanging Cords: Keep all cords from phones, answering machines, lamps and appliances out of reach of the children. Also keep cords from draperies tied up and out of reach.

Changing Table: Never leave a baby unattended on a changing table. The day that you turn your back will be when your baby turns over for the first time.

Cribs, Strollers and Walkers: Check the current safety standards. Make sure the equipment is sturdy and properly assembled. The American Academy of Pediatrics recommends forgoing the use of walkers because of the number of accidents they cause. Never use the carrier as a car seat. Do not place a crib near draperies or blinds where a child could become entangled and strangle on the cords.

Strings: To prevent strangulation, never put a pacifier or other items on a string around a baby's neck.

Choking: Avoid hard candy, hot dogs, grapes, nuts, popcorn, chips, and other small food items that your child could choke on. Learn CPR and know what steps you should take if your child chokes.

POTENTIALLY DANGEROUS HOUSEHOLD SUBSTANCES

- alcohol
- ammonia
- bleaches
- detergent
- floor wax
- furniture wax
- toilet cleaner
- lighter fluid
- medicines
- lye
- oven cleaners
- paint thinners
- pesticides
- gasoline
- turpentine
- weed killer

Contact the Poison Center for answers to your questions regarding these and other dangerous substances at 526-2121 or 800-732-6985.

❧ RESOURCES ❧

■ AUTO SAFETY HOTLINE
800-424-9393
This federal government hotline is staffed by members who can tell you whether your safety seat has been recalled. Part of the National Highway Traffic Safety Administration, they can provide registration forms if you never registered with the manufacturer to be alerted of any future recalls. When you call, have the manufacturer name, model number and the date the seat was made.

■ CHILDREN'S HOSPITAL RESOURCE CENTER
526-2201
4800 Sand Point Way N.E.
Seattle, WA 98105
Children's Resource Center offers a number of safety-related classes, workshops, and special events throughout the year. These include a program on injury prevention and a Car Seat Checkup Clinic (co-sponsored by the Safety Restraint Coalition). With the Childbirth Education Association of Seattle (CEAS), Children's offers two safety classes: Babysafe (infants) and Toddlersafe (1-5 years old). Call CEAS at 789-0883 for information. The classes are held at Children's in Seattle and in Bellevue. They cost $20 per family for a 3-hour session. Children's also co-sponsors a 3-hour infant and child CPR class ($20 per person, call CEAS to register).

Also call or visit Children's Resource Center for information on baby walker dangers, bike safety, and safe toys.

■ CHILDREN'S DROWNING PREVENTION HOTLINE
368-4990
Call the hotline and you can receive fun and fact-filled information about water safety, discount coupons for a child's life vest, and a list of life vest loan sites throughout King County. You can borrow a life vest free at 14 lifeguarded beaches during the summer. Children's also provides a booth at special Kid's Day events during the summer at Seattle Center. Kids can try on life vests and receive free water safety information and activity sheets.

■ CONSUMER PRODUCT SAFETY COMMISSION (CPSC)
800-638-2772
Office of Information and Public Affairs
Washington, DC 20207
This government commission reviews the safety of products in the market. They offer two free brochures called "Tips for Your Baby's Safety" and "The Safe Nursery." The only "mainstream" product CPSC does not regulate is car seats. If you question the safety of a children's product, please call the hotline number above.

■ MIDAS MUFFLER SHOPS
Throughout Western Washington
Midas has a special program called Project Safe Baby where they will sell you a car seat for $42 which can be used for children from 6-40 pounds. You'll receive a coupon with your purchase and if you return both the coupon and car seat after your baby has outgrown the car seat, you can get a voucher for $42 in car repairs at Midas.

■ **JUVENILE PRODUCTS MANUFACTURERS ASSOCIATION (JPMA)**
Two Greentree Centre, Box 955
Marlton, NJ 08053
The Juvenile Products Manufacturers Association (JPMA) affixes a logo on all products that it has tested in an independent laboratory to validate the product's safety. For information regarding the JPMA, safety standards and a list of the JPMA's Directory of Certified Products send a self-addressed business-size envelope to the address above.

■ **NATIONAL SAFETY COUNCIL**
National Safe Kids Campaign (NSKC)
(301) 650-8296
111 Michigan Ave. N.W.
Washington, D.C. 20010-2970
This group runs surveys to keep on top of safety issues. Parents can order a free safety checklist with tips on how to avoid injuries by sending a self-addressed stamped envelope. They also sponsor National Safe Kids Week in May. Local events include safety-seat inspections, drowning prevention seminars and smoke detector installations. Call the hotline to see what is happening in your area.

■ **SAFETY FOR TODDLERS**
885-3460 or 800-775-3460
12865 N.E. 85th St., Ste. 296
Kirkland, WA 98033
Hours: M-F   8:30 a.m.-6:00 p.m.
Safety for Toddlers offers a room-by-room consulting and installation of safety devices to help create a safe environment for your infant and toddler. Owned by two mothers, they also do safety presentations for parent groups, birthing classes, and conferences. Homes are customized with safety devices from a number of different manufacturers. Safety for Toddlers is well known for their outstanding service and willingness to customize safety products to any environment.

■ **SAFETY RESTRAINT COALITION**
828-8975 or 800-BUCK-L-UP
917 Kirkland Ave.
Kirkland, WA 98033
Hours: M-F   8:00 a.m.-5:00 p.m.
The Coalition is a nonprofit information and referral organization that answers questions about child car seats and state child restraint laws, and they recommend the best options for child passengers. They offer free training to health care professionals, parents, day care providers, and anyone interested in providing protection to kids in cars. They also distribute free materials about car seats and seat belts and maintain a current list of all child car seat recalls. You can call them for information on where to get short-term car seat rentals and loaners, too.

If you see an unbuckled child riding in a motor vehicle in Washington state, you're encouraged to call the toll-free number above and report the date, vehicle description, and license plate number, so the vehicle owner can be sent a reminder letter and educational information from the Washington State Patrol.

■ **SMART CHOICE**
800-444-6278
For the ultimate in security, parents can purchase a "Baby Cam" which is a portable video security system. For a purchase price of about $349, parents receive a small video camera that can be mounted over a crib or other furniture and a black and white monitor. The system works from about 150 feet between the two products. It even offers the sophistication of video taping in the dark. According to the manufacturer, the picture is clear and crisp. You can also hook the Baby Cam up to a VCR to tape your child's daily activities. This product is available at discount and specialty stores.

■ **TOT STOPPERS**
800-585-1988
Though based in Bellingham, Tot Stoppers serves the greater Seattle area, providing free in-home consultation on child safety. They offer a free catalog with over 400 products and can help parents identify safety risks in their homes and advise on the best safety products to use. They also can install the products for you and ensure that they are working properly.

■ **WASHINGTON TRAFFIC SAFETY COMMISSION**
(360) 753-6197
1000 S. Cherry St.
P.O. Box 40944
Olympia, WA 98504
The Commission provides information on child car seats, child passenger safety, and state seat belt laws.

■ **WINDOW COVERING SAFETY COUNCIL**
800-506-4636
Long window-blind cords can be a strangulation hazard in the home. To prevent this, furniture—especially cribs—should be moved away from windows, cords shortened or cut, and drapery cords anchored to the floor. This safety council is making available, at no charge, retrofit tassels to make existing cords safe. They can be obtained at participating retailers and more information can be obtained through the 800 number.

"SURVIVAL STRATEGIES"

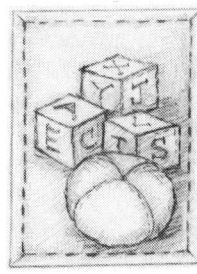

By Allison Blackham

❧

Sibling

arguments,

broken

windows

and lost

lunchboxes

are really

unimportant

things in the

whole scope

of what life is

about.

❧

I sat on my deck, nose pressed against the glass of the locked sliding door, watching my two-year-old, Laura, cavort around the room in her soggy diaper while eight-month-old Kirsten rocked happily back and forth on her bottom, gnawing away at my key ring. Unable to get in, unable to explain to my largely nonverbal toddler how to unlock the door she had so cleverly locked behind me, I sat fuming.

Alternating between a Mister Rogers-like gentle patience and insane shouting, I lured Laura back to the door again and again, coaxing her to open it. I could see both children and knew they were safe. Everything was okay, until the baby lost interest in my keys and crawled away into the unseen reaches of the hall. At that point I broke the bathroom window, struggled through, and rescued my wandering infant.

Later, as I painfully picked broken glass shards from the window frame, baby Kirsten watched, bouncing furiously in her jumper in the bathroom doorway, demanding to be held. Laura, free of mother's watchful eye, stripped all of the sheets from her sisters' beds and got stuck head first in a pillowcase. Quick to reach the scene of this latest household disaster, I watched the wildly screaming bundle of bedding on the floor for a moment. "This is funny," I thought. "This would make a great script for some dumb sitcom. Why am I not laughing?"

Catastrophe and crisis are a regular part of family life. There may be some robotic "wonder parents" out there with lukewarm children who never push the limits, but I have never met them. Every family I know has broken window days, trips to the emergency room, tantrums and general craziness from time to time. I, personally, am the mother of six children. I my early mom-work, I assumed that each crisis was a reflection of my own total inadequacy as a parent. After years of experience and a lot of commiseration with other frazzled moms and dads, I now know we all go through this stuff. Kids and chaos go together like bread and butter. From the non-sleeping newborn stage when we're all walking around like characters from "Night of the Living Dead" to the eerie episodes of hearing our mother's voice come out of our own mouths when we face off with a defiant teenager, these exciting times take their toll. I haven't uncovered any ways of avoiding the problems yet, because my husband insists that I live in the same house with the rest of the family, so I've had to deal with them. Here are some ideas that have helped at our house.

Save hysteria for life-and-death situations. Sibling arguments, broken windows and lost lunchboxes are really unimportant things in the whole scope of what life is about. When small things start to bug me, I stop and pull out my mental picture of myself at age 85 (still very peppy and active, by the way). At 85 will I care that my son lost four pairs of shoes in one year? Will it matter that my youngest child ate a worm? (I only found half.) Will my children blame me because we had cold cereal for dinner on Cub Scout night six years running? I hope not. I hope that what is important is that we said "I love you" and made cookies together and played pretend games. What doesn't matter in the long run is not worth getting tense about now.

Avoid out-of-body experiences. We tend to wish ourselves into another time or place when our current moment in life feels nasty. We think, "When the baby sleeps through the night/when the toddler is toilet trained/when my teenager gets through this awful phase, *then* everything will be better." Hey, by the time the kids are all perfect and out of our hair, we'll be dealing with Medicare and nursing home placement. There will always be challenges. No one is excused from the ups and downs of life. Even the Queen of England has to wear silly hats and put up with a lot of deranged relatives. Some day those shiny-eyed kids with their big mouths and sticky fingers will be grown

and gone. We need to live with the awareness that what we have and take for granted now changes and becomes a poignant memory tomorrow.

Seek joy. Life is jammed full of beauty and magic. A warm shower, sun shining on the grass, the smell of chocolate, a baby's smile—all of these things are miracles. Why wait for a trip to Disneyland or a letter of commendation from the President to feel like life is great? One of the best feelings I've ever had is seeing my daughter's face light up when I offer to read her a story, and that happens every day.

Treat yourself. Raising kids takes much more energy than any eight-hour-a-day job. Don't you work hard? Don't you deserve a reward? When was the last time your child kissed your hand and said, "Thank you, dear Mother, for all of your effort on my behalf?" It's not going to happen. Well, maybe at your funeral. We need to take time to reward ourselves. Go for a leisurely walk, eat an unshared candy bar, have lunch with friends, go to the pool and soak up the sunshine. Give to yourself so that you will have something to give away.

Sometimes on a really crazy day, I ask myself why I had children. And, after I answer that question, I ask myself why I had six children. Mostly, it's because I love kids, especially mine. And though I spend most of my days fishing the baby out of the cat food dish, fishing the cat food out of the baby, and pulling small people out of heating ducts and sofa cushions, I know I am actually making an investment, because love lasts, and broken windows can always be replaced.

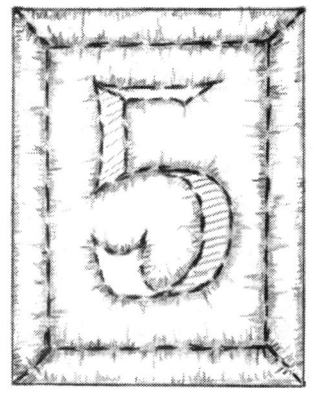

SPECIAL CONCERN RESOURCES

Life Experiences ...

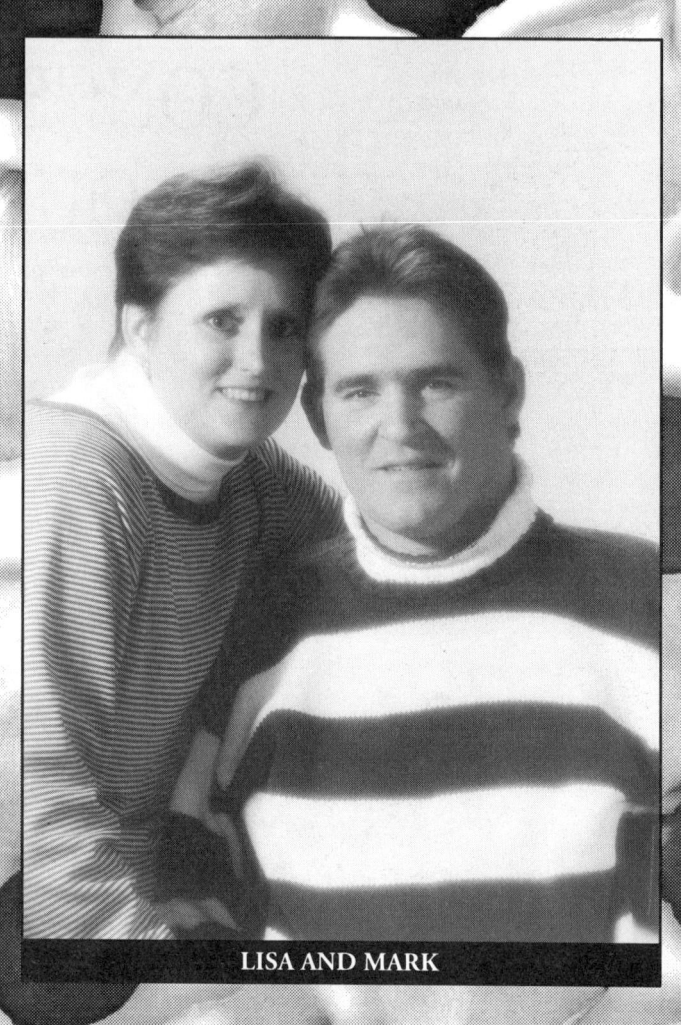

LISA AND MARK

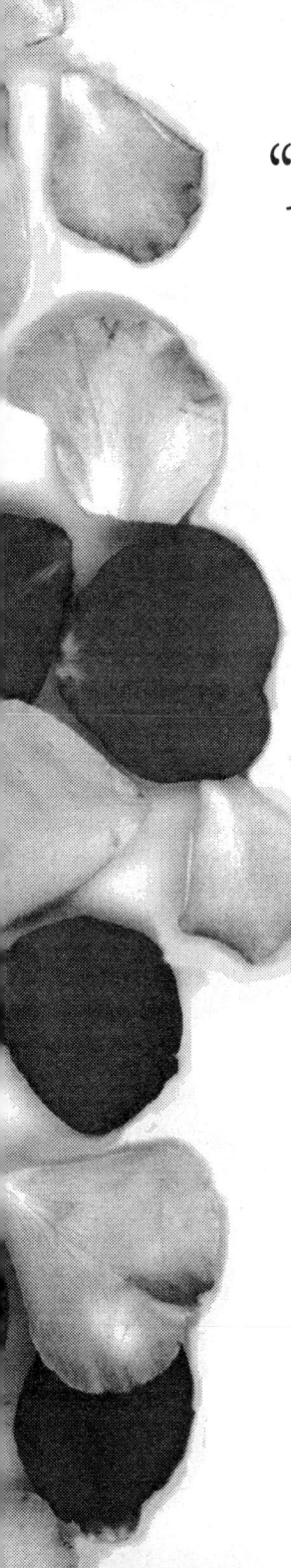

"ABILITY/ DISABILITY?"

by Lisa Farrell-Roberts

Our son, Austin, has brought us unspeakable joy. Mark describes the experience of parenthood as bittersweet: that it is the best thing that has happened in his life and it is the thing that makes him struggle with the disability the most. It is painful for him to see Austin fall and not be able to pick him up. When Austin recently moved into a "big bed," Mark told him how badly he wished he could toss him into bed and snuggle up with him. When Austin wakes up crying, Mark painfully wishes he could go pick him up.

When I watch the two of them, I see a father and son who love each other very much. When Austin was an infant, Mark would tickle him with his mouth wand (a stick held in his mouth to dial the phone, push remotes, and tickle babies!) while Austin sat on the kitchen counter in a bouncy chair. After Austin could sit, we would seatbelt him in with his Dad or put him in a backpack on the back of Mark's wheelchair. Now, Mark chases Austin on his riding toy and I hear Austin madly laughing as they go from room to room. In the mornings just about the time Austin and I are ready to go to child care and work, an attendant opens the bedroom door down the hall and we hear the click of Mark's wheelchair. And every morning Austin smiles and yells, "Daddy!"

The struggle of a disability cannot be understated. It is not an easy situation economically, physically, or emotionally. However, for us the rewards of parenthood far outweigh those struggles. I look at my husband with our son and I am proud of the relationship they have and I can see that Mark is a great father. I look at Austin and I wonder if he sees a disability at all. ❧

CHILDREN WITH SPECIAL NEEDS

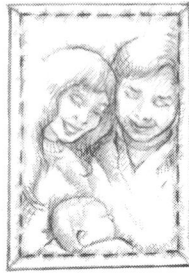

By Janet M. Hier

  Soft lights, romantic music, maybe a nice bottle of wine...and voila! Forty weeks later a squalling little child is presented to the world. Obviously, not every moonlit tryst creates another human being. All sorts of microscopic errors can occur between the candlelight and the cradle. Some fertilized eggs fail to implant in the uterus, while others have defects that cause them to be shed in the menstrual flow even before the woman may know she is pregnant. In fact, some statistics have shown that the awe-inspiring process that leads from conception to birth is so fraught with peril that as few as 25 percent of all successful conceptions actually end with the birth of an infant.

  Although these numbers may make it seem as though the chances for ever having a baby are pretty overwhelming, a glance at the birth rate proves that this simply isn't so. The vast majority of infants are born after having "beaten the odds" and come into this world in a healthy state. Unfortunately though, not all are. The number of newborns with some sort of congenital abnormality readily detected at birth has been estimated at three percent of the population, with another three percent being diagnosed within the first year of life.

  According to statistics from the American Medical Association Encyclopedia of Medicine, the twelve most common birth defects, in descending order, are:

- **Heart Defects:** Ranges from minor heart murmurs to severe heart valve errors requiring immediate surgical repair.

- **Mental Retardation:** This category includes cerebral palsy, a disorder that can be caused by developmental defects in the brain or trauma at birth. It also includes the effects of Fetal Alcohol Syndrome (FAS), which has been recognized as the most common cause of mental retardation in the United States. At first it was felt FAS only affected the babies of severely alcoholic mothers, but recent research has shown relatively small amounts of alcohol can cause birth defects.

❧

Statistics seem pretty irrelevant when the child in question happens to be yours, however.

❧

- ***Pyloric Stenosis:*** A narrowing of the muscle at the bottom of the stomach that causes vomiting and problems with eating. Surgical correction is necessary.
- ***Anencephaly:*** The brain fails to fully develop. Often detected during prenatal testing. Anencephalic babies carried to term die soon after delivery.
- ***Spina Bifida:*** The backbone does not fully fuse around the spinal cord. How severely a child will be affected depends upon the size of the opening and its location.
- ***Down Syndrome:*** A chromosomal defect that causes a characteristic appearance, heart problems, and often some degree of mental retardation.
- ***Cleft palate and cleft lip:*** Immediate surgery and intervention helps these children to breathe and suck properly. Later operations minimize disfigurement.
- ***Clubfoot:*** One or both feet are turned in an abnormal direction. Often corrected with special braces and shoes while little bones are still soft.
- ***Hypospadias:*** A malformation most often in boys that causes urine to flow from a second opening along the penis. Affected girls have an opening into their vaginas.
- ***Congenital dislocation of the hip:*** Possibly due to several genetic factors.
- ***Congenital deafness:*** Some children are now being fitted with electrical devices implanted into the inner ear that may enable them to perceive sounds.
- ***Cystic Fibrosis:*** A disorder in which the lungs fill with sticky mucus and other severe health problems occur. Some genetic markers for CF have recently been found, although there is no cure as yet.

Further down the list is Sudden Infant Death Syndrome, or SIDS. Nearly 7,000 healthy infants a year ranging in age from two weeks to one year are victims of SIDS. There is no known cause, and no cure. Records of SIDS deaths have been found as far back as writings in the Old Testament. Some SIDS infants have had severe blood pooling that has been mistaken for bruising, causing anguished parents to be accused of child abuse. The impact of losing a baby to SIDS can destroy families.

Statistics seem pretty irrelevant when the child in question happens to be yours, however. Although some prenatal tests can detect a few abnormalities in utero and surgical intervention has been successful at reversing certain problems even before birth, most parents have no warning their child will not be "born perfect."

Adjusting to this situation will take family members through a series of stages similar to those identified for the grieving process. Mothers, fathers, grandparents, siblings, and even extended family members will all experience the seven stages of reaction at different times and in different ways. These stages do not necessarily occur in order, but they can generally be considered as:

- ***Shock:*** A period of helplessness and numbness. It can be especially difficult to concentrate through this stage. Some parents have referred to it as "running on auto-pilot." Write down everything you need to remember, from questions to ask the neurologist to a reminder to feed the dog every day. A small hand-held tape recorder at the physician's office will give you something to refer to when it all seems to blur.

■ *Denial:* Disbelief; a sensation that it is all a bad dream, rationalizing a child's developmental patterns to "he'll (crawl, walk, roll over) when he's ready!"

■ *Sadness:* This stage can overwhelm parents at awkward times, causing them embarrassment or even paralyzing grief. It is of the utmost importance that you find non-judgmental help for this stage, either through a support group for parents of children with similar problems, or by seeking professional counseling.

■ *Anger:* Hair-triggering nerves, and a general feeling of rage. Many people find this stage affects their relationships with co-workers, family members, and spouses. Very few marriages are truly seamless unions, and this stage can amplify the tiniest flaws into tremendous conflicts. Tragically, some marriages do not survive the stress. Again, seek help.

■ *Anxiety:* Nervousness, sleeplessness, lack of appetite. The sense of isolation at this time is very strong. It may be difficult for outsiders to understand why you haven't "gotten over it." Hard as it may be to comprehend, it is vital for parents to take a break from the strain of coping with their child's needs. Other siblings also need a chance to "get away" without feeling guilty.

■ *Bargaining:* A faith in God may be restored at this point, although it may not resemble what it was prior to the birth of a special child. Many parents will find themselves trying any and all treatments they can find at this time, from the most conventional and aggressive to very nontraditional, alternative sources.

■ *Acceptance:* The ability to pull all the above together and still cope with your life. There is no set time as to how long these stages can take to work through, and not everyone feels them in the same order. Additionally, unexpected events such as an emergency surgery or milestones like entry into kindergarten can cause an emotional relapse.

ɷ RESOURCES ɷ

■ **ACCENT NURSING SERVICES, INC.**
546-2966
1306 N. 175th St., Ste. 101
Seattle, WA 98133
This is a private company led by nurses who believe in providing comprehensive home-based nursing services. Pediatric/maternal child health care, skilled nursing, respite care and hearing and speech assessments are just a few of the services Accent Nursing offers.

■ **ADVOCATES FOR RETARDED CITIZENS**
364-4645
10550 Lake City Way N.E., Ste. A
Seattle, WA 98125
ARC offers a Parent-to-Parent Program with weekly meetings to give support and guidance to parents of children with developmental disabilities. Facilitators are parents who have "been there," and offer understanding, resources, knowledge and group support. Family social events and a monthly newsletter are offered.

■ **AMERICAN DIABETES ASSOCIATION**
282-4616
557 Roy St., Lower Level
Seattle, WA 98109
This group offers educational meetings and support groups throughout King County, referrals to medical specialists, educational videos, and emergency insulin and medication for up to 30 days.

■ **AMERICAN HEART ASSOCIATION**
632-6881
4414 Woodland Park Ave. N.
Seattle, WA 98103
The Association promotes education, supports research, and trains CPR instructors.

■ **AMERICAN LUNG ASSOCIATION**
441-5100
2625 3rd Ave.
Seattle, WA 98121
They provide education and support for persons with respiratory problems, including a program for asthmatic children and their families and a camp for older children (6-12) with asthma.

■ **AUTISM SOCIETY**
368-0997
c/o Fircrest School
15230 15th N.E.
Seattle, WA 98155
The Society provides information, referral, and advocacy for children and adults with autism, and their families. They offer monthly support groups in Renton and Seattle, and volunteers to provide emotional support.

■ BIRTH TO THREE DEVELOPMENTAL CENTER
874-5445
35535 6th Pl. S.W.
Federal Way, WA 98023
A United Way agency, Birth to Three is "a special place for special children." Classroom and private sessions provide special needs children with physical, occupational and speech and language therapy in a playgroup setting. Toileting, feeding, and dressing skills are taught along with cognitive skills, sign language, and songs. Both handicapped and non-handicapped children participate in the program. Parent participation is encouraged.

■ BOYER CHILDREN'S CLINIC
325-8477
1850 Boyer Ave. E.
Seattle, WA 98112
The clinic provides diagnostic evaluation and treatment for children with developmental delays, cerebral palsy, neurological impairments, or other disabilities. Special evaluation and treatment for children birth to 3 is offered.

■ CAREGIVERS RESOURCE GUIDE
455-1603
P.O. Box 3734
Bellevue, WA 98009
The guide is a special loose-leaf workbook divided into sections addressing family, medical, daily living, personal, legal and financial information. It becomes both a fact file and personality profile. In case of a change in caregivers, residential situation or family emergency, all necessary information is available in one place.

■ CENTER ON HUMAN DEVELOPMENT AND DISABILITY (CHDD)
685-1251
University of Washington
Box 357920
Seattle, WA 98195
The CHDD provides assessment and diagnosis for developmental delays and retardation. They also offer high-risk infant follow-up.

■ CHILDREN WITH SPECIAL HEALTH CARE NEEDS (CSHCN)
296-4610
Seattle-King Co. Health Dept.
110 Prefontaine Place S. #500
Seattle, WA 98104
This federally and state funded program assists children up to age 18 who are disabled or at risk of becoming disabled. Evaluating the child's needs, planning for medical care and working with other professionals to help provide treatment are part of CSHCN's focus. Financial support for medical care is available, depending on eligibility.

■ CHILDREN'S CYSTIC FIBROSIS CENTER
526-2024
Children's Hospital
4800 Sand Point Way N.E.
Seattle, WA 98105
A parent support group for families coping with cystic fibrosis.

■ **CHILDREN'S HOSPITAL AND MEDICAL CENTER**
526-2000 (526-2223 TTY)
4800 Sand Point Way N.E.
Seattle, WA 98105

Children's Bellevue
454-4644
400-112th N.E. #110
Bellevue, WA 98004

Children's at Valley
251-5198 (228-3450 TTY)
400 S. 43rd St.
Renton, WA 98055
Children's Hospital provides general and acute in- and outpatient medical services for sick and disabled children. They offer special services for premature and critically ill infants, and for children with cystic fibrosis. Testing is available for specific health problems, including speech and language difficulties, developmental delays, learning disabilities, and other conditions. Branch locations offer more limited services.

■ **CHILDREN'S RESOURCE CENTER**
526-2500
Located at Children's Hospital, the Resource Center provides information and education on children's health issues. See chapter four (support groups) for more information.

■ **CHILDREN'S SERVICES OF SNO-VALLEY**
888-2777
1407 Boalch Ave. N.W.
N. Bend, WA 98045
An individualized education and therapy program for developmentally delayed children up to age 3, and their families.

■ **CHILDREN'S THERAPY CENTER OF KENT**
854-5660
10811 Kent-Kangley Rd.
Kent, WA 98031
The Center provides physical, occupational, and speech therapy for children from birth to 10 years who have developmental or other disabilities. They also provide an early childhood education program for children with disabilities, age birth to 3.

■ **COMMUNITY INFORMATION LINE**
461-3200
Hours: M-F   8:00 a.m.-6:00 p.m.
Operated by the Crisis Clinic's Resource Center, this phone line provides information and referrals to over 2,000 social services agencies in the area. The center maintains a current data base of agencies and also publishes an annual directory called "Where to Turn" which lists agency addresses and phone numbers. A larger "Where to Turn PLUS" directory includes more detailed information on agencies, including a service description, eligibility requirements, fees, and branch locations.

■ **COMMUNITY SERVICE CENTER FOR THE DEAF AND HARD OF HEARING**
322-4996
1609 19th Ave.
Seattle, WA 98122
Services are available in American Sign Language and include information and referral to community resources and to interpreters. The center also has a resource library.

■ COMMUNITY SERVICES FOR THE BLIND AND PARTIALLY SIGHTED

525-5556
9709 3rd Ave. N.E. #100
Seattle, WA 98115
This organization provides information and referral to community resources, as well as counseling and support groups.

■ CRISIS NURSERY—CHILD CARE SITE CHILDHAVEN

328-KIDS
The Crisis Nursery is a free, self-help program designed to keep families together while also preventing child abuse and neglect. When families are facing crises and have few or no other resources, parents voluntarily place their children into licensed respite provider homes for up to 72 hours.

■ CYSTIC FIBROSIS FOUNDATION

282-4770 or 800-647-7774
100 W. Harrison N. Tower #510
Seattle, WA 98119
Learn from peers how to be an advocate for your child with cystic fibrosis.

■ DEAF-BLIND SERVICE CENTER

323-9178
2366 Eastlake Ave. E. #206
Seattle, WA 98102
The center offers information and referral to community resources, and other services to assist deaf-blind persons. They also provide public education about deaf-blind people and issues.

■ DEVELOPMENTAL DISABILITIES, DIVISION OF DSHS

720-3300 (720-3325 TTY)
1700 E. Cherry
Seattle, WA 98122

545-6709
9620 Stone Ave. N. #204
Seattle, WA 98103

649-4211
15831 N.E. 8th
Bellevue, WA 98008

872-6490
1313 W. Meeker, Ste. 102
Kent, WA 98032
These offices coordinate state services for the developmentally disabled, including clients with mental retardation, cerebral palsy, autism, and epilepsy.

■ EASTER SEAL SOCIETY

281-5700
521 2nd Ave. W.
Seattle, WA 98119
The Easter Seal Society provides information and referral services for disabled children and adults. They also operate camps for children with disabilities.

■ EPILEPSY ASSOCIATION

623-4366
1306 Western Ave. #308
Seattle, WA 98101
This organization provides support and information for persons with epilepsy and for their families. They have a support group for parents of epileptics.

■ EXPERIMENTAL EDUCATION UNIT

543-4011
University of Washington
Box 357925
Seattle, WA 98195

The Experimental Education Unit offers the Early Childhood Home Instruction Program for Hearing Impaired Infants and their Families (ECHI), which works with families to assess children's auditory, communication, language and speech skills. Individual programs are designed for each family, usually including weekly home visits, and a center-based program with classroom experience for the children and support discussion group/sign language class for parents. ECHI covers children from the time of their diagnosis until age three. All services are at no cost to parents.

They also offer an Infant-Toddler Program—any child from birth to three with an identified developmental delay is eligible for this free program, which provides center- and home-based small group sessions, home visits, baby and toddler groups, and parent groups. The ITP is a training facility for UW graduate students in disciplines which emphasize working with handicapped children, from special education to audiology and social work. Supporting Extended Family Members (SEFAM) is a program for families of handicapped infants and children. (Call 543-4011, ext. 168 for more information.)

■ FOSTER GRANDPARENT PROGRAM

672-5552
19009 33rd Ave. W.
Lynnwood, WA 98036

Low-income elderly volunteers provide care to children with special needs. The volunteers receive training and then are paid a small, non-taxable stipend, as well as given meals, transportation, and other benefits.

■ HEARING, SPEECH & DEAFNESS CENTER

323-5770
1620 18th Ave.
Seattle, WA 98122

226-6111
305 S. 43rd St.
Renton, WA 98055

The Center offers evaluation and treatment for speech, hearing, and other communicative disorders. They provide therapy, information and referral, and parent support. A parent/infant program for families with hearing impaired children ages birth to 3 is offered.

■ JUVENILE DIABETES FOUNDATION

545-1510
1333 N. Northlake Way
Seattle, WA 98103
Hours: M-F   8:30 a.m.-5:00 p.m.

Volunteers provide support to parents whose children have been diagnosed with diabetes. The foundation also provides information and referrals.

■ **KID CARE, COMMUNITY HEALTH ACCESS PROGRAM**
284-0331
300 Elliott Ave. W., Ste. 300
Seattle, WA 98119
Referral and information is available, along with a resource guide, for families of developmentally disabled children. They can refer you to the Child Find office for your local school district so you can get free screening and evaluation for your child, and find out about special educational programs for preschoolers.

■ **KINDERING CENTER**
747-4004
16120 N.E. 8th
Bellevue, WA 98008
The school provides an educational preschool and home training for developmentally disabled or abused children. They also offer a support group for fathers, parent training, respite care, and foster home licensing.

■ **LEARNING DISABILITIES ASSOCIATION**
882-0792
7819 159th Pl. N.E.
Redmond, WA 98052
The association offers information on learning disabilities, screening and referral, tutoring, and parent support.

■ **LEARNING DISABILITIES HOTLINE**
621-9768
P.O. Box 46188
Seattle, WA 98146
This is a phone referral and information line run by volunteers. They can provide literature on learning disabilities, as well as someone to talk to who's learning disabled herself and can help address concerns.

■ **LEUKEMIA SOCIETY OF AMERICA**
628-0777
1001 4th Ave., Ste. 3714
Seattle, WA 98154
The Society provides information and referrals for persons with leukemia. They offer financial help for medication, blood transfusions, lab tests, and transportation.

■ **MARCH OF DIMES BIRTH DEFECTS FOUNDATION**
624-1373
1904 3rd Ave., Ste. 230
Seattle, WA 98101
The goal of the March of Dimes is to promote awareness about birth defects and reduce infant mortality. They accomplish this by community service programs, research, and legislative advocacy.

■ **MOM'S CASE MANAGEMENT (DSHS)**
721-2888
3600 S. Graham
Seattle, WA 98118
Through this program, pregnant women can receive free alcohol/drug treatment and support services. Besides services such as case management, inpatient or outpatient treatment, parenting education, transportation, and other services, program participants also get 2 years of follow-up support.

■ **MUSCULAR DYSTROPHY ASSOCIATION**
283-2106
701 Dexter Ave. N.
Seattle, WA 98109
MDA provides diagnosis and support for those with neuromuscular diseases. They offer medical treatment, social activities, and a summer camp; no fees are charged.

■ **NATIONAL FATHERS NETWORK**
Kindering Center
747-4004 or 284-2859
16120 N.E. 8th St.
Bellevue, WA 98008
A national organization that refers fathers of children with special needs to support groups throughout the country. They publish, on a twice-yearly basis, a free newsletter written for and by fathers.

■ **NATIONAL ORGANIZATION FOR RARE DISORDERS (NORD)**
800-999-6673
This is a clearinghouse for information on more than 900 rare disorders. NORD will send you information and articles and recommend other resources and networking possibilities. The first two articles are free; there is a $4.50 fee for additional articles.

■ **NATIONAL SIDS FOUNDATION**
(301) 322-2620
2 Metro Plaza, Ste. 104
8200 Professional Pl.
Landover, MD 20785
More information available for families coping with the loss of a child to Sudden Infant Death Syndrome.

■ **NORTHWEST AIDS FOUNDATION**
860-6241
127 Broadway E., Ste. A
Seattle, WA 98122
This agency provides support services, public information and education programs on AIDS.

■ **NORTHWEST CENTER CHILD DEVELOPMENT PROGRAM**
286-2322
2919 1st Ave. W.
Seattle, WA 98119
A child care program that integrates disabled and normally developed children 4 months through 5 years old. Includes parent education and support and a registered nurse is on site.

■ **NORTHWEST HOSPITAL SPEECH AND LANGUAGE SERVICES**
368-1848
1550 N. 115th St.
Seattle, WA 98133
This division of Northwest Hospital provides services, evaluation, individualized treatment, parent training, free screenings and community presentations for children with speech, language and hearing special needs. They offer a comprehensive program that can assist you and your child in areas such as stuttering, vocal cord problems, orofacial myofunctional disorders, delayed language, language learning disabilities and more. Parents who suspect their child has a speech, language or hearing problem may schedule a free screening at the above number.

■ **PARENT RESOURCE LINE**
259-2973
This phone line is operated by the Child Care Resource and Referral of Volunteers of America in Snohomish County. Besides providing phone referrals to agencies, parent support groups, and classes, a Parent Resource Guide is published quarterly which lists information on programs for parents. This publication is published by Lifenet in conjunction with the Volunteers of America.

■ PARENTS OF BLIND CHILDREN

823-6380

Volunteer groups of parents and sight-impaired people provide support for families of blind and visually impaired children.

■ PARENTS ARE VITAL IN EDUCATION (PAVE), WASHINGTON BRANCH

565-2266

800-5-PARENT

6316 S. 12th

Tacoma, WA 98465

One-on-one peer support for parents of children with disabilities. Program participants learn about the rights of children with special learning needs, so they can increase their skills in working with teachers, therapists, etc. to obtain appropriate educational services. Workshops, lending library, and quarterly newsletter make this a worthwhile program. Other programs offered through PAVE include the SSI Parent Mentor Program at 800-786-1620 and the Toddler-Infant Program at 800-298-3543.

■ PEDIATRIC INTERIM CARE CENTER

852-5253

233 2nd Ave.

Kent, WA 98032

This center provides care for drug-affected infants going through withdrawal. They also recruit and train foster families to care for drug-affected infants and provide support services and follow-up for people caring for these babies. A 24-hour hotline is operated to answer questions about care and also tell how to refer a baby that will be born drug-affected.

■ PUBLIC SCHOOL PROGRAMS

Auburn	931-4927
Bellevue	455-6077
Edmonds	670-7208
Federal Way	941-0100
Highline	433-2557
Issaquah	557-7500
Kent	859-7511
Lake Washington	822-9588
Mercer Island	236-3325
Northshore	489-6311
Renton	204-2200
Seattle	298-7805
Shoreline	361-4220
South Central	248-7590

To find out if your baby qualifies for assistance from a school program, call the school district serving your area and ask about its infant program. Free assessment is available. Services may include individual early intervention, weekly home visits, mother/child support groups, and speech and physical therapy. The services are free. Check with your school district's office for details of its program. The programs are designed for all developmentally delayed infants from birth to age 3.

■ SCOTTISH RITE CENTER FOR CHILDHOOD LANGUAGE DISORDERS

324-6293

1155 Broadway Ave. E.

Seattle, WA 98102

This center provides free assessments and therapy for children ages 2-8 with communication disorders. They help with obtaining support services within the community, and offer training for parents.

■ **SEATTLE AIDS SUPPORT GROUP**
322-AIDS
Free support groups for persons with AIDS or HIV and their families and friends are offered, as well as information and referral to resources, and support services (hospital and home visits, phone check-ups).

■ **SOCIAL SECURITY INCOME (SSI)**
800-772-1213
If your baby has a disability that is expected to last more than one year, you may be eligible for SSI. Your eligibility and financial assistance depend upon family income.

■ **UNITED CEREBRAL PALSY ASSOCIATION OF KING-SNOHOMISH COUNTIES**
632-2827
4409 Interlake Ave. N.
Seattle, WA 98103
Individuals with cerebral palsy are offered services including case management, information, and referral.

■ **WASHINGTON TALKING BOOK & BRAILLE LIBRARY**
464-6930
821 Lenora St.
Seattle, WA 98121
Hours:　M-F　　　8:30 a.m.-5:00 p.m.
　　　　Sat.　　　9:00 a.m.-1:00 p.m.
The library provides materials on cassettes, records, talking books, braille, and large print format.

ADDITIONAL RESOURCE

■ **EXCEPTIONAL PARENT MAGAZINE**
800-247-8080
P.O. Box 3000, Dept. EP
Denville, NJ 07834
A magazine geared for parents of children with special needs. A subscription is $18/year (9 issues). Topics include education, mobility products and technology.

SPECIAL RESOURCES

■ **ON-LINE SERVICES**
Most commercial on-line services offer a number of resources pertaining to special needs. Many have on-line "chat rooms" that can link up families in an electronic support group. Current theories and new treatment technologies can be found using search indexes and key words.

■ **DENTAL REFERRALS**
Check your local phone directory for the local Dental Society, or ask your personal dentist for a referral to a periodontist skilled in dealing with disabled children. Do not be afraid to "shop around" for a practitioner both you and your child are happy with.

INFERTILITY

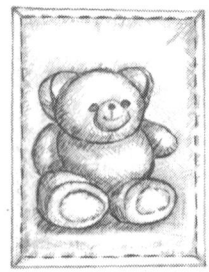

Having a family is a basic human desire that ranks near the top of most people's life dreams, and fortunately happens easily and naturally for most. A person gets married, gets pregnant, and then raises a family, right? Well, not always. Today, unfortunately, one in six couples has difficulty in conceiving. Each month, couples who are trying to get pregnant have a one in four chance of conceiving and in most cases, become pregnant during the first year of trying. As a general rule, if a couple has not been successful within a 12-month period, it is time for them to seek help.

When conception difficulties occur, couples often experience a wide range of emotions including feelings of frustration, anxiety, embarrassment, and disbelief. Because these feelings are so common, one of the first things a couple must realize is that they are not alone. Medical and emotional support is available to help you to overcome your fertility obstacles.

Medically, the first place to start is with your obstetrician/gynecologist. You will undergo a thorough physical examination and will be asked a series of personal questions that should help your physician make a determination about your case. At this point, a clear plan for testing will be outlined with your current physician or you may be referred to an infertility specialist or reproductive endocrinologist. The more difficult, advanced therapies are usually directed and administered by a reproductive endocrinologist who has had additional specialized training.

Emotionally, it is important that the partners support one another through this process and participate in the treatments together. Going through the medical procedures may be stressful at times, but hopefully the end result, a baby, will provide you with an incentive throughout the infertility evaluation and treatment process. You may ask your physician about support groups, such as RESOLVE, that may offer insight into others experiencing similar problems.

❧

As a general rule, if a couple has not been successful within a 12-month period, it is time for them to seek help.

❧

THE INFERTILITY EVALUATION

There are many factors that can have an influence on fertility, some of which are fairly easy to overcome and others that require much more effort. One of the most common causes of infertility is irregular ovulation, often manifested by irregular periods. Just because your menstruation is regular, however, does not mean you ovulate each month. One of the easiest and most inexpensive ways to determine whether or not a woman is ovulating is with the use of a basal thermometer and a temperature chart. The basal thermometer measures 1/10th degree changes in temperature. Because a woman's body temperature increases one-half a degree following ovulation, a typical "biphasic" graph is seen in those who are ovulating. Generally, it is recommended you track your temperature for two or three cycles.

You may also want to consider purchasing an ovulation predictor kit. This kit measures luteinizing hormone (LH) in the urine that signals ovulation.

Ovulation can also be monitored by obtaining a blood progesterone level at an appropriate time during the cycle. Lastly, development of the follicle (which contains an egg) can be monitored by ultrasound.

Once ovulation cycles are confirmed, your doctor may suggest that your partner have a semen analysis. Because 35 percent of fertility problems are due to the male, a semen specimen—which measures sperm concentration (count), motility (percent moving) and morphology (shape)—should be obtained as part of the initial testing.

The next step evaluates the fallopian tubes. Blockage of the tubes prevents the sperm from reaching the egg and is a common problem in women with infertility. During a radiologic procedure known as a hysterosalpingogram, a small amount of dye is injected into the opening of the cervix. The media, which is seen by x-ray, then passes into the uterine cavity and out the fallopian tubes (if they are open).

Laparoscopy may be necessary as a final part of the testing. In this outpatient surgical procedure (usually requiring general anesthesia), an incision is made in or just below the belly button, through which a small telescope is passed. The uterus, fallopian tubes, and ovaries are inspected, looking for adhesions (scar tissue), endometriosis or any other abnormalities. Many of these conditions may be treated with the use of laser and special instrumentation.

BEFORE YOU BEGIN YOUR TREATMENT

Once you've gone through the initial testing, your next step is determining the type of treatment that will best solve your problem. It is also important to check with your insurance carrier to find out what, if any, procedures are covered. To date, only seven states nationwide have mandated that fertility coverage is provided. Only in California, Texas and Connecticut is it required that insurance companies offer options to purchase policies with infertility coverage. The decision to purchase these options is usually made by the employer who frequently does not include this coverage. Fertility therapy is considered by many as a luxury, rather than a necessity.

If your insurance carrier does not offer coverage, talk with your infertility specialist and find out if any "package" plans are available. Several clinics now offer financial assistance and package plans that allow you to know exactly what and when you are paying for treatment.

Secondly, sit down with your spouse or significant other and talk about what you are about to embark upon. Are you ready to undergo tests and treatments that may not always occur around your work or social schedules, but rather are dictated by your body's schedule? Have this conversation often, even if you do proceed with treatments. Also, discuss what medical procedures you agree upon. And, figure out what you can afford financially. If possible, come up with a limit that has some flexibility, but also does not stretch indefinitely.

You may also want to talk with friends and family to see who they recommend for fertility treatment. Since infertility is common, you may be able to find several people who can offer their opinions of who to seek treatment from. Also, consider checking references from the fertility doctor or clinic you choose. Perhaps ask to speak to others who were and were not successful in conceiving with similar health conditions. The section on choosing your provider may also help you in making sure you and your fertility specialist make a good match.

Unfortunately, the success rate of the procedures may be difficult to predict. Although clinics and physicians can provide you with their overall pregnancy rate, remember each person has unique medical circumstances. Your physician should provide an individual plan that is designed to help solve your specific infertility problems.

THE COSTS OF FIGHTING INFERTILITY

The following are cost estimates of some of the commonly utilized medications and procedures:

Over the Counter

Basal Thermometer	$7
Ovulation Predictor Kit	$25-60

Medications

Clomiphene Citrate	$25-125 per cycle
Humegon and Metrodin (typically $1,000-3,000 per cycle)	$50 per kit
Lupron (enough for approximately 2-3 weeks)	$250 per vial

Procedures

Sperm Analysis	$100
Hysterosalpingogram	$400
Ultrasound	$100-200 each
Laparoscopy	$2,500-5,000
Intrauterine Insemination	$250-350 (per cycle)
Vasectomy Reversal	$5,000
Tubal Ligation Reversal	$9,000-12,000
In Vitro Fertilization	$7,000-9,000 (excluding medications)
GIFT	$8,000-10,000 (excluding medications)
Micromanipulation	$1,500 (in addition to the cost of IVF)

PRIMARY TREATMENT

OVULATION INDUCTION

Disorders of ovulation are commonly treated with clomiphene citrate (Clomid or Serophene). This oral medication is effective, with a low risk for a multiple pregnancy. Other medications (Pergonal and Metrodin) are given by injection and require ultrasound monitoring and blood estrogen level testing. Patients have a higher risk for a multiple pregnancy. Ask your physician about any side effects from these drugs and issues regarding prolonged usage.

ARTIFICIAL INSEMINATION

Placement of sperm (from the male partner or a sperm donor) into the uterus (intrauterine insemination) may be indicated for patients with sperm and/or cervical mucus problems. Donor sperm can be purchased from a sperm bank which rigorously screens the donors for medical and genetic problems. After collection, the sperm is frozen and quarantined for a minimum of six months. At the end of this time period, the donor is retested for infection before the sperm is released for use.

ASSISTED REPRODUCTIVE TECHNOLOGIES

The assisted reproductive technologies (ART) are a group of treatments performed in specially equipped centers. These procedures are indicated for specific disorders and for patients who have been unsuccessful with primary treatments. Before choosing an ART program, you should inquire about success rates and possibly speak with other patients who have undergone similar treatments. The procedures listed below are the current, most commonly performed ART procedures. New advances are continually being made. Check with your physician or support group for the most up-to-date information.

IN VITRO FERTILIZATION (IVF)

IVF is a nonsurgical procedure in which eggs are removed from the ovaries using a needle passed through the vagina. These eggs are then fertilized in the laboratory with the partner's sperm, and after three days the resulting embryos are transferred into the uterus by means of a small catheter placed through the opening of the cervix. The main advantage of IVF is that the fertilization process may be monitored in the laboratory from conception to formation of the early embryo. This allows the physician to choose the most viable and strongest embryo(s) to transfer to the womb. Patients find out if they are pregnant ten days after the embryo transfer. Indications of IVF include the following problems: (1) tubal blockage or dysfunction, (2) endometriosis, (3) sperm abnormalities and (4) unexplained infertility resistant to other treatments.

GAMETE INTRAFALLOPIAN TRANSFER (GIFT)

In contrast to IVF, patients undergoing GIFT have eggs and sperm placed into the fallopian tube(s) before fertilization occurs. This procedure requires a laparoscopy (minor surgery) and at least one healthy fallopian tube. Fertilization cannot be confirmed after a GIFT procedure unless a pregnancy results.

ZYGOTE INTRAFALLOPIAN TRANSFER (ZIFT)

ZIFT is similar to IVF except that the embryos are placed into the fallopian tube instead of the uterine cavity. Like GIFT, this procedure usually requires a laparoscopy and at least one healthy fallopian tube.

MICROMANIPULATION

Micromanipulation refers to a group of procedures, used in conjunction with IVF, in which the eggs and sperm are individually manipulated to enhance fertilization. Men with very low sperm counts and motilities may not fertilize their partners' eggs, even with IVF. A new procedure known as intracytoplasmic sperm injection (ICSI) has revolutionized treatment for these couples. This procedure requires special expertise and involves the injection of a single sperm into each egg under a microscope. Resulting embryo(s) are then transferred into the uterus after three days.

Another recent development, known as "assisted hatching," has also increased the success rate of IVF for some patients. Most people are unaware of the fact that human embryos must "hatch" out of a shell before they are able to implant and establish themselves within the uterine lining. By drilling a small hole in this shell just prior to the embryo transfer, the procedure enables embryos to hatch and implant more readily.

OTHER OPTIONS
OVUM DONATION

Many women may not be able to become pregnant with their own eggs due to poorly functioning or non-functioning ovaries, prior surgical removal of their ovaries, or because of genetic concerns. In this group of women, eggs obtained from a donor (by IVF) are fertilized with the male partner's sperm. Two or three days later, the embryos are transferred into the uterus. The woman then becomes the biological mother and is able to carry and deliver the baby. For most couples, this process is arranged anonymously and the couple and egg donor never meet. The couple, however, is provided with a detailed physical description of the donor and her complete medical and family histories.

SURROGACY

This option is indicated for women unable to carry a pregnancy because of uterine abnormalities, hysterectomy, or other medical problems. Embryos obtained from the eggs and sperm of the couple (IVF) are transferred into the uterus of another woman (the surrogate) who carries and delivers the baby. Laws governing surrogacy vary from state to state and expert legal advice is an important part of this procedure.

ADOPTION

It is important to realize that some couples may never conceive no matter what form of treatment is attempted. Other couples may be unable or unwilling to go ahead with some forms of therapy. Fortunately, adoption offers them another way to become parents. There are many adoption choices for parents. The adoption section of this guide may give you a good place to start, if this becomes your decision.

A FINAL WORD

Fighting infertility is often an emotional roller coaster ride. Most couples have high expectations following treatment. When conception does not occur, they may experience a huge "let down" at the first sign of a period. Many couples also have difficulty with scheduled sex. Normal, spontaneous and caring lovemaking often feels more like "show time!" Many facets of the infertility process hinge on the outcome of diagnostic procedures and decisions made by the couple with their physician. Choices are not always easy and sometimes there are no answers. Some of these patients may continue with fertility therapy while others may turn to adoption or choose to remain childless. These are very personal decisions that can only be made by you and your partner.

Contributing authors: Dr. John Gililland, M.D., Board Certified Reproductive Endocrinologist and Obstetrician/Gynecologist, Tandé Montez, Dr. Michael Soules, M.D., Patricia Marshall, RNC, and Laurie Guidry, RNC.

⁂ RESOURCES ⁂

■ FERTILITY & ENDOCRINE CENTER

(206) 548-4225
University of Washington
4225 Roosevelt Way N.E., Ste. 101
Seattle, WA 98105
University of Washington's Fertility and Endocrine Center (FEC) is the Pacific Northwest's largest fertility clinic, serving the Washington, Alaska, Montana and Idaho (WAMI) region. They consistently surpass the national average rate of IVF pregnancies.

■ GYFT CLINIC

475-5433
Puget Sound Hospital
3582 Pacific Ave., 3rd Fl.
Tacoma, WA 98408

■ REPRODUCTIVE TECHNOLOGY

386-2483
1229 Madison, Ste. 710
Seattle, WA 98104
Reproductive Technology is Seattle's largest sperm bank. You will need to be referred by a physician to utilize their services. Laboratory technicians and embryologists can also perform sperm testing, IVF, GIFT and ZIFT procedures.

■ RESOLVE

524-7257
Resolve offers support for individuals having difficulties conceiving. It offers a facilitated support group, information on a variety of medical procedures, referrals to fertility specialists, and adoption agencies. Resolve serves the greater Seattle area.

■ **SEATTLE FERTILITY &**
GYNECOLOGY CLINIC
Swedish Hospital
682-2200
1229 Madison, Ste. 1050
Seattle, WA 98104

■ **VIRGINIA MASON MEDICAL**
CENTER
223-6190
1100 Ninth Ave.
Seattle, WA 98111

■ **FAIRFAX CRYOBANK**
800-338-8407 or (703) 698-3976
3015 Williams Dr., Ste. 110
Fairfax, VA 22031

■ **PROCREATIVE**
TECHNOLOGIES, INC.
(310) 203-5453
11543 W. Olympic Blvd.
Los Angeles, CA 90064

■ **REPOSITORY FOR GERMINAL**
CHOICE
(619) 743-0772
450 S. Escondido Blvd.
Escondido, CA 92025

READING

Becker, Gay. *Healing the Infertile Family: Strengthening Your Relationship in the Search for Parenthood.* New York, NY: Bantam Books, 1990.

Harkness, Carla. *The Infertility Book: A Comprehensive Medical & Emotional Guide.* Berkeley, CA: Celestial Arts, 1992.

Johnston, Patricia Irwin. *Taking Charge of Infertility.* Indianapolis, IN: Perspectives Press, 1994.

Menning, Barbara Eck. *Infertility: A Guide for the Childless Couple.* New York, NY: Prentice Hall Press, 1988.

Salzer, Linda P. *Surviving Infertility: A Compassionate Guide Through the Emotional Crisis of Infertility.* New York, NY: Harper Collins, 1991.

Life Experiences ...

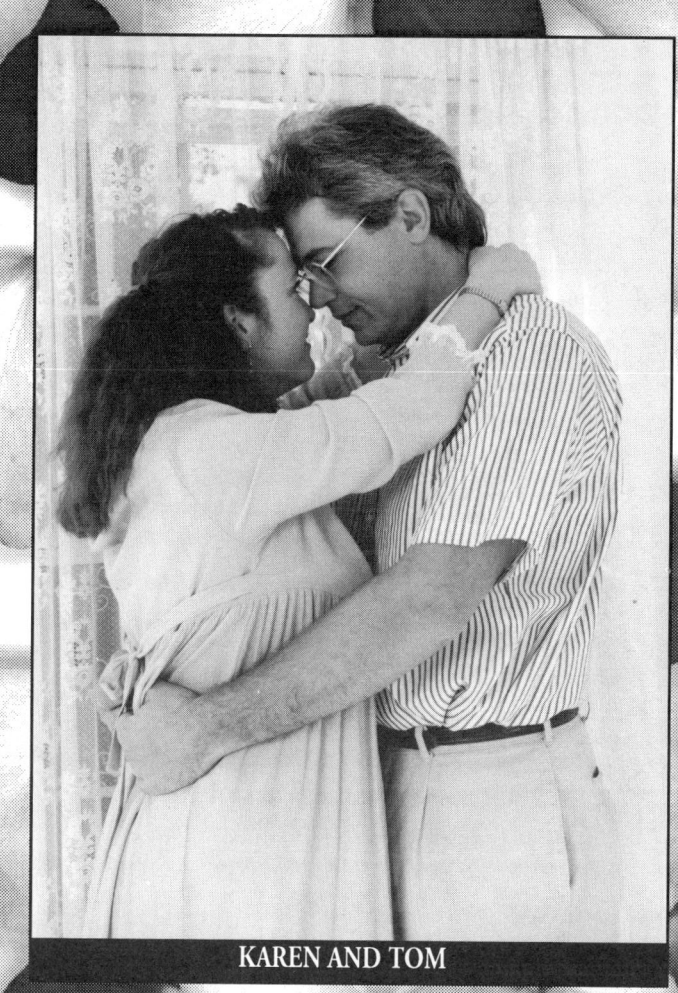

KAREN AND TOM

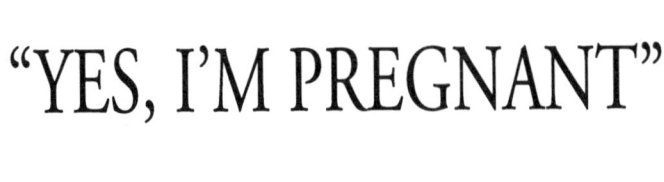

"YES, I'M PREGNANT"

By Karen Bauman-Mesich

All of my life I have been perfectly healthy, or so I thought. At 35, I learned not everything in my body was in order.

My husband Tom and I had been trying for some time to have a baby, with no success. After two years of hoping and failing, I made an appointment with a specialist. More time passed, with tests and interminable waits, until the laparoscopy showed my tubes were badly scarred from an illness I hadn't even known I had. With my damaged fallopian tubes, our only hope to conceive was through in-vitro fertilization (IVF).

We interviewed three IVF clinics before deciding to use a well-known fertility center with a high success rate. Our chance of success was estimated to be 30 percent per try (cycle). We chose the "Option Three" plan, for three cycles (embryo implantations) to be performed within one year. Sometime during the coming year I would either conceive or be childless for life.

My first cycle (30 days) started with no exercise, no caffeine and no sex. Tom gave me daily intramuscular injections of fertility drugs, which were followed by two vaginal sonograms which monitored my egg follicle maturity and uterine lining. Three blood tests indicated my estradiol (hormone) level. According to the textbooks, I was a model case. Six egg follicles were surgically retrieved under general anesthesia. Eggs and sperm were then combined (in vitro) for two days. Four picture-perfect embryos were gently transferred vaginally into my uterus. I spent seven days in bed, waiting for the embryos to attach to my uterine lining.

I was filled with hope and fear. I pleaded, begged and bargained with God for a baby. Wait ... wait ... ten days after embryo transfer a blood draw indicates pregnancy. The results: no baby. Failure. But my embryos, estradiol levels, uterine lining, were all perfect. No complications. Why not me? I was confused, angry and downright depressed. I felt I

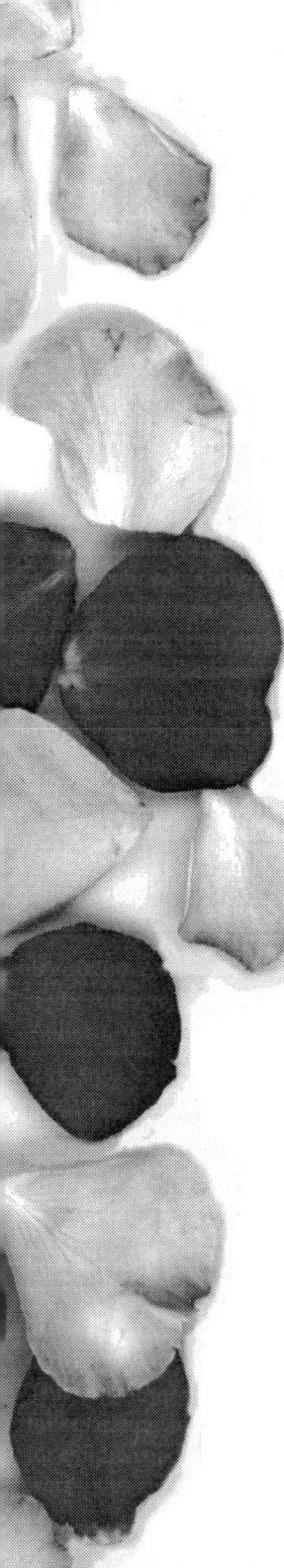

had lost control over my life. This couldn't be. It seemed like a big broken promise. It just wasn't fair.

My driving sense of purpose escalated. I became single-minded, putting all my energy into making the dream of a baby a reality. I read every birthing, parenting and IVF book published. I was determined to do whatever it took. I tried again.

The staff at the fertility clinic was positive and supportive from start to finish. One of the three nurses always returned my call within the hour. They were there for me 100 percent.

Cycle Two—I knew what to expect from the physical procedures from the first cycle, the shots and surgery. The biggest challenge was the total loss of control. There was absolutely nothing I could do to ensure pregnancy. The wait was painfully exhausting.

Cycle two was another perfect cycle with quality embryos, uterine lining, estradiol level. Again seven days bed rest was followed by a tenth-day blood draw—yes! I'm pregnant! Reproductive technology has blessed us with unfathomable joy! We won! Sheer bliss!

I carried pictures of my six-week-old embryo and showed them to everyone, recounting my miracle to anyone who would listen. I welcomed with delight sore breasts and fatigue. I started buying maternity and baby clothing.

In my seventh week, I suddenly doubled over with severe cramps. Tom immediately rushed me to the hospital's emergency room. My IVF doctor diagnosed an ectopic pregnancy in my fallopian tube. He immediately removed both tubes. I recovered at home...waiting for seven days for a sonogram to see if the baby in my uterus was still alive. I had a one in 40,000 chance. Yes! Alive! This baby survived the ectopic pregnancy and we deserved this miracle baby. The baby was the correct gestational size for eight weeks, with a normal heart beat. Two weeks later my IVF doctor released me to an obstetrician.

Three weeks later I woke up with an intuitive sickening feeling that something was seriously wrong. A sonogram that morning showed no heartbeat. There was no longer a miracle baby. I was in shock; I cried for days. This was the most

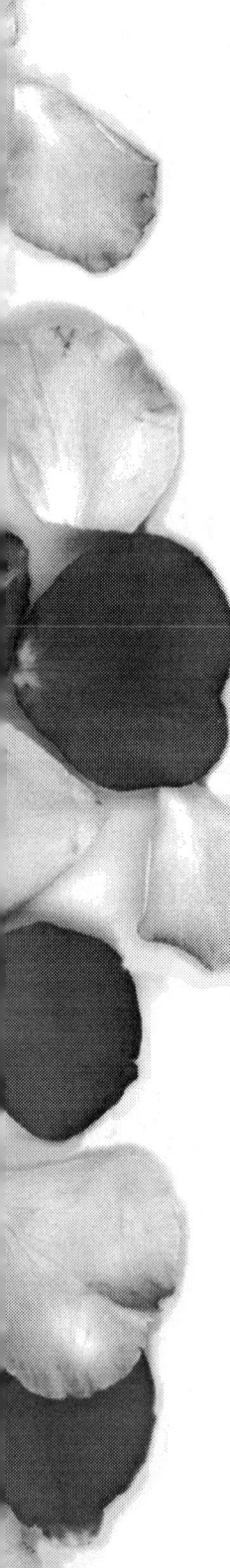

horrible experience of my life, a heart-wrenching ordeal. I felt an unbearable loss, and was overwhelmed by my grief. The worst part was how fast everything was erased. After imagining the baby, talking with new moms, planning the years ahead, my life suddenly collapsed in one second. My place in the world, my identity, was no longer the same.

My obstetrician explained it was just nature taking care of an abnormality. One in four women miscarry and it was "no big deal." Well, it was a very big deal to me! I searched out, and had every test done, to try to determine why I miscarried. Still no explanation. I'll never know why. It's an unsettling feeling.

Sometimes it seemed almost too painful to risk letting myself hope for a new pregnancy, and to risk being crushed again. But gradually the courage to try again grew. I had more hope than fear.

I joined a women's IVF group for eight weeks. That helped me immensely. Finally I found I wasn't alone. It was comforting talking with women who were having the same physical and emotional challenges. We gave each other hope and strength and confirmed the insanity of it all.

My friends were as supportive as they could be. They liked the happy, enthusiastic, positive Karen. (I prefer her also.) But with so many disappointments, coupled with massive amounts of hormones raging through my body, my energy was spent working overtime (IVF is very expensive).

Cycle Three—My last chance. The pressure was intense. I was hopeful, because I did get pregnant before. I tried to be realistic, understanding that getting pregnant is just the beginning of a very long process. There are many hurdles, and anything can happen.

Once again perfect embryos, estradiol, lining, bed rest, ten-day wait for a blood draw, then a five-week wait to see the heart beating. Pregnant! Fraternal twins! Two separate placentas, two beating hearts.

We are beaming with happiness. I am going to be a mother. We are going to be a family. I praise medicine. As my story goes to print, I am halfway to birth...22 weeks. Waiting...and enjoying every minute. ❧

❧ RESOURCES ❧

■ CENTERING CORPORATION
(402) 553-1200
1531 N. Saddle Creek Rd.
Omaha, NE 68104
This company publishes a "Creative Care Package" catalog that features several books and pamphlets on bereavement issues that deal with every part of the death of a child. They also offer some of the best published literature in children's grief literature.

■ CHILDREN GRIEVE TOO
246-6142
This program of Family Services offers counseling and support for children (and their parents) who have lost a loved one.

■ CLIMB
(907) 746-6123
Jean Kollantai
P.O. Box 1064
Palmer, AK 99645
The Center for Loss in Multiple Births publishes a quarterly newsletter called "Our Newsletter" for families who have experienced the death of one or more, or all, of their children during a twin or higher multiple pregnancy. Several parents share their stories, poems and ideas to help with this unique kind of grief. Special issues are published throughout the year that feature parents who have lost a multiple to SIDS; on raising/talking to surviving multiples; and one on the loss of a triplet or other supertwin(s); and material for parents who learn during pregnancy that one multiple will not live past birth.

■ COMPASSIONATE FRIENDS
241-1139 (Seattle-King County)
259-1048 (Everett)
(708) 990-0010 (National Office)
P.O. Box 3696
Oak Brook, IL 60522-3696
Compassionate Friends is a self-help organization offering friendship and understanding to bereaved parents. The purposes are to support and aid parents in the positive resolution of the grief experienced upon the death of their child, and to foster the physical and emotional health of bereaved parents and siblings. Healing is slowly and gently promoted as parents gain insight and understanding, have an opportunity to ventilate their feelings in an accepting atmosphere, and as they are able to reach out to the newly bereaved.

■ INFORMATION & CONSULTATION SERVICES
246-6142
Grief support for children who have lost a parent or sibling.

■ NATIONAL SHARE OFFICE
(314) 947-6164
St. Joseph's Health Center
300 First Capitol Dr.
St. Charles, MO 63301
The mission of SHARE (Pregnancy & Infant Loss Support Inc.) is to serve those who are troubled by the tragic death of a baby through miscarriage, stillbirth or newborn death. Six times a year, they publish a newsletter with information and ideas from parents and professionals to support and provide a sense of friendship for bereaved parents.

■ **NATIONAL SIDS FOUNDATION**
526-2110 or 800-533-0376
c/o Children's Hospital, CG-07
P.O. Box 5371
Seattle, WA 98105
The SIDS Foundation offers programs of emotional and informational support to those who have experienced a baby's death due to SIDS. Peer contacts offer personal visits and regular telephone contact, assisting in funeral planning, and visiting throughout the pregnancy and infancy of a subsequent child. The SIDS Foundation also has a speakers' bureau available for presentations and sends out a quarterly newsletter as well as targeted mailings. Crisis situations are handled on a 24-hour on-call basis.

■ **PAILS OF HOPE**
(702) 826-7332
P.O. Box 8738
Reno, NV 89507
PAILS of HOPE is a bi-monthly publication for parents who have battled through infertility and/or experienced pregnancy/infant loss and are contemplating pregnancy, are pregnant or have given birth and/or adopted a baby subsequent to loss or infertility. PAILS is sponsored by Pen-Parents.

■ **PEN-PARENTS**
(702) 826-7332
P.O. Box 8738
Reno, NV 89507
Pen-Parents is an international referral network for parents (grandparents and siblings) who have suffered the tragedy of pregnancy loss or the death of a child. Many bereaved find it healing to express their feelings through writing. Pen-Par-
ents fills the need for support and validation through correspondence with others in similar situations.

■ **P.S.**
772-5338
P.O. Box 5962
Bellevue, WA 98006
For those experiencing stillbirth, newborn death or miscarriage, P.S. provides telephone contact with a trained volunteer parent and monthly meetings to discuss common concerns and experiences and share information. Regular presentations by experts in various areas and a bimonthly newsletter are available for all in need.

■ **SWEDISH MEDICAL CENTER**
386-6133
747 Broadway
Seattle, WA 98114
The Women and Infants Social Work Services at Swedish offer the following support groups:
Difficult Decisions: If fetal testing reveals a genetic or developmental abnormality that results in your choosing pregnancy termination, this support group can offer help and support. Sharing and receiving the support of other couples who had made the same decisions can be helpful and assist in arriving at a comfortable resolution to your grief. The group meets monthly.
Pregnancy After Loss: For expectant parents who have experienced a miscarriage, stillbirth or the death of an infant, contemplating or celebrating a new pregnancy can be difficult. This group meets monthly to share experiences with couples in similar situations.

Support After Miscarriage: A master's level social worker presents a series of three one-hour sessions for women who have experienced a spontaneous miscarriage in the last 12 months, less than 20 weeks gestation. Sharing and receiving support from other women may validate your feelings. Coping strategies and information in grief loss are also presented.

■ **TWINLESS TWINS SUPPORT GROUP INTL.**
(219) 627-5414
11220 St. Joe Rd.
Fort Wayne, IN 46835-9737
Confidential e-mail: (only accessed by Dr. Brandt): BRANDT@mail.fwi.com
Office e-mail: twinless@iserv.net.com
Web page: http:\\www.iserv.net/twinless
This international organization has 14,000 members. Dr. Brandt heads up this group that is supported by memorial donations in the name of the lost twin (or multiple). They have many different parent contact groups, with many in the local area. Dr. Brandt himself is a surviving twin. Dr. Brandt also publishes *Twins World* magazine which is for twins and twinless twins. The back of the magazine deals specifically with grief management and loss. The cost for a subscription is $20 per year.

PREMATURE INFANTS

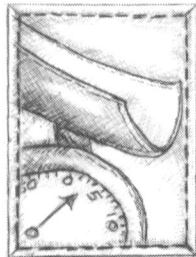

Babies born before the end of the 36th week of pregnancy are considered premature. According to the American College of Obstetricians and Gynecologists, eight to ten percent of all babies born in the United States are preterm. Preterm births, however, account for 60 percent of infant deaths, not counting those related to birth defects. Fortunately, the advances of modern technology allow for some premature babies to go home earlier and lead happy and healthy lives.

According to Washington State's Center for Health Statistics, during 1994, 5.5 percent of all babies born to residents residing in King County were considered to be low birthweight. Any infant that weighs less than five and a half pounds is considered a "low birthweight" baby. Yet, the smallest premature babies may weigh less than 24 ounces. One of the biggest risks to these newborns is their immature lungs. Since they leave the womb before their lungs are completely developed, they are missing surfactant, a substance that keeps the air sacs open. To prevent the lung from collapsing, doctors use surfactant therapy and high frequency ventilation. A preterm baby may also have problems swallowing, making it necessary for the infant to be fed through a tube. And when preterm babies lack body fat, they have difficulty maintaining adequate body temperature. Warming beds provide preemies with an environment as warm as the womb. These technological advances have saved thousands of premature infants' lives.

It is frightening for parents to see their newborn attached to monitors and special equipment. This chapter of the resource guide provides information from the American College of Obstetricians and Gynecologists on the causes, risk factors and warning signs of preterm labor. In addition, it gives an overview of hospital facilities and area resources available for parents of premature infants.

❧

Fortunately, the advances of modern technology allow for premature babies to go home earlier and lead happy and healthy lives.

❧

PRETERM LABOR CAUSES AND RISK FACTORS

What causes some women to go into premature labor is not completely understood. For about two-thirds of women who deliver prematurely, the exact cause is never known. However, what we do know is that women who receive little or no prenatal care seem to be at an increased risk for preterm labor. Regular prenatal care is vital to the health of your baby, and even more so if you are already at risk for preterm labor.

According to the American College of Obstetricians and Gynecologists, the following are risk factors for preterm labor:

- Previous preterm labor or history of preterm birth
- Current multiple pregnancy—two or more fetuses
- Several induced abortions—the planned ending of a pregnancy
- Abnormalities of the cervix, such as incompetent cervix, or of the uterus, such as malformations or fibroids
- Abdominal surgery in current pregnancy
- Serious infection in the mother
- Bleeding in the second trimester of current pregnancy
- Underweight mother; less than 100 lbs.

Having one or more of these factors does not necessarily mean that you will have preterm labor—only that you are at increased risk. If you are concerned about the risks of having a preterm baby, be sure to discuss it with your doctor.

WARNING SIGNS OF PRETERM LABOR

How do you know if you are actually in preterm labor? For first-time mothers, labor is a brand new experience and so it may be difficult to judge if you are really in labor or just having Braxton Hicks contractions. In any case, if you have the following signs, make sure you contact your doctor immediately. It is better to be sure of your labor condition than to wait

until it may be too late to reverse the situation. Bed rest, extra fluids, and/or a variety of medications may be prescribed to stop early labor.

The following are guidelines from the American College of Obstetricians and Gynecology on warning signs of preterm labor:

- Vaginal discharge: change in type (watery, mucous, or bloody) or increase in amount
- Pelvic or lower abdominal pressure
- Low, dull backache
- Abdominal cramps, with or without diarrhea
- Regular contractions or uterine tightening

Your doctor will determine if you are in preterm labor by examining your cervix for any changes. You may also have a fetal monitoring test to record the heartbeat of the fetus and to determine the contractions of the uterus. Ultrasound may be used to estimate the size, age and position of the fetus.

If you are actually in preterm labor, your doctor will make a medical decision about whether to try to stop your labor.

HOSPITAL FACILITIES

If your baby is born 8-10 weeks prematurely, he/she may be able to remain at the hospital where you delivered, if it has a Level II special care nursery. These hospitals include Evergreen, Group Health Central, Northwest, Overlake, Providence (Colby), Stevens, and Virginia Mason. The hospitals have neonatologists on staff or on call, and most offer surfactant therapy. For births more than 10 weeks early, or when other medical conditions require, babies are transferred to the Level III nurseries at Children's Hospital and Medical Center, University of Washington Medical Center, or Swedish Medical Center. These hospitals have staff and equipment capable of handling newborn emergencies. Children's Hospital is the only area hospital to offer Extra Corporeal Membrane Oxygen (ECMO) and is also the only place where newborn cardiac surgery is done.

The chart below compares premature infant facilities at three local hospitals.

Hospital Facilities

Children's Hospital and Medical Center • 526-2041   19 beds
Children's has an attending staff of 12 neonatologists, six from the community and six from the University of Washington's Medical Center. They handle the most complex newborn medical and surgical procedures and are the only hospital in the area to perform infant cardiac surgery. Children's does the most major infant surgeries in the area. They're also the only hospital that offers ECMO. Children's offers surfactant therapy and high frequency ventilation, as well as newer and experimental treatment. The staff at Children's and at UWMC work closely together in determining which of their two hospitals can best treat babies being transferred from other hospitals.

Swedish Medical Center • 386-2430   36 beds
Swedish has a comprehensive facility to care for premature infants born at 24-36 weeks. They have 11 neonatologists on their attending staff (5 at any given time). They offer surfactant therapy and neonatal surgery. Babies requiring cardiac surgery and certain other treatments are transferred to Children's.

University of Washington Medical Center • 548-4606   32 beds
The UWMC is considered the regional center for high-risk obstetrics and perinatal services. They offer surfactant therapy and high frequency ventilation and other new therapies as they are available. Six senior neonatologists are on staff. Babies requiring immediate surgery are transferred to Children's.

❧ RESOURCES ❧

■ PARENT CARE
(317) 872-9913
9041 Colgate St.
Indianapolis, IN 46268
An international organization of parents of premature and high-risk infants, Parent Care provides information through publications, videos and conferences. Membership categories range between $25 and $110. Once a year they organize a national conference that addresses high-risk neonatal care issues.

■ PARENTS OF PREMATURES
283-7466
P.O. Box 3046
Kirkland, WA 98083
Parents of Prematures is a voluntary organization made up of parents who have experienced a high-risk pregnancy and/or the birth and hospitalization of a premature baby. Helping others since 1973, they offer an outreach program, parent education meetings, a newsletter, guidelines for breastfeeding, clothing, and a lending library. Support groups are held at Providence Hospital (Colby campus) and Group Health Central.

■ SIDELINES NATIONAL SUPPORT NETWORK
522-5045 or (714) 497-2265
2805 Park Pl.
Laguna Beach, CA 92651
Sidelines of Seattle is part of a network of support groups across the country for women with complicated pregnancies and their families. The Seattle group telephone number is listed first. They offer educational information, a lending library, local resources, and emotional support.

PREEMIE CATALOGS
The following companies will be happy to send you a catalog listing of their line of premature baby clothes and items.

Preemie Wear	800-382-8469
T.L.C. Preemie	800-876-9071
Oh So Small	770-BABY
Le Petite Baby	(770) 475-3247
Simply Premie	800-382-8469

DIAPER SERVICES
Many diaper services offer premature baby sizes. Review the diaper service chapter of your resource guide for reviews and prices on the various services.

■ PAMPERS FOR PREMATURE INFANTS
800-543-4932
Hours: M-F 8:00 a.m. -5:30 p.m. (EST)
To order Pampers disposable diapers directly you may call their toll-free number. Within ten days after placing an order, a case of 180 preemie diapers will be delivered to your home. The cost is between $33 and $37 depending on how you pay. These diapers will fit infants up to 6 pounds, and they are all white with no elastic. They also offer and "improved" diaper that fits infants up to 5 pounds. They come in a case of 240 and the cost is between $45 and $48.

BEDREST: A PRESCRIPTION, NOT A SENTENCE

You're at a routine obstetrical appointment. Expressing concern, your doctor recommends bedrest. "I can't be on bedrest!" you immediately think. But if you're like thousands of women each year, you won't have a choice. For the safety of your unborn child, a period of bedrest will decrease the chance of premature labor.

You will survive bedrest. We suggest calling Sidelines, a support group dedicated to helping women through bedrest and complicated pregnancies, at 522-5045. They will send you information to make this time easier for you and your family.

It is important to be equipped to cope with the stresses of bedrest. Be prepared to be totally dependent on others, and expect feelings of inadequacy. You can fight feelings of isolation by calling friends and relatives, and having people come and visit. People may tell you how "lucky" you are to "lay around all day." Know that bedrest is serious work for a confined mother, and the focus is on keeping you and the baby healthy through your pregnancy. Find friends who will be supportive and caring, and let them help you!

Some suggestions:

■ Be sure phone, phone book, television remote control, reading and writing materials and projects are within reach on the bed or next to it. At night, put everything into a laundry basket and set up your "nest" first thing in the morning.

■ Have a small ice chest within reach, packed with the day's supply of drinks and snacks.

■ Open your window—weather permitting—to let the outdoors in and get some fresh air.

■ Make a list of things people can do for you, so that when they ask, you can easily respond and even give them a choice.

■ Work on long-put-off projects: update photo albums, write letters, finish stitchery projects, mend clothes, update your phone book and holiday card list, reorganize files.

■ Consider renting a sliding side table (similar to the ones used in hospitals) to make it easier to eat or write while in bed.

■ Have a "date" with your husband—gourmet take-out food and candles.

■ Invite another couple for a game of cards or trivia or to watch a video movie on Saturday night.

If you have other children in your household, find creative ways to interact with them. Play bed-basketball with rolled-up socks and a laundry basket. Keep building blocks, board games, coloring books and crayons, puzzles, playdough, children's books, paper, scissors, paste and old magazines in a laundry basket near your bed. Include paper towels for spills.

Thanks to Sidelines for providing information for this article.

Life Experiences...

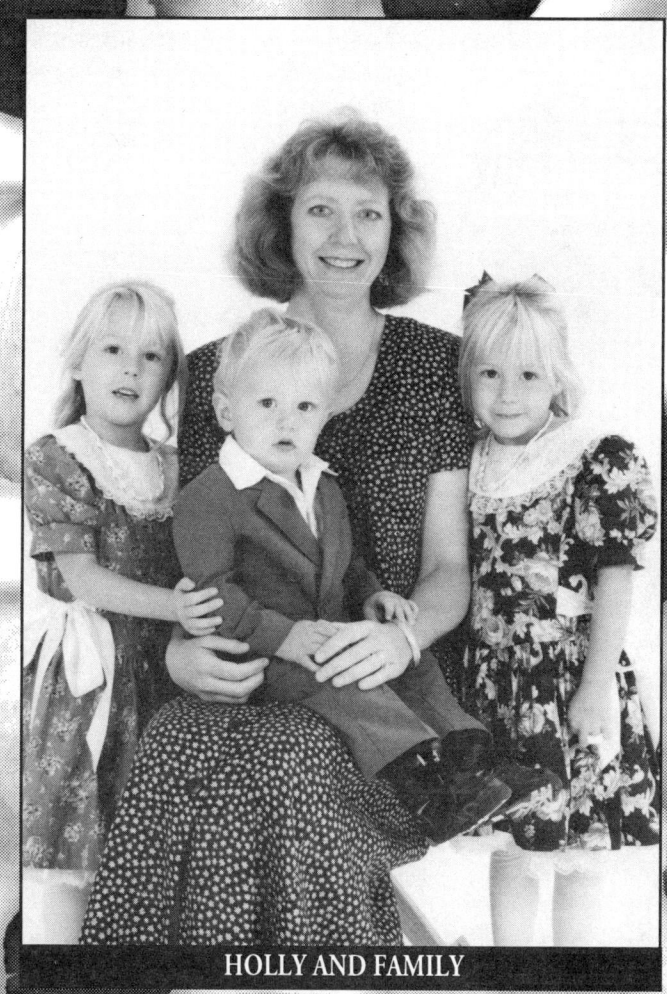

HOLLY AND FAMILY

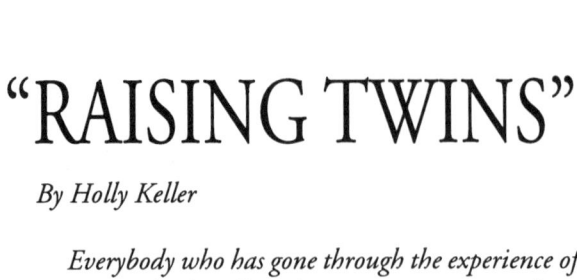

"RAISING TWINS"

By Holly Keller

Everybody who has gone through the experience of having a multiple birth will say that at one point or another, they felt like a strange sideshow at a circus. When people ask me if I knew I was going to have twins, I usually respond with, "Not really, but I knew something was wrong!" My doctor suspected that something was going haywire with my pregnancy around my 18th week. I, of course, had figured this out much earlier. I was huge, felt terrible, and looked awful. So needless to say, when the ultrasound showed two babies, my husband turned pale, almost fainted, and nearly went into shock.

Life became stranger after this discovery. I gave in and told the new company that I was working for that I was pregnant. Then I expanded the news and explained I was having twins. Imagine their surprise! Our friends and family were thrilled, and my mother thought this was extremely funny (payback for my wild teenage years, I guess).

The newness of the "twins" wore off when I went into premature labor at 24 weeks. I was hospitalized for two days, and took a variety of medications which made me feel sick. After that, I was sent home for complete bed rest, and I was hooked up to a contraction monitor with computer feed to a nurse's station. I had to monitor my contractions three times a day. By this time, I was so huge I could hardly even stand up.

At 33 weeks I got the flu. My husband raced me to the hospital. They admitted me, and since the labor wouldn't stop this time, they prepped me for a C-section and gave me one more hour to see if the drugs to stop the flu would work. Amazingly they did and my labor stopped. Back home we went, to be on bed rest again, for what the doctor said should only be two to three weeks. Well, I stayed pregnant until my 39th week, when the doctor scheduled a Cesarean. He couldn't believe I made it that long ... of course, neither could I. The twins were so active, it looked like "aliens" were about to pop out of my stomach.

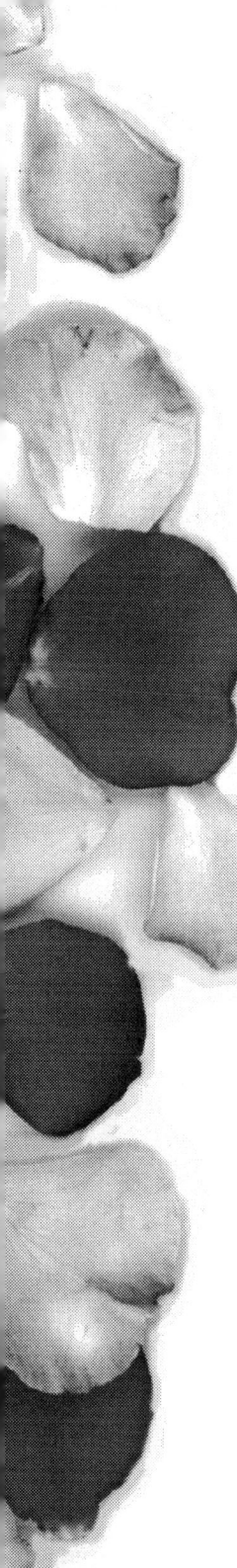

Healthy babies were born as scheduled. The identical girls were each almost seven pounds and they were 20 inches long. We named them Allison and Sherry.

Once I found out my babies were healthy, the whole experience went much better. I was extremely frightened during my pregnancy that something would go wrong and I would lose one or both of the babies. The birth was such a relief, I didn't know what to do next. I had put off setting up their room, washing bedding and clothes, and buying diapers and wipes. Thank goodness my mother came when they were born and helped us out. With all of the contacts I had made at the local twins club, I have since found out that the fears and strange experiences I had during my pregnancy were completely normal for moms of multiples.

Once we brought our beautiful girls home, the challenges of day-to-day activities seemed incredible. Should I wake them both to feed them? What about breastfeeding both of them? How should I dress them? Should I put them in the same crib? The same room? Who could I trust to baby-sit two babies? And last but not least, how could I stay nice to the public (even after being asked, "Are they twins?" for the hundredth time).

We found our own answers to many of these questions. I chose to breastfeed both twins until they were six months old, but I also supplemented. My husband would bottle-feed one baby, and I would nurse the other. At the next feeding, we would switch. This made it extremely important to be able to tell the twins apart during their first year. We used the toenail polish method of differentiating them. Allison had no nail polish and Sherry had bright red nail polish. (The only problem with this came after a year, when Allison wanted her nails painted too!) Even if one of the girls was sleeping, we always woke her up and fed them both at the same time.

We also decided to let both girls share the same crib, until they were two months old and started to roll over onto each other. We assembled the other crib, and put them side by side in the same room.

One of the things we couldn't believe was how quickly the twins developed their motor skills. They rolled over at two months, crawled at four months, and walked at eight months.

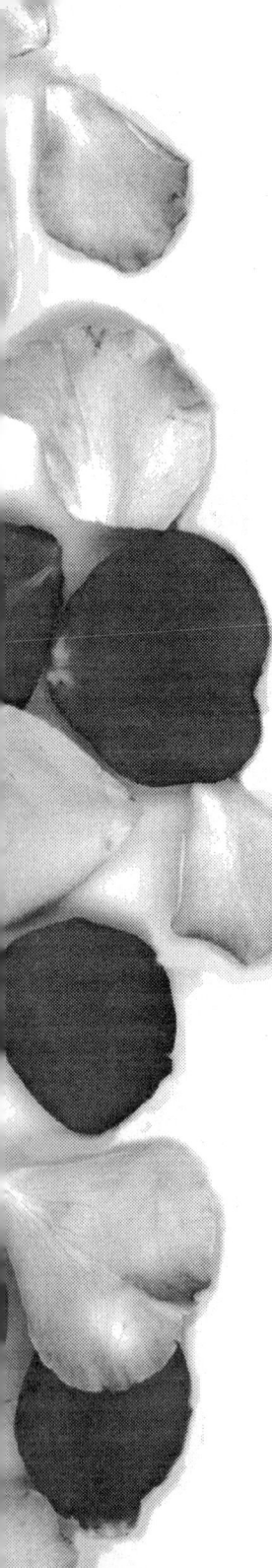

The most unbelievable fact was that both girls' milestones occurred on the same day!

As for dressing, Allison and Sherry always wear similar clothing, like shorts and tops, but usually in different colors. I would put them in identical clothing if they received it as gifts, but I usually varied something—their hair, shoes, or socks.

Trying to find child care for one baby is difficult enough, but for two it is even harder. We found friends and family to be great baby-sitters. We found that we trusted relatives who had children of their own best to baby-sit our girls. We figured they knew what to do if they had managed with their own. Once I went back to work, when Allison and Sherry were three months old, we hired a nanny through a local agency. It was cheaper to pay for one nanny than to pay for two kids in child care. This was also great because we didn't have to get them ready and take them out.

And last but not least, what do we do when people ask us, "Are they twins?" I usually answer that question with a long-winded answer about Allison and Sherry and all of their statistics, in hopes that the person asking, will become bored, and not ask any more questions. It usually works!

As our twins got older, we decided to have another child (only one this time!). Allison and Sherry were actually mad that I was only going to have one baby, and not one for each of them! But once our son Spencer was born, they were thrilled. They told us that he was the "best pet they ever had."

Through the years, we have always tried to recognize Allison and Sherry as different children, and not lump them together as "the twins." They do develop as individuals and even though they may look identical, they each have their own special personalities. It takes some effort to always see them as individuals, but it's worth it in the long run. ❧

ᾳ RESOURCES ᾳ

■ **MOTHERS OF MULTIPLES**
Eastside: 821-5911
This organization operates branches throughout the area. Groups offer family social events, as well as monthly meetings that feature a guest speaker. They encourage pregnant women to join, so they can have the support of others early on.

■ **M.O.S.T.**
(MOTHERS OF SUPERTWINS)
(516) 434-MOST
P.O. Box 951
Brentwood, NY 11717
A nonprofit group that provides information, resources, empathy and support to families with triplets or more.

■ **N.W. ASSOC. OF MOTHERS OF TWINS CLUB**
For general information:
Janice Totey, 235-1702
Eastside Moms (East King Co.):
Kathy Morehead, 392-5689
Halls Lake Mothers of Twins (N. King & S. Snohomish Co.):
Lisa Alfi, 776-9330
North Seattle Families of Multiples (North Seattle):
Velvet Eko-Bronson, 937-9535
Snohomish "Pair"ents of Twins (E. Snohomish Co.):
Sandy Ellis, 794-6552
South Seattle See-N-Double (West and South Seattle):
Shirley Laycock, 922-5208
Valley Mothers of Multiples (Renton, Kent, Auburn):
Rhonda Angevine, 432-4609
Clubs listed above are members of the

N.W. Assoc. of Mothers of Twins but are operated individually. Clubs serve as both a social and support group for families containing multiples. Groups sponsor activities such as clothing and toy sales, and offer resources on parenting.

■ **N. SEATTLE FAMILIES OF MULTIPLES**
937-9535
Olympic View Community Church
425 N.E. 95th St.
Seattle, WA 98115
Meetings are the second Tuesday of every month at 7:30 p.m. Activities include children's parties, summer picnics, clothing, toy and equipment exchanges, and a monthly newsletter. If you have questions or just need to talk to someone who's been there, the members of this group can help.

■ **TRIPLET CONNECTION**
(209) 474-0885
P.O. Box 99571
Stockton, CA 95209
The Triplet Connection maintains what is perhaps the world's largest data base of multiple births. Information packets and networking opportunities are available for parents who are expecting or who have had three or more babies, as well as a quarterly newsletter, and a resource list.

■ **TWIN SERVICES**
(510) 524-0863
P. O. Box 10066
Berkeley, CA 94709
They have a complete listing of services including multiple birth information and referral, parenting publications, and consultations with multiple birth experts.

■ **TWINS WORLD MAGAZINE**
(219) 627-5414
11220 St. Joe Rd.
Fort Wayne, IN 46835-9737
Dr. Brandt publishes Twins World magazine. This is a magazine for twins, parents of twins, and twinless twins. The magazine has sections on twin research studies, entertainment, social functions, and twin loss. The cost is $20 per year.

RECOMMENDED READING

Alexander, Terry Pink. *Making Room for Twins*. New York: Bantam Books, 1987.

Noble, Elizabeth. *Having Twins: A Parent's Guide to Pregnancy*. Boston: Houghton Mifflin Co., 1991.

Novotny, Pamela. *The Joy of Twins*. New York: Crown Books, 1988.

Twins Magazine
800-821-5533
P.O. Box 12045
Overland Park, KS 66282-2045

SINGLE PARENTING

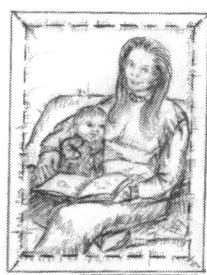

In addition to the resources listed in this chapter, hospitals, churches and synagogues also offer special workshops or support groups dealing with single parenting. Also, investigate Parents without Partners to find out more about ongoing single parenting activities.

■ APPLE PARENTING CLASS
Highline-West Seattle Mental Health Ctr.
248-8226
1010 S. 146th St.
Seattle, WA 98146
On a quarterly basis, Highline-West Seattle Mental Health Center offers a course which involves an educational presentation on parenting issues to help people cope with the stresses of parenting. This is a nonprofit parenting program for families who are having a challenging time with their children or for those simply wishing to make parenting a more fun and rewarding experience. Children are incorporated into the learning process by means of parent-child lab activities.

■ CHILDREN'S HOME SOCIETY
524-6020
3300 N.E. 65th
Seattle, WA 98115

854-0700
4338 Auburn Way N.
Auburn, WA 98002

453-5698
1240 116th Ave. N.E.
Bellevue, WA 98008
This non-profit organization provides multiple services to children and families. Single parent workshops, support groups, and counseling are offered.

■ DIVORCE LIFELINE
624-2959
This organization offers support groups for separating and divorced persons, and for children of divorce. They also provide workshops and seminars.

■ NATIONAL ORGANIZATION OF SINGLE MOTHERS

(704) 888-KIDS
P.O. Box 68
Midland, NC 28107-0068
This national organization helps members form or locate local support groups. They publish a bimonthly newsletter called SingleMOTHER.

■ PARENTS WITHOUT PARTNERS

270-7797 (Regional Office)
388-9859 (Everett)
776-5811 (S.Snohomish/N.King Cty)
440-7596 (Seattle Metro)
270-7666 (So. King County)
631-0927 (Auburn, Renton, Kent)
454-9997 (East King County)
PWP is an international nonprofit, non-sectarian education organization, devoted to the interest and welfare of single parents and their children. To be eligible, one need only be the single parent of at least one living child; custody is not a factor. An orientation meeting must be attended before joining PWP. There is a fee of approximately $30 to join. They offer social events for single parents, as well as education and referral services.

■ SINGLE PARENT NETWORK

233-1152
Dedicated to helping single parents build effective parenting and life management skills, the Single Parent Network sponsors conventions and workshops, and links individual families to area support groups. SPN's goal is to abolish the stigma and stereotypes associated with single parent families by redefining the single parent family.

■ SOLO PARENTING ALLIANCE

720-1655
139 23rd Ave. S.
Seattle, WA 98144
Solo Parenting Alliance is a grassroots, nonprofit organization created by and for solo parents to strengthen their community by promoting self-sufficiency. This group offers a unique Family Home Share program bringing together single parent families to share expenses and experiences in the same house. A resource center in Seattle's Central District and a quarterly newsletter are two other benefits of membership. The Alliance sponsors support groups and parenting classes at family support centers and other community locations.

Life Experiences...

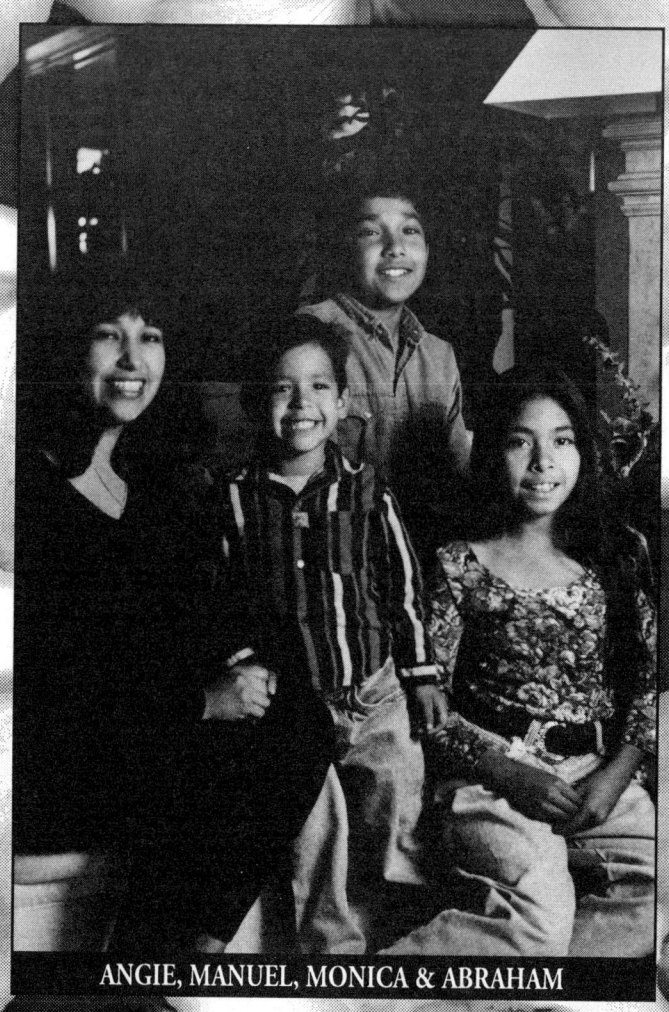

ANGIE, MANUEL, MONICA & ABRAHAM

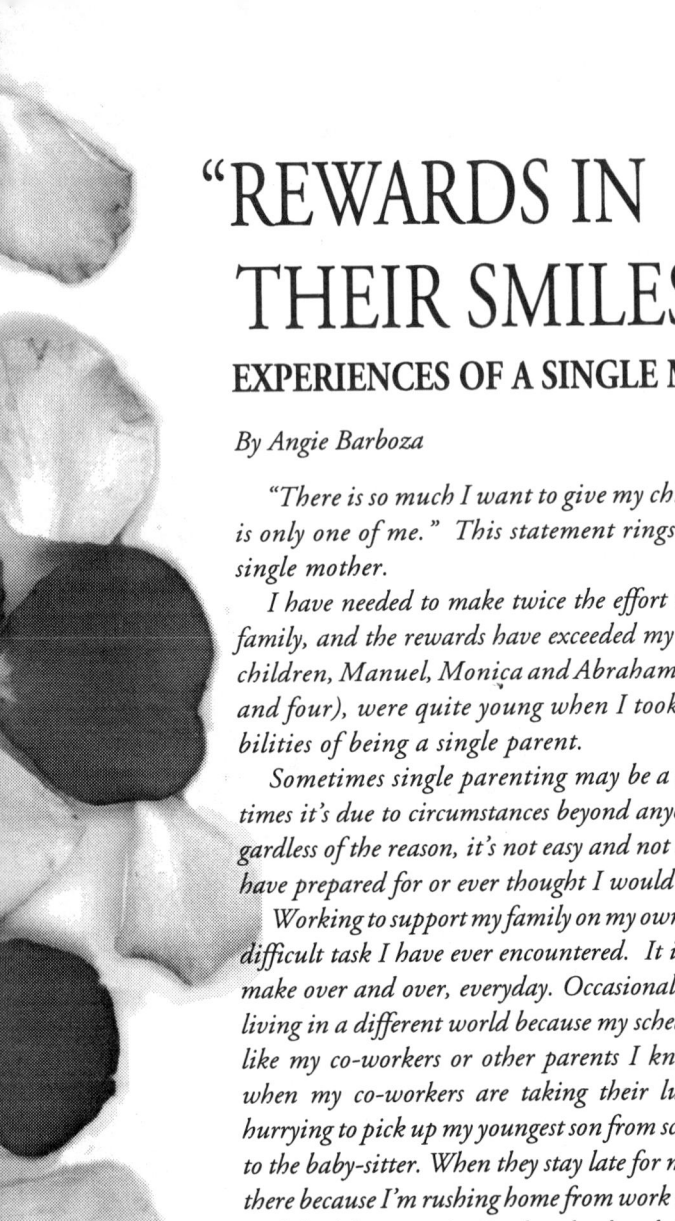

"REWARDS IN THEIR SMILES"

EXPERIENCES OF A SINGLE MOM

By Angie Barboza

"There is so much I want to give my children, and there is only one of me." This statement rings true for me as a single mother.

I have needed to make twice the effort to provide for my family, and the rewards have exceeded my expectations. My children, Manuel, Monica and Abraham (ages nine, seven and four), were quite young when I took on the responsibilities of being a single parent.

Sometimes single parenting may be a choice, and sometimes it's due to circumstances beyond anyone's control. Regardless of the reason, it's not easy and not something I could have prepared for or ever thought I would be doing.

Working to support my family on my own has been the most difficult task I have ever encountered. It is a commitment I make over and over, everyday. Occasionally, I feel like I am living in a different world because my schedule does not seem like my co-workers or other parents I know. For example, when my co-workers are taking their lunch hours, I am hurrying to pick up my youngest son from school and take him to the baby-sitter. When they stay late for meetings, I can't be there because I'm rushing home from work to get dinner ready and check homework. On the other hand, I can't always leave work to be with my kids at special school activities.

Trying to meet the needs of my work, my children and myself has proven to be a real challenge, and quite a balancing act. Somedays, it's both tiring and lonely, even with my very busy schedule. But every time I feel I have had enough and can't keep going, I get a smile or hug from my children. The help I get from my family gives me the energy and courage to go on. I have found that when sharing my experiences with other single moms, I gain advice that might help me or encouragement for the things I have accomplished. Seeking out mothers in similar situations reinforces my confidence in myself as a parent.

The good feelings about my role as a single parent come back again and again in knowing I am doing my best and that my children are learning from me. I am teaching them that facing challenges and working hard at overcoming obstacles can make them appreciate what they have even more. I see the rewards in my kids' smiles. I am proud of the family we have become, especially when they sit and talk to me about their day. Or when they are lying in their beds, looking so adorable. Or when they kiss me good-bye. When they run home from school, knowing that I am there to meet them. And when they tell their friends they can't do certain things because their mother told them so … it makes me feel proud.

This is when I feel it's working. I am doing the right thing, and all this positive influence is coming from me, just me! 🍃

BAPTISM

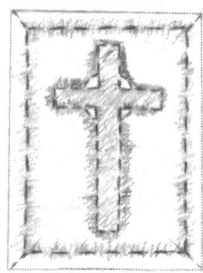

By The Reverend Dennis R. Odekirk
St. Michael's Episcopal Church

WHAT IS BAPTISM?

Baptism is the ceremony with water by which persons become members of the Christian Church—in New Testament language, "members of the Body of Christ"—and receive the life-giving gift of God's Holy Spirit. This second meaning is sometimes symbolized by the anointing of the baptismal candidate on the forehead with water or oil. This part of the ceremony is called the *christening*. Baptism signifies that we accept God's call to be a people chosen to serve God and to manifest God's goodness and love to the world. Baptism requires repentance of sin and confession of faith in Jesus Christ. Some traditions reserve baptism for those who have attained an age which allows them to be able to make a profession of personal faith. This is called *believer's baptism*. A greater number of traditions practice the baptism of infants. In this case, the commitment to repentance and a life of faith is made by the parents and godparents on behalf of the child.

✺

Baptism is the ceremony with water by which persons become members of the Christian Church.

✺

WHAT IS THE "RIGHT TIME" TO HAVE YOUR CHILD BAPTIZED?

At one time, it was thought that infants should be baptized as soon as possible after their birth. Such thinking placed special emphasis upon the baptismal ceremony as the key saving element. Without lessening the importance of the baptismal rite, there exists today a growing focus upon the development of an environment which will enable the child to be nurtured in, and to grow into, the Christian life of which baptism is only the beginning. Increasingly, families are being asked to become active members of a church community before planning a baptism. Support groups are always helpful, and no less so for Christians.

HOW DO WE CHOOSE GODPARENTS OR SPONSORS AND WHAT DO THEY DO?

Godparents (or sponsors) are persons who take on the baptismal vows of repentance and faith on behalf of the child and promise to see that their godchild is raised in that life of Christian faith and practice. Although godparents sometimes can (and do) serve as legal guardians, there is no direct connection between the two responsibilities. Godparents' responsibilities are *spiritual.* For this reason, primary consideration should be that they are, themselves, committed and active Christians who are willing to take an active role in their godchild's Christian upbringing. No special number of godparents is required.

HOW DO WE ARRANGE TO HAVE OUR CHILD BAPTIZED?

Reaching a decision as to whether or not to have a child baptized is not only an important and serious matter for the child, but also an occasion when parents can reexamine their own spiritual life and values. For many, especially with the first child, it is a time to "get back to church" following those normal unsettled years of young adulthood. "Getting back to church" is really the first step toward the baptism of a child. And so the answer to this question is: Consult your telephone directory to locate a church of your tradition or simply one that is conveniently located. Connect with the church. Make some friends there. Take some classes. Get to know the pastor. Attend a service of baptism (many are now performed as a part of the Sunday service). After that, the "arrangements" are easy.

PLACES TO PURCHASE BAPTISMAL GOWNS

The stores listed below offer a wide selection of baptismal and christening gowns. A variety of other department stores and children's clothing stores offer a smaller supply of baptismal clothing. The stores chapter notes individual stores that carry baptismal gowns.

- Baby Express
- Brat Pack
- Country Cradle
- La Preciosa

- Merry Go Round Baby News
- Nordstrom/Bon/JC Penney
- Stars
- The Tree House

JEWISH BABY-NAMING CEREMONIES

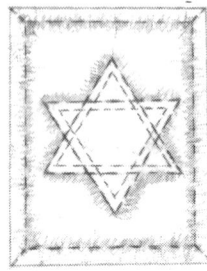

By Rabbi Simon Benzaquen

BRIT MILAH

The mitzvah of Brit Milah (ritual circumcision) was the first commandment given to the first patriarch Abraham. Circumcision is the mitzvah that the Jewish people, no matter what level of observance, still practice. Brit Milah was a covenant given to Abraham out of love and affection for him by Almighty God. This ceremony continues to be one of the foundations of the Jewish religion and has taken deep root in the soul of Jewish people. The scripture that Brit Milah is based on reads: "God then said to Abraham, As far as you are concerned, you must keep My covenant, you and your offspring throughout their generations. This is My covenant between Me and between you and your offspring that you must keep: you must circumcise every male. You shall be circumcised through the flesh of your foreskin. This shall be the mark of the covenant between Me and you." (Gen. 17:9, 10) Brit Milah, also called a Bris, takes place on the eighth day after the birth of the baby. This is mandated by Jewish law.

ﺑﻌ

Brit Milah, also called a Bris, takes place on the eighth day after the birth of the baby.

ﺑﻌ

Brit Milah is a mitzvah that everyone who is involved in any part of it becomes honored. The Mohel, a specially trained and certified expert, performs the ceremony, usually in a home environment. The sandak, who holds the baby while the circumcision is performed, and those who bring the baby into the room and out again after the ceremony and the one who holds the baby while he is being named immediately after the circumcision are all considered honorees of the day. The ceremony ends with a festive meal.

The Brit Milah ceremony performed by a Mohel takes literally only seconds to complete. The infant experiences pain that lasts only seconds, similar to that of a routine immunization. Just as there may be some swelling that lasts a few days from an immunization, there may be some minimal discomfort for a comparable length of time following a Brit Milah.

PIDYON HABEN
REDEMPTION OF THE FIRST BORN

This is a ceremony that fulfills the Biblical obligation (Numbers 18:15-16, Exodus 13:2) to redeem every Jewish male child who is a first born to his mother, when he becomes a month old. On the 31st day, (or after when the 31st day falls on Sabbath or a holiday) his father must redeem him by giving five silver shekels to a Kohen (Priest), a descendent of the priestly family of Aaron. In today's currency, five silver dollars is adequate to fulfill this commandment.

By slaying every Egyptian first born with the last plague in Egypt, God laid claim to every Jewish first born. All this is to teach man to dedicate his very first achievements, the culmination of much yearning and sacrifice, to God, and to recognize that even a first born, like first fruits, are a gift from God and should be dedicated to His service.

The redemption ceremony is done in the form of a dialogue between the father and the Kohen (Priest), thus increasing the love of the father for his son, and culminating with the Kohen invoking the priestly benediction on the child. Like the circumcision ceremony, the redemption is celebrated with a festive meal.

ZEBED HABAT
NAMING A BABY GIRL

The naming of a girl traditionally takes place in the synagogue or at home, when the mother has recovered and feels up to joining in the ceremony. In the synagogue it is held usually after birth, at a time when the Torah scrolls are read, namely Monday, Thursday, Sabbath or Rosh Hodesh (the beginning of the lunar month.) At that time the father is given the honor to be called up to the reading of the Torah scroll. After the reading, the baby is given her name and a special blessing is recited which includes prayers for the recovery of the mother and the hope of her parents to see her in turn at her wedding, as a mother of a family, with all God's blessings to live to a healthy and ripe old age.

When it is held in the home, the child is brought in on a pillow either by a young relative dressed as a junior bride or by the parents. Special verses 2:14 and 6:9 from the Song of Songs by King Solomon are sung by those present to welcome the newborn daughter.

Then a special blessing and prayer is recited by the Rabbi for the mother and baby, and the naming of the girl takes place. Following, a psalm is recited and the formal ceremony is followed by a festive meal amidst singing and joy.

❧ RESOURCES ❧

■ CERTIFIED MOHELS

Rabbi Simon Benzaquen
721-2275 or 723-3028

Dr. Ze'ev Young
228-4450

■ JEWISH TRANSCRIPT
441-4553
2031 3rd Ave.
Seattle, WA 98121
The Jewish Transcript is a local paper which provides comprehensive information regarding the Jewish community.

TEEN PREGNANCY

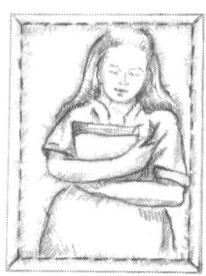

Every day hundreds of Seattle teenagers discover they are pregnant. If you or someone you know is a pregnant teen, you'll be glad to know that there are many local resources dedicated to meeting your needs.

■ **CAMPFIRE TEEN PARENTS PROGRAM**
461-8550
8511 15th Ave. N.E.
Seattle, WA 98115
Campfire holds three-day retreats twice a year to Vashon Island for teen parents and pregnant teens. Seminars are also offered on leadership, employment, and education opportunities.

■ **CATHOLIC COMMUNITY SERVICES**
323-6336
100 23rd Ave. S.
Seattle, WA 98144
This agency provides housing, health, and referral services for pregnant and parenting teens.

■ **CENTRAL AREA MOTIVATION PROJECT**
329-4111
722 18th Ave.
Seattle, WA 98122
This organization offers a mentoring program where pregnant women and new mothers are matched with community volunteers who provide guidance and support. CAMP services are for residents of central and southeast Seattle.

■ **CENTRAL AREA YOUTH ASSOCIATION**
322-6640
119 23rd Ave.
Seattle, WA 98122
CAYA offers teen parent housing for girls 14-17 years old. Program participation requires a 2- to 3-year commitment.

■ **CHILDREN'S HOME SOCIETY**
322-8918
339 22nd Ave. E.
Seattle, WA 98112
Single moms, 14-18, are housed in a foster home setting, work on self-esteem and nutrition, and attend weekly parenting classes to encourage the best possible future for themselves and their children.

■ **COLUMBIA HEALTH CENTER**
296-4650
4400 37th Ave. S.
Seattle, WA 98118
Medical exams and tests, counseling, family planning, adoption referrals, and obstetrical services are provided on a sliding scale as part of Columbia Health Center's confidential services.

■ **DSHS FIRST STEPS PROGRAM HEALTHY MOTHERS, HEALTHY BABIES**
800-322-2588
Call the toll-free number for more information on state medical and support services for teens who are pregnant or new parents. Services include child care, education, financial assistance, case management, transportation, and family planning.

■ **EASTSIDE HEALTHY START**
869-6658
This family support program offers voluntary, home-based support services to young families with a mother 21 years or younger who is pregnant or parenting her first infant. The program serves young parents in Bellevue, Bothell, Issaquah, Kirkland, Mercer Island, Redmond, Skykomish, and Woodinville. Parents are provided support, information, and referrals to help them make healthy choices

for themselves and their families. This early intervention program is provided until the child reaches school age. There are no fees charged. Services include social/support groups (including child care and transportation to the group) and linkage to community resources. Eastside Healthy Start is a joint program of Northshore Youth and Family Services, Youth Eastside Services, Friends of Youth, Children's Home Society, and Seattle-King County's Public Health.

■ **FRIENDS OF YOUTH**
392-6367
414 Front St. N.
Issaquah, WA 98027
Eight-week long parenting classes are offered quarterly in Systematic Training for Early Childhood Issues, counseling, teen parent support, and a Teen Shelter Line are provided by this organization.

■ **GROUP HEALTH EASTSIDE HOSPITAL**
883-5151
2700 152nd N.E.
Redmond, WA 98052
The hospital offers a teen pregnancy program with prenatal and postnatal support groups.

■ **KING COUNTY WORK TRAINING PROGRAM**
296-5220
506 2nd Ave., Ste. 305
Seattle, WA 98104
Pregnant teens and teen parents (ages 16-21) who live in King County, outside of Seattle, can participate in an integrated program of employment services, medical care, parenting training, counseling, and case management.

■ **MEDINA CHILDREN'S SERVICES**
461-4520
P.O. Box 22638
Seattle, WA 98122-0638
This interagency group offers school-site classes and GED assistance, as well as counseling and crisis intervention at no charge for parents 14-18 years old. Child care is provided for participants. They offer a program for teen fathers called Project Mister and a program called TAPP (Teenage Pregnancy, Parenting, and Prevention) at four Seattle locations.

■ **PROGRAM FOR EARLY PARENT SUPPORT (PEPS)**
547-8570
4649 Sunnyside Ave. N.
Seattle, WA 98103
PEPS offers support groups for teen parents and their children, birth to 3. Groups are held at schools, community centers, and private homes throughout the community.

■ **TEEN PARENT CHILDCARE HOTLINE**
329-3481
1265 S. Main St. #210
Seattle, WA 98144
This organization, funded by the city of Seattle, provides free assistance to teen parents in finding child care so they can attend school.

■ **TEEN PARENT WIC PROGRAM**
296-4627
Teen parents are considered to be at nutritional risk under the guidelines of the Women, Infants and Children (WIC) program. They can receive vouchers for food, as well as nutrition education and other services.

■ **TEENS LOVING THEIR CHILDREN**
258-9211
Everett YMCA
2720 Rockfeller
Everett, WA 98208
This support group focuses on pregnant and parenting issues and community services geared to teens. Child care is provided on site. The program is sponsored by Deaconess Children's Services, Everett YMCA, Camp Fire, and Family Opportunities Council.

■ **YOUNG PARENTS SUPPORT GROUP**
364-7930
North Seattle Family Center
13540 Lake City Way N.E. #5
Seattle, WA 98125
Come together to share your stories, ideas and opinions while giving and receiving support from each other. Volunteer facilitators lead the drop-in group which is continuous throughout the year. The program is free, and free child care is available for participants.

■ **YOUTH FAIR CHANCE AMERICORP RESOURCE MOTHER'S PROGRAM**
Southwest Community Career Center
932-7901
6335 35th Ave. S.W.
Seattle, WA 98126
This program offers support services to promote and protect the health and well-being of teen parents and their infant children. It serves teen parents and young adults, ages 14-29, who live in West Seattle, including High Point, Parklake Homes, Roxbury Village, White Center, and Southpark. Services include referrals, advocacy, outreach, emergency food and clothing assistance. Also available through the Career Center are G.E.D., high school reentry, and ESL classes.

Life Experiences...

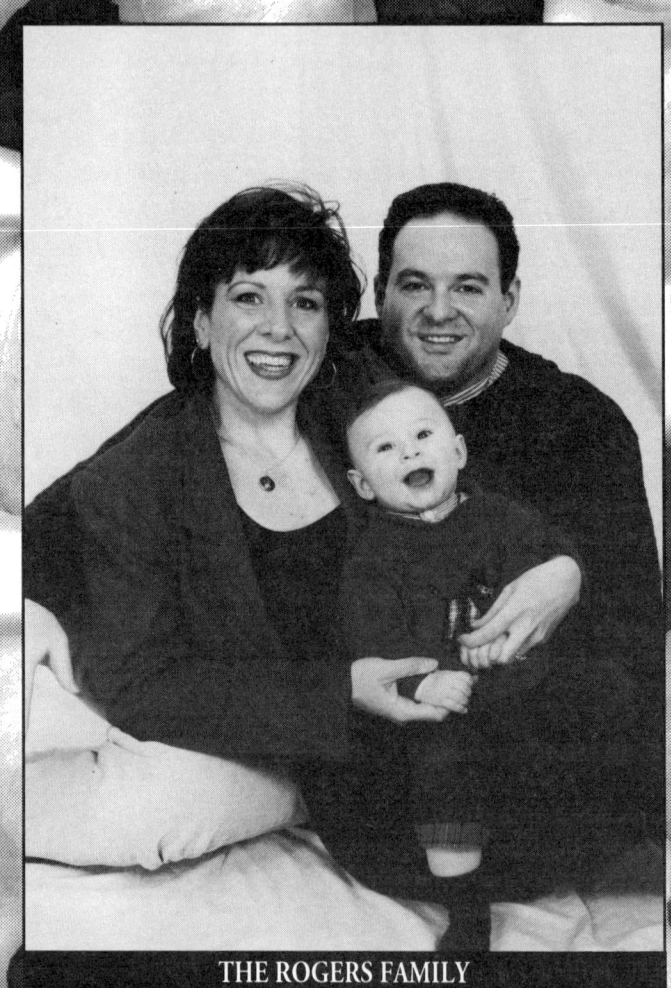

THE ROGERS FAMILY

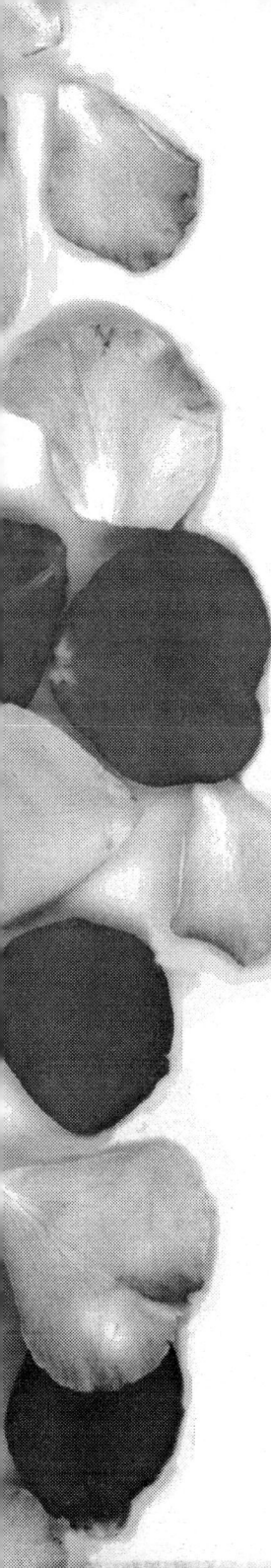

"NEW WINDOWS OF LOVE"

By C. Rogers

Ten years ago, when my husband and I married, we were just out of college and had endless energy for our careers and our new life with each other. We always knew we wanted a family, but had strong feelings about where we wanted to be regarding our finances and our relationship with one another. As a couple we enjoyed setting a well-planned course for our future and then worked together to achieve the desired outcome.

Our plan was to wait at least five years and then spend a short and enjoyable time trying to conceive. Although our plans were somewhat calculated, they were nonetheless filled with hopes and dreams of sharing ourselves with our child. After trying unsuccessfully to conceive for over one year we found that all the best laid plans could not overcome fertility problems. We had absolutely no control, or so was our thinking at that time. Upon further investigation, we found that with the help of in vitro fertilization we could conceive. This route is an extremely viable option for many couples. It is also not the one we chose to take.

My husband and I had been Christians for a long time, but I must say that all of our self-reliance left little space for God in our lives. This all was about to change. Not knowing what to do next, we were brought to our knees. Soon we were praying about and discussing adoption. We examined our reasons for wanting a family in the first place. What we found is that our motivation to have a child had very little, if anything, to do with genetics. Our desires had everything to do with the love we had within us. Feeling completely comfortable with adoption, we went about the process of researching all the variables. We read books, we sent out questionnaires to agencies, we went to adoption forums, we analyzed everything about every option.

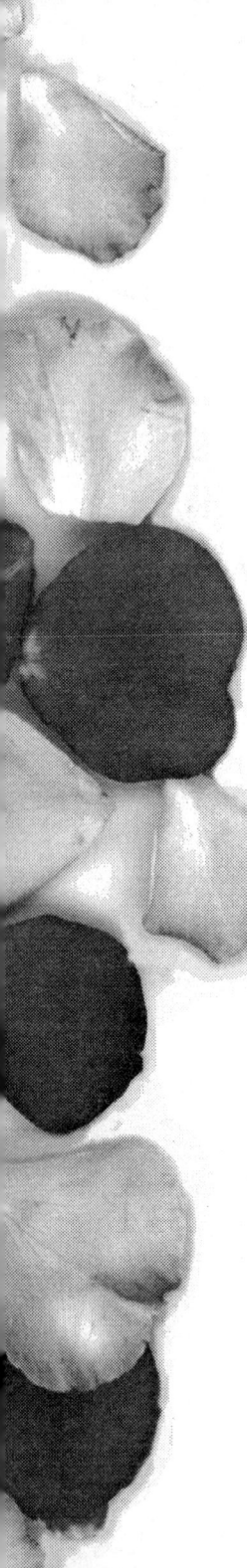

Our decision was to enlist the help of a private Christian agency. This was the beginning of the biggest adventure of our lives. There was money to consider; there were family and friends to educate about the challenges we were about to undertake; and then there was the start of the process itself— lots of interviews and paperwork and referrals. To say adoption dominated our lives would be an understatement.

After all the probing and interviewing our agency and the state requires to qualify us, we started the hard part: the waiting. Throughout this waiting, our countenance was changing. We actively sought God's purpose versus our own. We also learned compassion for the difficult decisions birth parents face when choosing adoption. This time of waiting was painfully long, yet completely productive.

It was only about four months until we were notified that a birthmother had chosen us. When we met her we had immediate rapport. We followed her pregnancy for three months, when she changed her mind. We were so disappointed; we thought this was definitely the perfect match. Amazingly, two weeks later we were chosen by another birthmother. This time the birthfather was also involved. They were such a nice couple and so determined to make a good decision for their unborn child. We were scared to make an emotional commitment to this couple for fear of disappointment. We felt as if we were on an emotional roller coaster. We were advised to approach this situation with concern for the birthparents. This is what we did. We spent our energy praying for this unborn child, and ministering to the needs of the birthparents. As the due date approached, the birthparents became more committed to their decision. We slowly became excited. We thought, "This is really going to happen." We wallpapered the baby's room. We chose names. We started making plans, all sorts of exciting and wondrous plans. We couldn't help loving this baby. Then came the news the baby was born and the birthmother had decided to parent. Just conveying this experience is painful. I can only say this experience has been equated to the death of a child.

Over the next four months we focused on finding God's purpose in this pain. Why were we having to suffer not one loss,

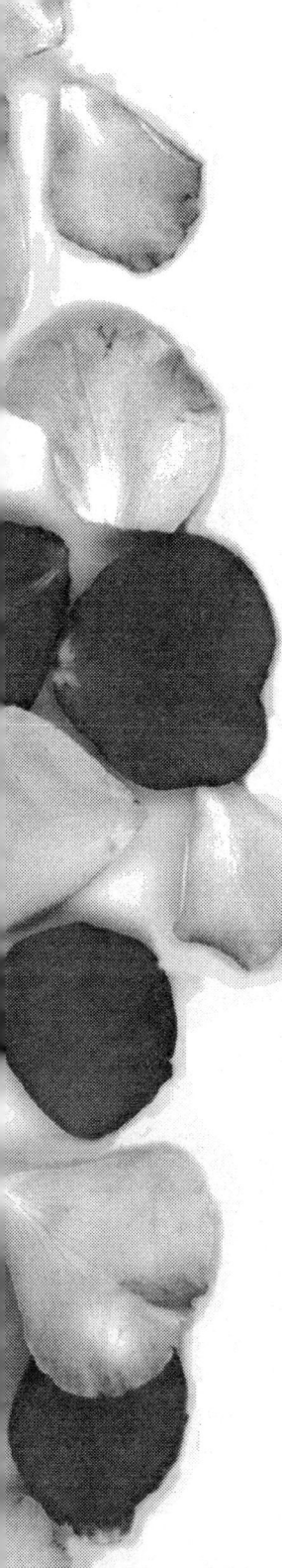

but two? We were experiencing all the stages of grief. My husband and I found solace in good friends and family. Several weeks after our loss we found out that the baby we were supposed to adopt had a hole in its heart and that the birthmother may have lied about her involvement with drugs. In a strange way we took comfort in seeing God's protection of us. We refocused on each other and tried to have fun again. We continued waiting, but our intensity waned.

Just when we felt we had been left in the valley of darkness forever, we were chosen again. Once again we were excited, feeling sure this was the one. Our birthparents were perfect. We felt a peace the moment we met them. They were young and so honest about themselves and their circumstances. I say we were peaceful about them, but we were still scared. It was impossible to completely relax. We met several times in the weeks to follow. The more we learned about our birth family, the more fondness we felt toward them. We knew it would be very important to our family in the future to be able to share with our child the wonderful people who helped bring him into this world.

Our son was born a long six weeks after our initial meeting. We received the call early in the morning. "Your son was born at midnight the night before." This was the most exciting moment of my life. We rushed to the hospital. First we visited with our birthmother and her family. She was doing fine and looking forward to getting out of the hospital. There were tears of joy and sadness. Within 30 minutes I was holding our beautiful, handsome son. Motherhood—what an amazing feeling! It was as though all of the time spent waiting for this moment melted away in that instant. New windows of love were flying open in my heart. My husband's face had a joy and softness that radiated.

We learned through this incomparable experience that we are not to have control; God is. We learned that there is a perfect plan for our lives. These were hard lessons for us, but well worth the work. Our son is four months old now and we love him more each day.

Would we do it all over again? You bet. ❧

ADOPTION

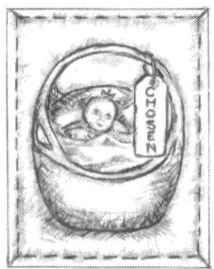

By Mark Demaray, J.D.

The adoption process in the State of Washington is governed in part by state statutes and regulations. The current system allows three basic but distinct types of adoption. The first type involves the adoption of a child in the custody of the State of Washington Department of Social and Health Services (DSHS), usually through the foster care system. The second type is adoption through licensed child placing agencies. The third type is through an attorney or doctor, commonly referred to as private placement or independent adoption. Each type of adoption may have different procedures followed, yet they all accomplish the same result: the termination of parental rights of the birth parents, either voluntary or involuntary, and subsequent recognition of the child as a legal member of the adoptive family.

Washington law provides that any person who is legally competent and is 18 years of age or older may be an adoptive parent. However, prior to a child being placed in an adoptive home, the parent must have successfully completed a pre-placement report or home study as it is more commonly called. Depending the type of adoption a parent chooses, the home study may be conducted by one of four entities or individuals: a licensed adoption agency, DSHS, an individual approved by the court or a qualified salaried court employee. In the latter two cases, certain minimum qualifications and training are required to perform a home study.

🙠

The current system allows three basic but distinct types of adoption.

🙠

A HOME STUDY

A home study is a written document that provides relevant information about the person(s) who wish to adopt a child. The home study includes an investigation of the home, family life, health, facilities and resources of the adoptive parent(s). A criminal background check is also included.

The home study is necessary for any person who wishes to adopt a child. The court will not grant custody to adoptive parents without a favorable home study report.

TERMINATION OF PARENTAL RIGHTS

Before any child can be adopted, that child must be "legally free" from the custody of the birth parents. This can take place in two basic ways. The parental rights of the birth parent(s) may be terminated involuntarily or against their will. This usually happens when the state steps in because of concern for the child's safety and well-being, perhaps in an abusive or neglectful home situation, and removes the child from the birth family's home and places the child in foster care. If the court finds after a trial that the birth parent is unfit and terminates the parental rights, the state then becomes the legal custodian of the child.

Independent adoptions usually don't involve involuntary termination of parental rights. Instead the birth parents usually consent and agree to give up their parental rights.

CONSENT TO ADOPTION

In any Washington adoption, the rules, procedures, and form of a consent to adoption by a birth parent are similar. A consent to adoption can be signed by a birth parent before or after the child's birth, at the option of the birth parent, and must be witnessed by someone of the birth parent's choosing. However, once signed, the consent to adoption form has no force or legal effect unless and until it is presented and approved by the court. It also cannot be presented to the court for review and approval until a minimum of 48 hours has passed since the child's birth, or since the time the document was signed, whichever is later.

And, until the court accepts and approves of the consent, the birth parent has the right to revoke or take back the consent and stop the adoption. After the parental rights have been terminated, however, a birth parent cannot revoke his order of consent to adoption unless they can show some type of fraud in the consent procedure, coercion or duress, or mental incompetency at the time the consent was signed. Even those three grounds, which are generally very difficult to prove, cannot be raised more than one year after the consent is accepted by the court. (If the child is American Indian there are certain limited exceptions to this rule.)

FINALIZATION OF THE ADOPTION

Once the parental rights of the birth parents have been terminated by court order, the court will grant temporary custody to the adoptive parent(s) and appoint them as the child's legal guardian pending further order of the court in an independent adoption. In an agency adoption, the agency is generally granted legal custody of the child. Washington's adoption laws require a post-placement or follow-up investigation be done, usually by the case worker or agency who performed the pre-placement report. The purpose of this report is to make sure that the adoptive family and child are adjusting well to each other, that there are no problems or concerns, and usually involves a recommendation to the court as to whether or not the finalization of the adoption would be in the child's best interest. State law currently requires that the post-placement report be completed within 60 days of the child's placement.

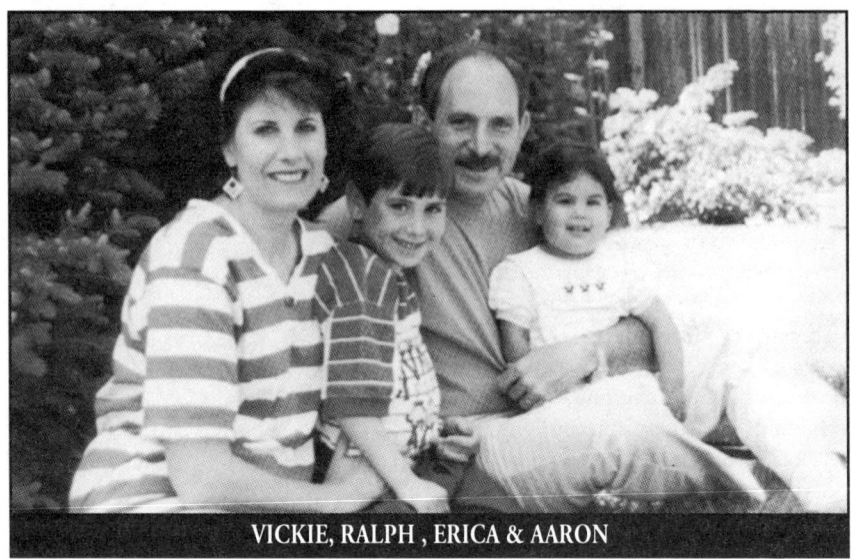

VICKIE, RALPH , ERICA & AARON

IF YOU CHOOSE TO ADOPT

This article only briefly touches on the different procedures which take place in an adoption and is only intended to be used as a general reference tool. There are many other circumstances, such as if the birth parent(s) are under 18, interstate adoptions, birth father's rights, American Indian adoptions, and much more that have specific procedures and laws that may vary from the text provided. If you choose to adopt, contact as many resources as possible to help you fully understand the adoption process and to determine the type of adoption that is right for you.

The above article was written by Mark Demaray, J.D.

A PRIVATE ADOPTION STORY

Vickie and Ralph, along with their son Aaron, went through a labor of love to add another child to their family. After four years of trying unsuccessfully to have a second child, they believed adoption to be their best alternative.

The couple says that, for them, there were three keys to successful adoption:

❶ Participation in a support group
❷ Use of the expertise of an attorney or agency
❸ Listening and trusting yourself and your intuition

Without the help of Vickie's support group, they would have found the adoption process much more difficult. The support group did far more than give her a shoulder to cry on and an ear for listening. The infertility group also served as a guide, with participants sharing an abundance of knowledge.

Vickie and Ralph strongly believe that going to a private adoption attorney was the best route for them. They contacted an attorney who specializes in adoption and works alongside his wife, who is a counselor. The couple had also adopted children of their own.

Adopting a child can be quite costly, ranging from $5,000 to more than $15,000 in legal fees and the birth mother's medical expenses. Vickie and Ralph learned that the more they were willing to do themselves, the less the lawyer needed to do—and less lawyer time equalled less cost.

Fortunately for Vickie and Ralph, the wait was not long. They began to send out letters in June, and they learned of their daughter in December. It is said that the wait for a Caucasian baby is the longest. There are also other factors that come into play. When going through a private adoption process, the final decision is the birth mother's; she will choose parents who fully meet her expectations. She may determine this through the initial letter of introduction (which is not unlike a resume), by the couple's photo, through a phone conversation, or during a face-to-face meeting. There is no way for the adopting parents to know exactly what the birth mother is looking for. It is crucial to listen to your intuition and trust yourself.

It is also important to communicate openly and honestly with all the involved parties. Vickie and Ralph both felt an immediate connection with the birth mother, and they knew once they met her that "this was it." They had talked to other birth mothers, but during these conversations there were too many questions and too many obstacles. And they knew in the long run that it would not work out. Throughout this process Vickie kept reiterating: "The more open and honest we are, the better. Build trust."

Vickie wrote down a list of questions to ask a birth mother if and when one called. She knew that she would be nervous and that having the questions in writing would help keep her focused. A sample of these questions:

- Birth mother's name?
- Her city and state?
- Her phone number?
- Her age?
- How far along in pregnancy/expected due date?
- Is she married?
- Has she given up children for adoption before?
- Does the birth father know about the pregnancy? Will he sign a consent form for the baby to be adopted?
- Does she have medical insurance? Is she on public assistance?
- Does she have a job?
- Is she living on her own or with a family?

This story has a happy ending. They talked with the birth mother by phone. As soon as they spoke with the birth mother, they immediately made arrangements to meet in person. Since the birth mother was not fluent in English, they brought along an interpreter. "We instantly had this rapport," recalls Vickie. The birth mother actually came and moved into their home for three weeks before the birth of the baby girl. Vickie was there for the birth. She got to hold her baby daughter, Erica, immediately. After the baby was born, the birth mother stayed for one week with Vickie's mother and they, too, became very close. She became like part of the family. They still continue to write and send pictures to each other.

Now they are a family of four. They love their little girl with the same intensity and passion that they have for their genetic son. When asked about bonding, Vickie said with a smile and twinkle in her eye that it began immediately. As their daughter grows, they want her to know about her birth mother. And Erica will always know how much she is loved by all of them.

ADOPTION THROUGH A LICENSED AGENCY

The role of the licensed adoption agency is to provide services to all parties in an adoption. The guiding notion of agency-based services is an emphasis on serving the best interests of the child.

The public adoption agency in Washington State is the Department of Social and Health Services. Parents are trained and licensed to provide foster care for children in state custody. From there, fostering can move into a legal adoption. There are sometimes opportunities for adoptive parents and birth parents to exchange information. Most of the children in state foster care are aged beyond infancy and have special medical, emotional or behavioral needs.

Private agencies also arrange special needs adoptions, again, most usually on a foster/adopt basis. The fees for special needs adoptions are minimal, and there are sometimes subsidies available to help with any ongoing and/or extraordinary expenses.

Private adoption agencies also place infants. Typically, the woman or couple who wish to plan an adoption for a child select adoptive parents from biographical information. The sets of parents may choose to meet before the placement, and may continue to be in contact as the child grows.

Once a match is made birth parents sign papers terminating their legal rights as parents. At least 48 hours after the birth, the papers are presented to court, severing the legal relationship between genetic parents and infant. The custody of the child is transferred to the child placing agency.

The adoptive parents undergo a home study or pre-placement report done by their agency social worker, usually long before the baby is born. The result of the home study is a document submitted by the court terminating birth parent rights and endorsing prospective adopters' decision to adopt. After the agency transfers the custody of the child to the adoptive parents. A period of post-placement supervision follows, culminating in a document that again goes to court. At that point the adoptive parents finalize the adoption.

The fee for adopting an infant through an agency generally ranges from $8,000 to more than $20,000. Each agency charges different fees and follows its own selection process.

Some adoption agencies only handle adoptions within the United States, while others work overseas as well.

❧ RESOURCES ❧

■ **ADOPTION INFORMATION
SERVICES**
325-9500
Information about adoption and agencies is available at this number. Leave a message on the answering machine and an adoptive parent will return your call.

■ **ADOPTION RESOURCE
CENTER**
524-6020
Children's Home Society of Washington
3300 N.E. 65th St.
Seattle, WA 98115
This resource center offers a variety of services designed to assist those whose lives are touched by adoption. Information, education, support and counseling are available, as well as training and consultation for professionals. They offer a resource line and data bank of services for special needs adoptive families post-placement, as well as a book store stocking hard-to-find adoption titles. The Center does not place children for adoption. It's designed to be an objective source of information and education for people interested in adoption and offers the area's only staff of psychotherapists who specialize in adoption issues.

Many workshops and courses are offered at the center throughout the year. They include Adoption: A Lifelong Process, Intercultural Adoption, Sharing the Birth, Adoption for Gay and Lesbian People, Childbirth Education for Prospective Birth Parents, and more. Fees depend on services provided. Ongoing support groups are also held, including Birth Parent Support Group, Multi-Ra-

cial Family Group, Support Group for Gay and Lesbian Parents, Adoptive Parent's Support Group, and The Kid's Group.

■ **AMERICANS ADOPTING
ORPHANS**
524-5437
800-467-7426
12345 Lake City Way N.E., Ste. 2001
Seattle, WA 98125
This agency offers assistance with adopting children from China. After adopting two children from China, the owners began this business as a way to share the knowledge they gained from the experience as well as to help all the children they had to leave behind. The agency is licensed by the State of Washington and accredited by the People's Republic of China. Their program is unique in that they make it a point to have parents really participate in the process so that it becomes "their adoption." They allow parents to do as much or as little of the work as they want as they feel it is empowering to conquer the bureaucratic obstacles to reach one's child—not to mention the fact that it saves the prospective parents money when they do the work themselves. As an added bonus, the agency distributes a newsletter to interested parties and holds monthly support group meetings for parents wishing to adopt.

■ BETHANY CHRISTIAN
   SERVICES
367-4604
19936 Ballinger Way N.E., Ste. D
Seattle, WA 98155
This agency offers complete pre- and post-placement services to families and individuals interested in adoption and provides orientation and training for people interested in domestic, international, and special needs adoptions. Through their "Partners in Placement" program, Bethany Christian Services is also able to assist in adoptions where a birth mother has already independently chosen an adoptive family for her child and in certain situations, can place a birth mother in a licensed "Shepherding Home" as an added service.

■ CATHOLIC COMMUNITY
   SERVICES
323-6336
100 23rd Ave. S.
Seattle, WA 98144
The agency provides complete pre- and post-placement services to families and individuals interested in adoption. They provide orientation and training for people interested in special needs, international, and domestic adoptions. Classes and training are included in the cost of the home study.

■ JEWISH FAMILY SERVICE
461-3240
1601 16th Ave.
Seattle, WA 98122
This agency provides many different services focused on the Jewish community, including licensed adoption services.

■ LDS BIRTH PARENT
   PROGRAM
624-3393 or 228-0074
220 S. 3rd Pl.
Renton, WA 98055
This program is operated by the Church of Jesus Christ of Latter Day Saints and offers free counseling, information, referral, and other support services for girls and women with unplanned pregnancies. They also offer adoption placement for church members.

■ LUTHERAN SOCIAL SERVICES
672-6009
6920 220th St. S.W.
Mountlake Terrace, WA 98043
They provide counseling for women with unplanned pregnancies, and adoption planning and placement for infants and special needs children. Open adoption is available and services are customized to meet individual needs.

■ MEDINA CHILDREN'S
   SERVICES
461-4520
123 16th Ave.
Seattle, WA 98122
Medina Children's Services provides free counseling to pregnant women and their partners. They also offer special programs for families adopting older children, disabled children, African-American, Native American and biracial children of any age, and Caucasian infants.

■ NEW HOPE CHILD AND FAMILY AGENCY

363-1800
2611 N.E. 125th #146
Seattle, WA 98125

This agency provides counseling for expectant mothers, birth fathers, and families considering adoption. They provide a support group and residential facility for pregnant mothers. Adoption services for prospective adoptive parents are offered.

■ NORTHWEST ADOPTION EXCHANGE

292-0082
800-927-9411
1809 7th Ave., Ste. 409
Seattle, WA 98101

This agency specializes in special needs adoptions. They not only facilitate adoptions but also give information on a wide range of adoption issues, and advocate for and develop projects to expand support services for families throughout the adoption process. They also provide consultation, training, and technical assistance to adoption agencies, caseworkers, and adoptive parent groups.

■ ONE CHURCH, ONE CHILD

723-6224
4412 S. Myrtle St.
Seattle, WA 98118

This organization recruits prospective African American foster and adoptive parents for children waiting for placement throughout the state. They also provide training and seek to recruit at least one family from every church congregation to adopt or foster parent a child.

■ OPEN ADOPTION & FAMILY SERVICES

723-1011
P.O. Box 18795
Seattle, WA 98118

Open Adoption and Family Services provides a full range of counseling and adoption services, including home studies, preplacement adoption reports, seminars on adoption, support groups for birth and adoptive families and ongoing research. They are a licensed child placing agency in Washington and Oregon. Services to birth parents are free, as is counseling for expectant parents on pregnancy options. There is no arbitrary screening of prospective adoptive parents based on age, religion, marital status, gender, etc. Birth parents choose an adoptive family for their children.

■ PLANNED PARENTHOOD

Seattle: 328-7700 or 328-7738
Bellevue: 747-1051
Everett: 339-3389
2211 E. Madison
Seattle, WA 98112

Planned Parenthood provides comprehensive family planning services, referral for adoption, family counseling, birth control exams and supplies.

■ **POLISH ADOPTION
PROGRAM**
283-7092
3 Crockett St., Ste. H
Seattle, WA 98109
e-mail address:
72754,3144@compu-serv.com
This agency offers assistance in adopting
children from Poland. They offer two
avenues to adoption: first, allow the agency
to handle all aspects of the adoption, or
second, to handle the adoption oneself
using this service as an information resource. Those opting for the second option can purchase a manual through this
agency that directs parents through the
steps necessary for adoption and, for an
hourly fee, parents can request consulting
help as needed.

■ **WORLD ASSOCIATION FOR
CHILDREN AND PARENTS
(WACAP)**
575-4550
315 S. 2nd
Renton, WA 98055
This is a licensed nonprofit adoption
agency that specializes in the placement
of infants, special needs children, and
children from overseas. They offer pre-
and post-adoption counseling, classes for
adoptive parents, and free evening lectures for prospective adoptive parents.

ADOPTION ATTORNEYS

In Washington, as well as nationally, in excess of 60% of all newborn
placements of children born in this country are placed through independent or
private placement means, not through an adoption agency. The following
attorneys are members of the American Academy of Adoption Attorneys.

■ **RITA BENDER**
623-6501
1301 Fifth Ave., Ste. 3401
Seattle, WA 98101

■ **MICHELE GENTRY HINZ**
682-4000
1420 5th Avenue #3650
Seattle, WA 98101

■ **MARK M. DEMARAY**
682-4000
1420 Fifth Ave., Ste. 3650
Seattle, WA 98101-2387

■ **ALBERT LIRHUS**
728-5858
2200 Sixth Ave., Ste. 1122
Seattle, WA 98121

■ **ERIC GUSTAFSON**
(509) 248-7220
222 North 3rd St.
Yakima, WA 98901

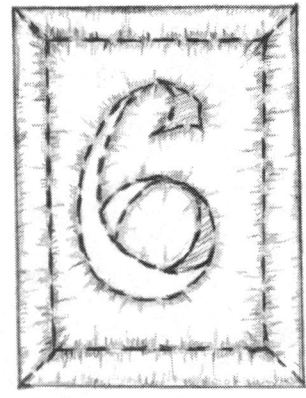

TAKING
CARE
OF
YOURSELF
AND
YOUR
FAMILY

KEEPING YOUR RELATIONSHIP ALIVE

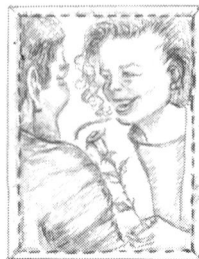

FROM A MOTHER'S POINT OF VIEW

By Kari E. Hazen

THE BALANCING ACT

Friday night arrives again. A week full of demands, deadlines and stress is coming to a close. I think I saw the father of my children about five hours this week if I was lucky. Now, another round of demands and duties arrive for the weekend...laundry, bills, and picking up this house. We, my husband and I, will take our daughters to the park, read stories, and give them the love and encouragement they need. Balancing the day-to-day responsibilities of work, home, and children, we search to find time for one another. And this, at times, can be challenging.

Having a good relationship, and children at the same time, may be difficult for today's parents. Difficult, yet very possible once you come to terms with the conflicting feelings that say: "I want to be a good parent" and at the same time "I want our relationship to stay strong and intimate...and even a little spontaneous."

Some may laugh at the idea that there is even the slightest possibility the two roles are compatible. Others will cheer, pop the champagne bottle and say yes! I too believe this is possible. Not only possible, but also extremely important. I think we all want a life filled with love from our significant other and love from our children. The real question lies in how to make it work for us.

And as a woman, at times this is not easy. No, let's face it, most of the time it's not, I repeat, not easy. Many of us were raised in families where our mothers kept a clean house, helped with science projects and were there to greet us when we stepped off the school bus. No parenting task was too difficult for our mothers.

Today, sixty percent of mothers with children under the age of five are working. It is nearly impossible to try to emulate our role models. As working mothers, we are faced with many factors limiting the amount of time we really have with our children. We hear many working moms say if they can spend three hours a day with their child they think it's great! Once home, you eat dinner (if you are lucky), go to Little League practice, pick up your daughter from ballet, help with homework and finally put the children to bed. Then, after all your parenting duties, you may still find an hour's worth of household chores to accomplish before you can call it quits for the day. A busy schedule leaves little time for long, fulfilling conversations in a relationship. Many times, depending on your jobs, it is difficult to have much energy to even start a conversation, let alone carry one on for more than five minutes.

Keeping a relationship growing is not only difficult for working moms, but for moms who stay at home as well. Most of their satisfaction and daily interaction comes from their children and what is done around the house. Often, stay-at-home moms find they don't receive praise from anyone other than themselves for what they accomplish. No one says, "Gee Mom, the bathtub looks great" or, "Thanks for taking Jason to the doctor." When you stay home, many times it is just what is expected of you. You are giving to your child and your family in a way that no one else can. The rewards must come from within, unless you are in a relationship with a husband who truly appreciates what you are doing. For those moms who do not receive any feedback, often resentment and anger can build up, making it difficult to achieve intimacy in a relationship.

PRIORITIZE YOUR RELATIONSHIP

Whether you are a working mom or a stay-at-home mom, it is clear you are giving a lot to your children. It is something that is instinctive and that moms do well. Because we may give so much to our families, it makes it that much more challenging to give to the relationship that started the family. So, how do we make our relationship a priority again? By simply doing that...making it a priority. Pick it up from the bottom of your to-do list and move it to the top. Make a commitment to your relationship again. Focus on the time, or lack of time, you're spending together and decide to make it better. To many, it may sound too simple; yet there are some simple, small steps that can be taken to get the relationship rekindled again. Set up strategies that work for both of you. Here are some practical ideas that many mothers suggest to help keep your relationship strong. Take a look:

- Try to get a baby-sitter at least once a month. It doesn't matter what you do, just that you leave the house and spend time with one another. If you like to dine out, consider purchasing an entertainment book. This allows you to eat out affordably. It also gives you quiet time with one another plus the opportunity to talk.

- Take a walk. This may keep your children occupied and gives you a chance to talk with little interruption. Walking also releases stress and provides good exercise.

- Try a vacation alone. This one is difficult for most moms, especially the first trip. Yet, once you enjoy a trip away and alone, you will find how good it is for your relationship. Nothing brings intimacy back better than complete and utter silence to enjoy with your partner.

- Celebrate! Celebrate your anniversary, your birthdays, and even your small triumphs. It's the little things that keep a relationship growing strong.

- Surprise one another. Put a small note in a lunch bag, car or coat pocket, telling one another how important you are...and really mean it. It will make you smile all day.

- Take a nap or just be lazy together. Many times when you have the opportunity to be lazy together, it seems like the perfect time to do what really needs to be done. That usually means chores and household duties. Every once in a while...don't do it. Just relax, watch a movie together, take a nap, snuggle, eat a bag of chips or candy, and forget the rest of the world. This is wonderful for the mind and refreshing to the soul.

- Take an individual time-out. Even if it is just an hour or two, do something you really want to do with a friend, or alone, and enjoy it. The happier you are, the better partner and parent you'll be. Leave the guilt behind.

- Kiss passionately and I mean really passionately, just as you did before you had a child. There's a great country western song that woos, "Hold me tighter, don't kiss me like we're married, kiss me like we're lovers." Good advice!

- Give yourself credit. Know you can't do it all without support from your family. The whole family structure doesn't have to revolve around one person. Remember it took more than one of you to make a family, and it takes more than one of you to care for a family.

- Know that having a good relationship with children isn't easy. Things have changed. At times, things may seem incredibly wonderful and other moments may seem bleak. It's just life. By committing to work on your relationship, you are one step ahead of many of us. It's hard work. It's frustrating, but in the long run, when your children are grown and gone at least you'll *have a relationship* and the silence won't frighten you.

QUESTIONS & ANSWERS
Postpartum Depression

This information is provided by Abby Myers, ARNP, and Dawn Gruen, ACSW, psychotherapists who work with women experiencing prenatal and postpartum disorders. Kathe Pratt, of the Postpartum Health Alliance of Sacramento, California, also contributed.

Q: *What are postpartum mood disorders (PPMD)?*

A: Having a child is one of the most challenging experiences in life. Expectations are that one be happy, overjoyed and content. Yet it is also normal to have feelings of being overwhelmed, upset or angry, disappointed or disillusioned. These conflicting feelings may be especially confusing if women and their partners are not prepared for their possibility.

The postpartum phase (up to one year) is one of the most vulnerable times for women and their partners. Giving birth is a physical, psychological, and emotional challenge during which everything is in upheaval. Because of this, it is difficult to know when normal transitional issues become problematic. In this culture, the turmoil surrounding childbirth is minimized so that many people ignore or deny any negative distress associated with it. The difficult emotions that many experience are often attributed to feelings of

exhaustion, with the hope that they will just disappear. But if a woman or couple is experiencing problems, it is important to acknowledge even the mildest forms of distress. Awareness of these adjustment problems can alert the family to seek information and possible evaluation for a postpartum disorder. If the distress continues unrecognized, postpartum disorders can progress to more severe dysfunction.

It is important to recognize that postpartum difficulties are not within your control, not your fault, and not due to a weakness of character. Postpartum disorders may affect up to 15 percent of women giving birth, and impact fathers, single moms, as well as adopting parents. The most common causes are many:

- hormonal and possible thyroid changes
- tremendous exhaustion
- lack of emotional support
- feelings of isolation
- unrealized expectations of birth and feelings of isolation
- unrealized expectations of birth and self
- feelings of being overwhelmed by change
- the unpredictability and constancy of baby's needs
- having a high need baby
- a family or personal history of depression or anxiety

Q: What are the signs and symptoms of PPMD?

A: "Baby blues" is the most familiar, affecting up to 80 percent of new mothers. Baby blues usually happen within the first two weeks after birth. The symptoms vary from the physical—such as headaches, tingling in limbs, hyperventilation—to the emotional, whose signs include development of new fears, constant worry about the baby or not wanting anything to do with the baby, confusion, memory loss, lack of interest or energy, and crying spells. Many of these are normal, transient adjustment reactions to the postpartum phase, but if the symptoms persist for one or two weeks, a qualified health professional should be consulted.

Postpartum depression, anxiety and panic disorders may manifest as more intense symptoms than the ones above. More severe symptoms may include increased anxiety, poor concentration, obsessional thoughts, guilt, insomnia, new phobias, anger and irritability, hypersensitivity, scary thoughts of hurting oneself or the baby, not eating, isolating oneself, being unable to relax, and experiencing panic attacks. Again, if these symptoms persist a woman may be experiencing a postpartum mood disorder and if the disorder is not recognized or treated, the person may progress to more severe incapacitation.

The most severe and rarest form of PPMD is postpartum psychosis. This affects one in a thousand women and includes symptoms of mania, hallucinations, persistent obsessions, bizarre beliefs, suicidal ideation, and possibly thoughts of harming the baby. The mother requires immediate treatment and possible hospitalization. It is important to remember that postpartum psychosis is very treatable and the sooner intervention occurs, the greater the likelihood for earlier recovery.

Q: How long do PPMDs last?

A: Depending on the degree of severity and type of treatment, postpartum depression may last only a few months or up to a year (with proper treatment). One unique factor differentiating PPMD from other types of depression or anxiety is its "mercurial" quality. This means that feelings can come and go, often within hours. As recovery progresses the number of good days increases steadily. Long-term studies indicate, however, that without treatment, it may take up to three or four years to recover. If left untreated, children and the couple relationship may experience irrevocable impact.

Q: How do I get help?

A: If you think you are having symptoms (even mild ones) that have continued for more than two weeks, it is important to mention these to your health care provider as soon as possible. Unfortunately, some providers are not trained to recognize signs and symptoms of postpartum disorders. They may minimize the problem, telling you to just get some exercise or take a break from the baby. This is good advice, but it may not be enough to help with your discomfort. If your provider minimizes your symptoms and you still feel distressed, find another health care provider who has experience with postpartum disorders. You should request a medical evaluation (including a thyroid exam). Once medical "causes" are ruled out, a referral to a qualified mental health professional should be made.

For some women, information about postpartum disorders and strong emotional support from family or from a support group may be enough. Others may need individual or group psychotherapy to help understand the contributing factors to their postpartum difficulties, to learn more effective stress reduction and coping skills, and to rebuild self-esteem. Many women benefit from medication in addition to psychotherapy. There are antidepressants which have been researched and approved for use while breastfeeding. Medication should always be monitored under the supervision of a physician or nurse practitioner.

It is important to involve your partner in your treatment as emotional support is one of the main factors in an earlier recovery. Postpartum disorders are quite treatable and with early intervention, recovery and stability for you and your family will be forthcoming.

TIPS FOR COPING WITH POSTPARTUM DEPRESSION

- Learn and identify the symptoms of postpartum distress as early as possible.
- Understanding and awareness help alleviate the guilt and confusion that can arise. Don't try to deal with this by yourself. Isolation only makes things worse. Talk to others, join a support group to know that you are not alone and that you are experiencing something that many other parents go through. Consult a health professional who is experienced in postpartum disorders.
- Get your thyroid checked.
- Explore with a health professional the possibility of using medicines that can reverse chemical changes in your body which may have contributed to the depression.
- See a professional you trust who has knowledge about postpartum disorders.
- Counseling can help you learn how to cope and care for yourself during this time.
- Obtain help with domestic chores and care for the baby. This will help relieve pressure and increase the likelihood of a quicker recovery.
- Allow yourself to grieve about your feelings of loss.

🙢 RESOURCES 🙢

■ DEPRESSION AFTER DELIVERY
800-944-4773
P.O. Box 1282
Morrisville, PA 19067

■ DEPRESSION AFTER DELIVERY
283-9278
P.O. Box 59973
Renton, WA 98058

This nonprofit group provides support to women with postpartum mood/anxiety disorders, and their families. They provide education to the public concerning the nature and management of this disorder, and promote related research. The number above connects you to an information line that provides names and numbers of women who have experienced postpartum mood/ anxiety disorders.

The listing below provides you with support group meetings. Infants, husbands, and other support persons are welcome at the meetings.

■ SOUTH KING COUNTY
Good Neighbor Center
305 S. 43rd
Renton, WA 98056
1st & 3rd Tuesday of every month at 7:00 p.m.

■ NORTH END-KING COUNTY
North District Multi Service Center
10501 Meridian Avenue N., Rm. C-110
Seattle, WA 98133
2nd & 4th Wednesday of every month at 7:00 p.m.

■ EASTSIDE
Overlake Hospital
1035-116th Ave. N.E.
Bellevue, WA 98004
3rd Thursday of every month at the SW Conference Room at 7:00 p.m.

■ EVERETT
Everett-Providence General Medical Office Building
14th and Everett
Everett, WA 98206
1st and 3rd Tuesday of every month at 7:00 p.m.

■ TACOMA
Tacoma General Hospital
315 S. K St.
Tacoma, WA
4th Tuesday of every month at Mary Bridge Children's Health Center small board room.

POSTPARTUM THERAPY GROUPS

■ DAWN GRUEN, ACSW
281-7610
222 Etruria, Ste. 130
Seattle, WA 98109

■ ABBY MYERS, ARNP
522-3543
4026 N.E. 55th, Ste. A
Seattle, WA 98105
Postpartum therapy groups meet weekly, focus on adjustment to the new role as parents, relief of symptoms, teaching of coping and relaxation skills, and medication education if needed. Babies are welcome. Every fourth session your partner is encouraged to attend a multi-couples session.

POSTPARTUM HELP

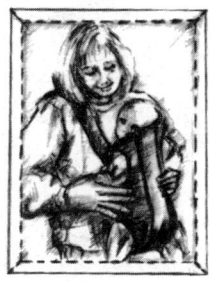

One of the most exhilarating and exhausting time periods of your life is right after your baby is born. Whether it is your first or third, during this time it seems as if "just living" may be truly overwhelming. The following resources should give you some relief during the postpartum period. This is only a partial listing, but the general rule is to look for as much help as possible. And, consider using any business that delivers and/or goes the extra mile for you during your recovery.

Whether it is your first or third baby, during the first few months, it may seem as if "just living" may be overwhelming. The following resources offer trained professionals dedicated to providing relief during the postpartum period.

DOULAS

Doulas, also called postpartum caregivers, are women who give non-medical support and hands-on help to the new mother and her family. Doulas are trained in breastfeeding, new baby care, and postpartum depression. They cook, make sure the mother gets to rest, do laundry, and help with older children. A doula's service is especially helpful in today's transient society where relatives are often too far away to help. Most doulas charge an hourly rate and have hourly minimums. Here are several Seattle services:

■ BEGINNINGS
486-5164
Beginnings offers in-home postpartum care for parents. Owned by two registered nurses, Carol Crow and Karen Cucera, the service offers well newborn and sibling care, light housekeeping, meal preparation and breastfeeding support. The hourly rate is about $25 per hour.

■ MOTHERCARE OF AMERICA DOULA SERVICE

672-8011

MotherCare was Washington State's first doula service, and is owned by Dorothy Harrison. As a mother of six children and a grandmother, Dorothy uses her own practical experience in hiring support care for mothers during the postpartum period. MotherCare provides infant care, new mother support, sibling care, breastfeeding support, light housekeeping, errands and family meal preparation. You can pick and choose what services you want during a pre-delivery interview with a care provider. The cost for this service is $20 per hour with a 12 hour minimum.

■ NEW FAMILY NURSE

867-0678

Barbara LaFayette, R.N., is your "New Family Nurse." She is available to teach baby care and breastfeeding. She will also do your errands, chores, prepare gourmet meals and do virtually anything you need her to do to make your life easier with baby. The cost for her service is $25 per hour with a 4 hour minimum.

■ SEATTLE MIDWIFERY SCHOOL

800-747-9433

322-8834 (Seattle area)

The Seattle Midwifery School offers training for both birth and postpartum doulas, and their training meets the requirements for certification through the National Association for Postpartum Care Services. This training provides doulas with the knowledge to provide wisdom and practical information to new parents. Doulas will care for a new baby while mom naps, prepare meals, straighten up a bit, read to an older sibling and teach the family how to bathe and care for a newborn. The Seattle Midwifery School keeps a listing of certified doulas they have trained and can give you names and numbers of doulas in your area.

Life Experiences ...

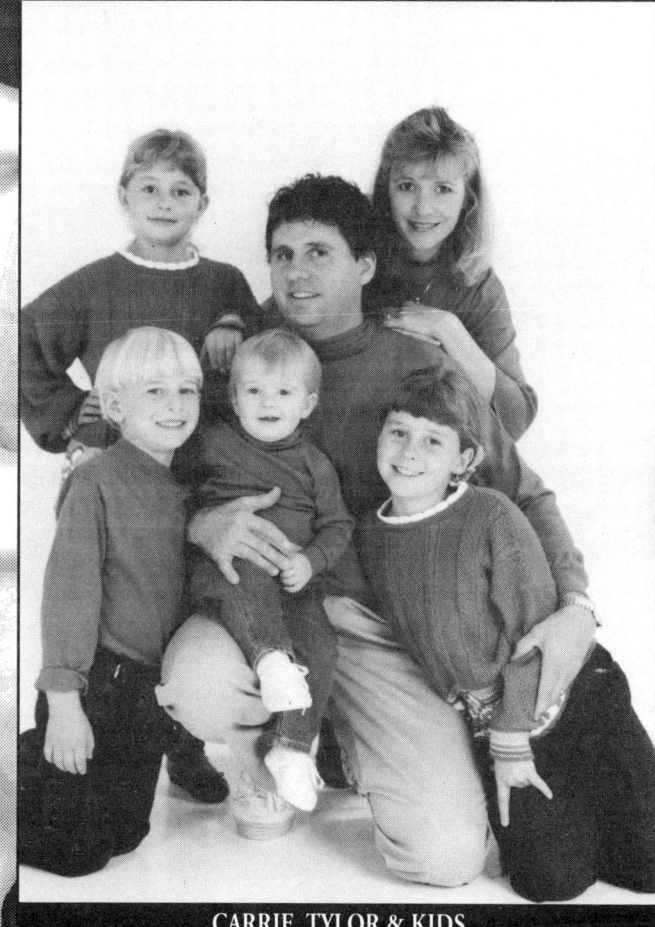

CARRIE, TYLOR & KIDS

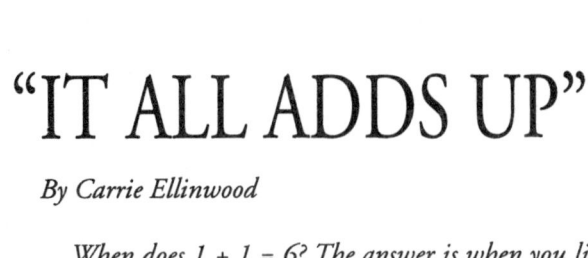

"IT ALL ADDS UP"

By Carrie Ellinwood

When does 1 + 1 = 6? The answer is when you live in a blended family! My husband, Tylor, and I married two years ago. Along with exchanging vows, we also exchanged children that we both had from previous marriages. He had two girls and I had one son. It may seem that two adults who love each other would be able to manage the "instant family" syndrome. After all, they're just children. Right? Maybe. Sometimes. Always prayerfully.

Many things come into play in a blended family. Some of them are more financial challenges, more scheduling considerations, more parenting questions, and also possibly more children together. The most important thing we found is that each partner must be committed to each other, and the marriage, and willing to accept a lifelong challenge of being a referee.

Financially, blended families deal with child support, possible attorney costs related to custody battles, and trying to duplicate the needs of the children in both homes. Not because we try to keep up with the ex-spouse, but rather so the children feel that they are a part of the family, even if they are not always a part of your home. It can also be difficult getting used to shopping for five one weekend and two the next. It takes considerable planning in the area of groceries—so there are not gallons of spoiled milk and lots of mushy bananas!

Scheduling for blended families sometimes means that not only are you blending in your family, but you may also be dealing with the schedules of two ex-spouses and their new families. Just when you think you have the routine down, the school offers a special program you must attend which is on the "other ex-spouse's" night. A slight deviation from an arranged schedule finds you wondering what effect it may have on the schedule next week.

Another scheduling nemesis of blended families is the holidays. Everyone has to be willing to give and take at a time

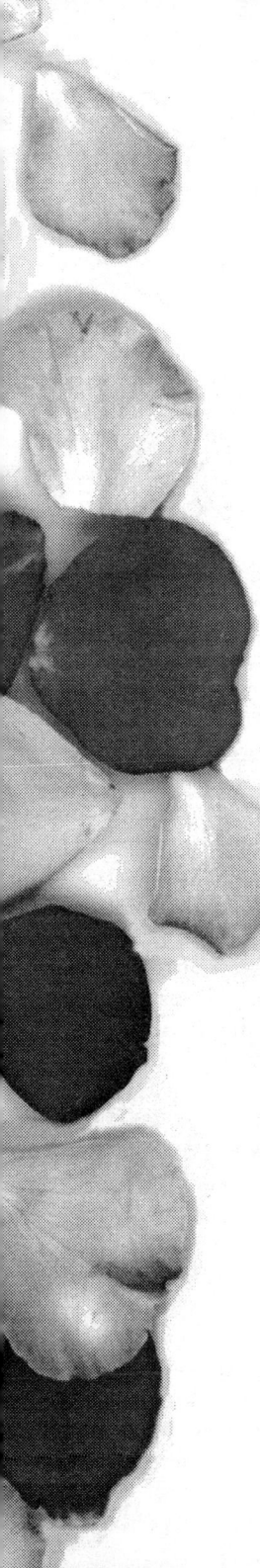

when you just want to be a family. Some families rotate holidays by years, some split them, and some just wish they would go away. In any case, you have to deal with them.

When you sign your marriage license, there is also the hidden line that says you are now a stepparent. This creates challenges, especially when the children are older and if the family life styles vary greatly between the children's two homes. We have found that the key for us in dealing with the kids is that we do our best to treat each as our own. If there is a disagreement on parenting we discuss it after the event when the children are not present. Most important to the kids is to see that they have two loving parents who care for them and care for each other.

Of course for some, the next inevitable step is children together. More blending...for us, that happened quickly and more than once! After two years of marriage we now have one child together with another on the way. The most difficult part of this is entertaining a one-year-old the "day after"—the day after a fun-filled, entertaining weekend packed with three other brothers and sisters who have doted on, carried around, and basically spoiled their little sister. Our daughter often wanders the house looking for her siblings and gazing up at us, wondering why it is so quiet.

I have given you a glimpse of life in one blended family. We are committed to each other and our faith. In our new life we believe that these are the keys for our success.

Sometimes things are challenging, but with every challenge comes a reward. For us it is the blessing of seeing our children grow, seeing their ability to love and accept us and one another beyond the capacity dreamed of, and seeing that there are second chances at happiness in life. ❧

FAMILY ACTIVITIES

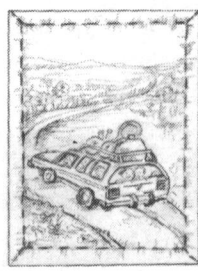

Take time out of your busy schedule to enjoy family life. Here are a number of activities and outings in the greater Seattle area... go explore.

Take time out of your busy schedule to enjoy family life. Here are a number of activities and outings in the Seattle area...go explore. You may want to check out four useful guidebooks for Seattle families: *Out and About Seattle With Kids*, by Ann Bergman and Colleen Carroll ($12.95); *Going Places: Family Getaways in the Pacific Northwest*, by Ann Bergman and Rose Williamson ($16.95); *Discover Washington and Seattle With Kids*, by Rosanne Cohn and Suzanne Monson ($16.95); and *Places to Go With Children Around Puget Sound*, by Elton Welke ($9.95). The free monthly newsmagazines, *Seattle's Child* and *Eastside Parent*, also offer up-to-date information on the many wonderful events and activities happening nearby. The daily Seattle Times lists children's activities in their Saturday edition, so you may want to check that out as well. The resources listed below are only a partial listing of what you'll find as a family in the greater Seattle area. Like everything else, the hours or prices may change throughout the year, so make sure you call ahead to verify this information. Have fun!

■ AQUA BARN RANCH
255-4618
15227 S.E. Renton-Maple Valley Hwy.
Renton, WA 98058
Swimming and horseback riding are the main activities at Aqua Barn. It's also a good place to take your young child for a pony ride since you get to walk the pony around in a small area, rather than having it hooked up to a "pony merry-go-round." The Aqua Barn is open different hours

each day for swimming and horseback riding, so its's a good idea to call and check times before you go.

■ **BAY PAVILION**
624-5673
Pier 57, Alaskan Way
Seattle, WA 98101
Hours: Daily   11:00 a.m.-9:00 p.m.
You'll find the only indoor carousel in Seattle here, along with some fun, touristy shops with souvenirs and great munchies. Stop by Seattle Fudge, where they often have free samples. The Pavilion is just a short stroller ride from the Aquarium, and outside there's a bright observation deck with walkways and benches.

■ **BELLEVUE DOWNTOWN PARK**
(South end of Bellevue Square)
A great place to visit during a shopping trip to Bellevue Square. Fountains, waterfalls and a play area make this a fun place for children.

■ **CHILDREN'S MUSEUM**
298-2521
Seattle Center House, Lower Level
Seattle, WA 98109
Hours: Daily   10:00 a.m.-5:00 p.m.
Cost: $4.50 per person, free for children under 1
The Children's Museum more than doubled in size with its 1995 expansion and offers many wonderful hands-on exhibits for children and families. A child-sized neighborhood, toddler play center, Imagination Station art studio, regularly scheduled hands-on workshops, and much more await visitors.

■ **CHILDREN'S MUSEUM OF TACOMA**
627-6031
925 Court C
Tacoma, WA 98402
Hours: T-F   10:00 a.m.-5:00 p.m.
         Sat.   10:00 a.m.-4:00 p.m.
         Sun.   12:00 p.m.-4:00 p.m.
Cost: $3.25 per person; under 2 free
The museum has hands-on exhibits, creative play areas, and special activities and workshops. The "Oh, Baby!" exhibit features a newborn nursery where kids can take care of baby dolls.

■ **COULON BEACH PARK**
235-2568
1201 Lake Washington Blvd. N.
Renton, WA 98055
Hours: Daily   10:00 a.m.-dusk
At the newest major park on Lake Washington, you'll find a big swimming beach, boat rentals, trails for walking, biking, and jogging, and a large playground with modern equipment. There's also an Ivar's Seafood Bar in the park, open seasonally.

■ **DECEPTION PASS STATE PARK**
(360) 675-2417
Whidbey Island, WA 98278
Hours: Daily   6:00 a.m.-dusk
This park has beaches, lakes, camping, fishing, meadows, trails, beautiful views. Take I-5 north to the Anacortes exit and go west on State Highway 20, following signs to Whidbey Island. The park actually begins on Fidalgo Island and continues on Whidbey Island, which is accessed by crossing Deception Pass (an inlet of water, crossed by a very high bridge). At Rosario Beach (on the Fidalgo side), you'll find tidepools to explore and a 30-foot tall wooden carving of Ko-Kwal-Al-Woot ("Maiden of Deception Pass").

■ **DISCOVERY PARK**
386-4236
3801 N. Government Way
Seattle, WA 98199
Hours: Daily   Dawn to dusk
         Visitors Center:
         Daily   8:30 a.m.-5:00 p.m.
A great place to introduce your kids to the
outdoors, Discovery Park has acres and
acres of forests and meadows to walk
through. Trails are well-marked, but it
helps to stop by the Visitors Center and
get a map too. Nature walks led by park
rangers are offered frequently on the weekends. There are beaches and a lighthouse,
but both are a bit of a hike to get to. You'll
also find some nice playground equipment near the Daybreak Star Art Center,
which is a great place to see Native American art. The best part—it's all free!

■ **EDMONDS PUBLIC FISHING
   PIER**
At the foot of Dayton St.
Edmonds, WA 98020
Even if you're not fishing, this is a wonderful place to take kids. Check the tide
tables in the newspaper or Yellow Pages,
and come close to the low tide. Kids will
likely find shells and interesting rocks on
the beach, and during low tide you can
walk from the pier north to (and under!)
the ferry dock. Besides the splashing waves,
you'll hear the sounds of seagulls, ferry
boat horns, and trains going by. There's a
large grassy area for picnicking just north
of the pier, and you can't beat the views of
the Olympic Mountains on a clear day.
On the other side of the ferry dock is
another beach park adjacent to Edmonds
Underwater Park, where you'll often see
divers descending into the deep. (They
even carve pumpkins underwater at Hal-
loween!)

■ **ENCHANTED VILLAGE &
   WILD WAVES WATER PARK**
661-8001
36201 Enchanted Pkwy. S.
Federal Way, WA 98003
Hours: April-Labor Day; call for hours
Cost: $11, $9 for kids over 10, $7 for
         kids 3-9 (Enchanted Village
         only); $18.95 (combination ad-
         mission)
Enchanted Village is a great place to bring
a picnic and enjoy amusement rides,
bumper boats, wading pools, puppet
shows, magic shows, the Antique Doll
and Toy Museum and mini-golf, all of
which are included in the price of admission. Wild Waves is geared for older children but there are some small slides and
water rides for younger kids.

■ **FOREST PARK**
259-0300
802 Mukilteo Blvd.
Everett, WA 98203
Hours: Daily   Dawn-10:00 p.m.
         Animal Farm (April-Sept.):
         Daily   9:00 a.m.-5:00 p.m.
This is a big park with trails, picnic areas,
fields, tennis courts, a swimming pool,
concessions, and a playground. There's
also a sprinkler pool that's open on hot
summer days. If you come at the right
time (2:00 p.m.-3:00 p.m.) and the
weather and ponies are cooperating, line
up for a free pony ride at the Animal
Farm. Besides the ponies, the farm area
has geese, pigs, sheep, and more.

■ **FUN FOREST**
728-1585
Seattle Center
Seattle, WA 98109
Hours: Daily   June 1-Labor Day;
        Weekends only, remainder of
        the year
The Fun Forest has lots of rides and carnival temptations for the kids, with special rides for little children on the south side of the park.

■ **KELSEY CREEK COMMUNITY PARK AND FARM**
455-7688
13204 S.E. 8th Pl.
Bellevue, WA 98005
Kelsey Creek Park is a perfect picnic spot, with a wonderful playground, as well as a big barn and lots of farm animals. Call for directions—it can be hard to find the first time!

■ **KING COUNTY LIBRARIES**
462-9600 or 800-462-9600
The best and most inexpensive way to interest your children in reading is to visit the library. Quick information, story times, lectures, books and videos are all available for free!

■ **LAKE SAMMAMISH STATE PARK**
455-7010
20606 S.E. 56th St.
Issaquah, WA 98027
Fishing, a sandy swimming beach, playground and picnic areas make this a great destination for families. Food concessions available.

■ **MATTHEW'S BEACH**
N.E. 93rd and Sand Point Way N.E.
Seattle, WA 98115
A great playground for.kids and a nice swimming area highlight this beach. Very popular with families during the summer months.

■ **MOLBAK'S GREENHOUSE AND NURSERY**
483-5000
13625 N.E. 175th
Woodinville, WA 98072
Hours: Daily   9:00 a.m.-6:00 p.m.
        F   9:00 a.m.-9:00 p.m.
        Call for expanded spring hours.
Molbak's is a fun place to visit any time of year, with its beautiful flowers and plants inside and out. Kids especially enjoy seeing the birds and waterfalls in the atrium, and parents will marvel at the selection in the garden center and gift shops. Our favorite time to visit is in October, when Molbak's presents free live performances of a fairy tale. Adding to the fun, Molbak's decorates the store with story page scenes from the play.

■ **MOVIE THEATERS WITH SOUNDPROOF "CRYROOMS"**
The Crest: 363-6338
Guild (45th): 633-3353
Metro: 633-0055
Northgate: 363-5800
Varsity: 632-3131
If you're not sure your toddler can make it through a feature without a fuss, these glass booths are a lifesaver. The Northgate's cry room is good-sized; most others are small. You'll need to call to find out if the movie you want to see is being shown in the "cryroom" in multi-screen theaters.

■ **MUSEUM OF FLIGHT**
764-5720
9404 E. Marginal Way S.
Seattle, WA 98108
Hours: Daily 10:00 a.m.-5:00 p.m.
         Th 10:00 a.m.-9:00 p.m.
Cost: $6, $3 for ages 6-15, free for children 5 and under
Located at Boeing Field, this terrific museum is home to a helicopter, monoplane and biplane, and lots of aviation "stuff." You can even climb into the cockpit of a Northrop F/A 18 mockup and move the joystick, and check out the control panels and radar screens. Family workshops available for children over 5 and their parents.

■ **MUSEUM OF HISTORY AND INDUSTRY**
324-1126
2700 24th Ave. E.
Seattle, WA 98112
Hours: Daily 10:00 a.m.-5:00 p.m.

Cost: $5.50, $3 for ages 6-12, $1 for ages 2-5, free for under age 2
Discover the history of Puget Sound! The Seattle Fire, national traveling exhibits, and a children's hands-on history area are some of its features. The museum offers special family programs on many weekends and holidays throughout the year. When the weather is nice, enjoy a picnic or walk on nearby Foster Island.

■ **NORTHWEST PUPPET CENTER**
523-2579
9123 15th Ave. N.E.
Seattle, WA 98115
Cost: $7.50, $5.50 for children
Seattle's only permanent puppet theater presents several productions between October and April of each year. Several of the shows are geared to younger children, making it a fun experience for toddlers. An ASL performance is held once a month. Call ahead for show times.

PARKS AND RECREATION DEPARTMENTS

Local Parks and Recreation Departments offer a treasure trove of activities for families. Free concerts, parent/child classes, playgroups, swimming, dancing, gymnastics, arts and crafts, seasonal programs, and much more are offered year-round by these communities, all for a very affordable price. Several now offer drop-in indoor playgrounds for young children and their parents; read about them in the "exercise" section of this chapter.

Bellevue	451-4106	Renton	277-5536
Edmonds	771-0230	Seattle	684-4075
Everett	259-0300	(See blue pages of phone book	
Kent	859-3991	for community center listings)	
Kirkland	828-1217	Northeast King Co.	296-2964
Lynnwood	771-4030	Northwest King Co.	296-2976
Mountlake Terrace	776-9173	Southeast King Co.	296-4281
Redmond	556-2350	Southwest King Co.	296-2956

■ **PACIFIC SCIENCE CENTER**
443-2001
200 Second Ave. N.
Seattle, WA 98109
Hours: M-F   10:00 a.m.-5:00 p.m.
        Sat./Sun.10:00 a.m.-6:00 p.m.
Cost: $6.50, $5.50 for ages 6-13,
        $3.50for ages 2-5
Part of the vast Seattle Center, the Pacific Science Center makes science fun for kids. There are many permanent hands-on exhibits that appeal to all ages, as well as changing exhibits and special events. Those 48" and under are welcome in the Just For Tots playground. IMAX movies and laser shows are available for an additional $2 charge. The Laser Nutcracker show during the holidays is especially popular with families.

■ **PIED PIPER PRODUCTIONS**
722-7209
Mt. Baker Community Club
2811 Mt. Rainier Dr. S.
Seattle, WA 98144
Cost: $2 donation
On Saturdays (except during summertime) watch for puppet shows, storytellers, dancers and sing-alongs at Mt. Baker Community Center. Shows appeal to 2- to 8-year-olds and their families.

■ **POINT DEFIANCE PARK, ZOO
   AND AQUARIUM**
591-5335
5400 North Pearl St.
Tacoma, WA 98407
Hours: Labor Day-Memorial Day:
        10:00 a.m.-4:00 p.m.
        Memorial Day-Labor Day:
        10:00 a.m.-7:00 p.m.
Cost: $6.50, $4.75 for ages 5-17,
        $2.50 for ages 3-4, free for under 3. (No charge for park only.)

Point Defiance Zoo and Aquarium is home to 5,000 animals, including whales, penguins, polar bears, and many Pacific Rim-species animals. Other features include: Never Never Land, which is an additional charge; Fort Nisqually, a restored trading fort complete with blacksmith shop; and Camp 6 Logging Museum, which features steam locomotive rides during the warmer months.

■ **REMLINGER FARMS**
451-8740
32610 N.E. 32nd
Carnation, WA 98014
Open mid-March to mid-December
This working farm is best known for its pumpkin patch and related activities—hay maze, covered wagon rides, and storytelling—but during the other months you can visit the petting zoo, take farm tours, and harvest everything from strawberries to Christmas trees.

■ **ROSALIE WHYEL MUSEUM OF
   DOLL ART**
455-1116
1116 108th Ave. N.E.
Bellevue, WA 98004
Hours: M-Sat.   10:00 a.m.-5:00 p.m.
        Sun.   1:00 p.m.-5:00 p.m.
Cost: $6, $4 for children 5-17, free
        for children under 5
Over a thousand dolls from Rosalie Whyel's collection grace this 13,000 square-foot mansion. Preschoolers are welcome; glass cases protect all the dolls. Adults will enjoy everything from antique dolls to Barbie, including two Egyptian tomb dolls.

■ **SEATTLE AQUARIUM**

386-4320

Pier 59, Waterfront Park

Seattle, WA 98101

Hours: Labor Day-Memorial Day:
10:00 a.m.-5:00 p.m.
Memorial Day-Labor Day:
10:00 a.m.-7:00 p.m.

Cost: $7.15, $5.70 seniors, $4.70 for ages 6-18, $2.45 for 3-5, free for 2 & under. Fees slightly lower for King Co. residents

See the only aquarium-based salmon hatchery in the world, walk underwater in the Dome, and explore the tidepool exhibit and Discovery Lab which recreates Washington's rocky outer coast and features a 6,000-gallon wave.

■ **SEATTLE CHILDREN'S THEATRE**

441-4488

Charlotte Martin Theatre

Seattle Center

Seattle, WA 98109

Hours: F   7:00 p.m.
Sat.-Sun. 2:00 p.m. & 5:30 p.m.

Cost: $17, $11/children

Housed in an elegant yet inviting theater, the Seattle Children's Theatre is considered one of the best children's theaters in the country. SCT presents a range of plays throughout its October-May season. Several are offered through the "Doorway to Theatre" series that introduces young children to the theater. Performances are followed by a question and answer session with the actors. Though not inexpensive, SCT's productions are a wonderful way for families to experience the magic of theater together. Season tickets are available at a reduced per-play cost.

■ **SEATTLE MIME THEATRE**

324-8788

915 E. Pine

Seattle, WA 98122

You can catch the mimes during one or two performances a year at their Capitol Hill theatre; the rest of the year the troupe performs for schools and private groups and participates in King County's Summer Day Camp program. Definitely entertaining for kids!

■ **WASHINGTON ZOOLOGICAL PARK**

391-5508

19525 S.E. 54th St.

Issaquah, WA 98027

Hours: Mar.-Oct.:
W-Sun. 10:00 a.m.-5:00 p.m.
Feb. & Nov.:
F-Sun. 10:00 a.m.-4:00 p.m.
Dec. 1-23 (Santa's Reindeer Farm) Daily 5 p.m.-8 p.m.

Cost: $2.50-$4.50, under 2 free.

This small, 14-acre zoo features threatened or endangered animals and birds. This is a perfect place for a low-key, up-close look at animals for your young ones.

■ **WOODLAND PARK ZOO**

684-4800

5500 Phinney Ave. N.

Seattle, WA 98103

Hours: 9:30 a.m.-various closing times

Cost: $5.75-7.50, $5 for ages 6-17, $2.75 for ages 3-5, free for 2 & under. Parking is $3.50.

This 92-acre zoo features a tropical rain forest exhibit, temperate forest exhibit, northern trails exhibit, African savannah and Asian elephant exhibits, Nocturnal House and Reptile House, and a family farm. Kid-sized animals' homes are found along the Habitat Discovery Trail.

EXERCISE

■ **GYMBOREE**

Federal Way: 661-7205
Seattle (Crown Hill): 523-8011
Seattle (Laurelhurst): 522-2045
Other areas: 800-520-7529

Gymboree believes that one of the most important parts of a child's day is play time—not only to enhance key early developmental skills, but also to promote positive interactions with others. Gymboree's movement play program is geared to seven developmental stages for newborns through 5-year-olds. With tyke-sized equipment, parachute time, bubbles, songs, and Gymbo the Puppet Clown, every Gymboree class offers fun for parents and children. Children learn socialization, physical and emotional development, and about the world and how to relate to it. Gymboree's goal is to offer "a rich environment where children's own 'ah-ha' experiences contribute to the building of their self-esteem." And to have fun! You can register at any time. A 12-week session costs $89 and other options are also available. Check it out at a free preview class. Gymboree also does birthday parties. Overall, we found Gymboree a fun, diversified program for parents and their children. Reasonable prices and esteem building are just a few of its assets.

■ **KID SWIM**
364-7946
14540 Bothell Way N.E.
Seattle, WA 98155

Kid Swim offers parent-tot classes for infants starting at six months through toddler age. Classes are taught by American Red Cross standards. A series of six half-hour classes cost about $45.

■ **KING COUNTY POOLS**
296-4258

This is the number for the public swimming pools in King County. The county offers swim instruction for all ages throughout the year. Prices are reasonable. For swimming lessons and pool information in other areas, see "Parks and Recreation Departments" in the previous section of this chapter.

■ **LITTLE GYM**
885-3866
1800 130th Ave. N.E.
Bellevue, WA 98005

347-0522
1203-O S.E. Everett Mall Way
Everett, WA 98204

869-5496
16315 N.E. 87th, Ste. D
Redmond, WA 98052

524-2623
7777 15th Ave. N.E.
Seattle, WA 98115

481-5889
6728 N.E. 181st #C
Kenmore, WA 98155

859-8301
10427 S.E. 240th
Kent, WA 98031

This developmentally-based, fun exercise program is designed to offer your child a variety of activities at every age. Programs begin for infants as early as four months. Activities include stretching, aerobics, songs and games, parachute games and ball play. When we did our research, we found prices reasonable, averaging about $40 per month. Little Gym offers classes for children through the grade school years. Gymnastics, sports skills development, karate, swimming programs, and summer camps are all a part of the activities for your growing child. Two other unique features of Little Gym include a parents' survival night and birthday parties. The parents' survival night is available for children ages 4-12 at varying times and weekend nights. In Bellevue, for example, it's offered every Saturday night from 6:00-10:00 p.m. Kids enjoy an evening filled with games, gymnastics, snacks, and a G-rated movie. If you're looking for an out-of-the-house birthday party, Little Gym does that too! Packages are available for almost any size party and are held on Saturdays and Sundays.

■ SAFE 'N SOUND SWIMMING
285-9279
2040 Westlake Ave. N.
Seattle, WA 98109
One-on-one swimming lessons, beginning with children at age 13 months, are based on infant swimming research. Children are encouraged to focus on the safety and respect for the water. Classes are offered in 11-week series. They last 15 minutes and cost $11 each.

INDOOR PLAYGROUNDS

There are several types of indoor playgrounds available to families in the area. The larger, privately-owned places such as Discovery Zone feature some assortment of giant Habitrail-like tubes, slides, balls to jump in, air bouncing areas, rope-climbing apparatus, and more. They also offer birthday party packages. Except as noted, parents are required to stay with their children while they play. This is especially true for the under 40" play areas. The playgrounds are an excellent workout for parents too, but you'll enjoy

it more if you borrow knee pads (which most places have available)—all that scooting through the tubes can be very hard on the knees. There's no extra charge for parents. Kids (and parents) are required to wear socks while in the play areas. For very small children, some of the places have rocking horses and ride-on toys and/or a mini-version of the big playground for children 40" and under.

Another type of indoor playground is more low-key but offers a great opportunity to interact with other parents and young children. These playgrounds are located at local parks and community recreation centers. You won't find tri-level tubes and slides here, but you'll always find a nice assortment of ride-on toys, balls, mats, bouncing toys, toddler slides, and indoor toys. These play areas are usually open just one or two mornings a week and just for toddlers and preschool age kids. Parents or caregivers must stay and supervise. Cost is minimal, usually $1-$2 per child.

Kids also love the indoor playgrounds under the golden arches. McDonald's has adopted these play areas in a big way in recent years and taken our local weather into consideration, too. Many of the newest play areas are completely enclosed, including the "McBoat" at the McDonald's on Aurora Ave. N. in north Seattle, and several other new or remodeled ones. Burger King is also picking up on this trend. Both chains do birthday parties too!

■ **DISCOVERY ZONE**
290-8325
West Mall Drive
Everett, WA 98208
Hours: M-Th   10:00 a.m.-8:00 p.m.
      F   10:00 a.m.-9:00 p.m.
      Sat.   9:00 a.m.-10:00 p.m.
      Sun.   11:00 a.m.-7:00 p.m.
Cost: $5.99 per child (ages 3-12),
      $3.99 per child (12-24 mos.)
Filled with large play equipment, parents and children go on an exercise adventure through tunnels, slides, and more. The Discovery Zone also offers a play area for kids 40" and under which offers slides, a moon jump, a small water walk and more.

■ **FAMILIES AT PLAY**
(Formerly Discovery Zone)
363-4844
Lake Forest Park Towne Centre
17171 Bothell Way N.E.
Seattle, WA 98155
Hours: M   12:00 p.m.-8:30 p.m.
      T-F   9:30 a.m.-8:30 p.m.
      Sat.   9:00 a.m.-8:30 p.m.
      Sun.   11:00 a.m.-6:00 p.m.
Cost: $5.99 per walking child on weekends; weekdays the cost is $4.99. Babies not walking yet are free!
First known as Discovery Zone, then Energy Zone, now it's called Families at Play. The equipment hasn't changed through the name transitions. A "zone" area for kids under 40" tall is available with blocks, slides, balls and more.

■ **MERLYN'S MAGIC CASTLE**
747-2020
4051 Factoria Square Mall S.E.
Bellevue, WA 98006
Hours: M-F   10:00 a.m.-7:00 p.m.
      Sat.   10:00 a.m.-6:00 p.m.
      Sun.   10:00 a.m.-6:00 p.m.
Cost: $3.75 for unlimited play when parents stay on-site. Free for under 18 months with a paying child; $2.95 per hour for ages 3-7 for a maximum of 3 hours.
Merlyn's Magic Castle is at the former location of Tube Town, but has added new equipment. They cater to younger children—in fact, kids over age 7 are not allowed. They have a real magician on-site and do birthday parties too.

■ **PLAY CLUB**
778-4009
19723 Hwy. 99, Ste. F
Lynnwood, WA 98036
Hours: Sun.-M   11:00 a.m.-6:00 p.m.
      T-Th   10:00 a.m.-8:00 p.m.
      F-Sat.   10:00 a.m.-8:30 p.m.
Cost: $3.95 weekdays, $5.75 weekends
A mini play area for toddlers (ages 1+) includes a slide, balls, and jumping area.

■ **PLAYSPACE®**
644-4500
Crossroads Shopping Center
Bellevue, WA 98008
Hours: M-Th   10:00 a.m.-9:00 p.m.
      F-Sat.   9:30 a.m.-10:30 p.m.
      Sun.   10:00 a.m.-6:00 p.m.
Cost: $5.95 per child for unlimited time when parent is on-site $7.95 for first hour, $1.49 for every hour after that, plus $1 for pager if parent drops off

631-0966
Kent-Lake Meridian Market Pl.
Kent, WA 98032
Hours: M-Th   11:00 a.m.-8:00 p.m.
       F   11:00 a.m.-9:00 p.m.
       Sat.   10:00 a.m.-9:00 p.m.
       Sun.   11:00 a.m.-7:00 p.m.
Cost: $5.95 per child (ages 4-12) for unlimited time when parent is on-site; $3.95 per child (ages 1-3), $5.95 per hour, plus $1 for pager if parent drops off (must be 5 years or older)

Bellevue's Playspace® offers licensed child care for children 3 years and potty trained up to 12 years. For toddlers, there's an open space play area with soft toys and a baby slide. Kids 17 months and under play free when accompanied by a paying sibling and parents are always free! Parents night out is every Friday and Saturday night. Children receive dinner, a G-rated movie, a guided crafts project and unlimited fun in the play room. No reservations are required and kids can be dropped off as early as 5:30 p.m. Cost is $18.50.

Playspace® in Kent offers similar equipment and drop-off care. They don't have the parents night out option. Both locations offer birthday party packages.

■ COMMUNITY INDOOR PLAYGROUNDS

Edmonds Playzone
771-0230
700 Main St.
Edmonds, WA 98020
Cost: $2 per 1-hour visit
Ages: 1-6

Everett
259-0300
Everett Community College Gymnasium
Everett, WA 98203

Cost: $1 first child, $.50 each additional 90 minute session
Ages: 1-6

Green Lake Community Center
684-0780
7201 E. Green Lake Dr. N.
Seattle, WA 98103
Hours: M-F   10:00 a.m.-9:00 p.m.
       Sat.   9:00 a.m.-4:00 p.m.
Cost: $1 per child
Ages: Toddler-5

Mountlake Terrace
776-9173
5303 228th St. S.W.
Mountlake Terrace, WA 98043
Hours: T & Th 10:30 a.m.-1:00 p.m.
Cost: $1.50 first child, $.50 second, $1 each additional through 6 kids per adult.

North Kirkland Community Center
828-1105
12421 103rd Ave. N.E.
Kirkland, WA 98033
Hours: T & Th 10:00 a.m.-1:00 p.m.
Cost: $1 per visit (up to 3 hours), no charge for babies
Ages: 1-5

Shoreline
296-2976
Shoreline Center Gym
N. 190th & 1st N.E.
Shoreline, WA 98155
Cost: $1.50 per visit (90 minutes)
Ages: 1-6

Schedules at all centers except Green Lake vary seasonally so it's best to call first to find out the current dates and times that they operate.

SIBLING PREPARATION

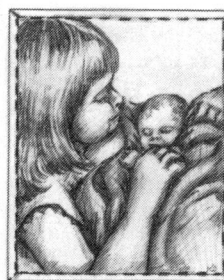

By Shelly Bokman Elia

By carefully considering your child's age, temperament and individual needs, you can help ease the transition into the role of older sibling. Here are some tips:

- Plan a time to inform your child of the pregnancy, preferably sometime after 20 weeks. Take time to answer your child's questions.

- Include your child in discussions and activities to prepare for the baby's arrival. What will you name the baby? How will you decorate the nursery? What do you need to buy for the baby?

- Use children's books to prepare your child for the baby's arrival.

- Spend some time around other infants—friends', relatives', the infant room at your child care center. Look at your child's own baby photos.

- Include your child in some of your prenatal visits. Hearing the fetal heartbeat makes the experience more "real," even for a child. Let your child feel the fetal movements through your abdomen.

- Enroll your child in a sibling preparation class. Visit the hospital or birthing center before your due date so that your child will see where Mom will be when the baby is born. This is a nice time to see other newborns. Your child can also help pack your suitcase and choose an outfit for the baby to wear home.

- Have a doll and baby items available for your child to play with. By acting out the care and holding of a baby, your child can relieve some of the anxiety that may accompany the impending birth.

- Stress that the new baby will not take your older child's place in the family, but will add more love to your family.

- Any changes that are necessary in your child's life—starting preschool, moving into a "big bed," potty training—should happen well before the baby's due date.

- Make arrangements for your child to be cared for by a familiar relative or friend who can be sensitive to your child's feelings and need for reassurance at this time.

- Try to maintain as much of your older child's usual routine as possible when the baby arrives. Familiar routines—bedtime stories, going to preschool, feeding the dog with Dad each morning—will reassure your child that life as he knows it has not completely changed.

- Plan some one-on-one time for your older child and Dad while Mom is away. Take advantage of the telephone to maintain contact with Mom. Your child really needs to know that Mom is safe and well and will be returning soon.

- You may consider having your older child give the baby a gift and receive one in return.

- Allow your child to come along to pick you up from the hospital and bring you and the baby home.

- Emphasize the role of "big" sister or brother. A snapshot of the new baby to take to school or a T-shirt proclaiming "I'm the Big Sister" establishes your older child's firm place in the family.

- Allow your child to help care for the infant. Explain safety and caregiving procedures. Have the child talk to the baby and call him/her by name.

- Schedule individual time for both mom and dad with the older child. "Clinginess," temporary developmental regression or acting out are normal reactions of a sibling to a new baby in the family. Give your child time and lots of love and the adjustment to "big" sister or brother will be made easier.

THE VAST ADVANTAGES OF PARENTHOOD

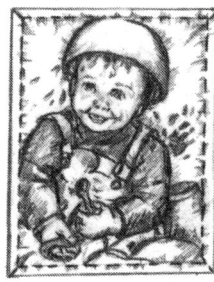

By Joyce Armor

In trying to explain the deep and lasting significance of our wedding anniversary to our almost five-year-old son, I said, "If we hadn't gotten married, we never would have had you." He thought about this for a moment, then replied, "You mean Judie and Stephen (our very married but childless next door neighbors) aren't married?" I had obviously painted myself into a corner and tried to paint myself back out by explaining the differences between married couples with children and married couples without. He interrupted my riveting explanation to ask where lightning comes from, and I gave him my sage answer to such questions: "Go ask Daddy."

That was the end of the children vs. childless comparison for him, but not for me. My first thought was that Judie and Stephen have things that we don't. A new car, for one. Light (and clean) carpeting, for another. Time. But we have things they don't have, too. Toys, for instance. A refrigerator art gallery. Fruit by the Foot. Then again, they don't have to drag a bar stool outside, pry the screen off their bedroom window and somersault onto the bed, all in full view of passing traffic, because some little guttersnipe thinks it's funny to lock Mommy's bedroom door with the key inside at least once a week. They haven't changed enough diapers to cover the planet or broken up fistfights over a grain of sand. On a chilly, drizzling day, my son ran out of a friend's house into her front yard and sat on a huge pile of wet poop that had obviously been left by an elephant. I made the mistake of exclaiming, "Oh no! Look what you just sat in!" So he, naturally, scraped both hands across his backside and came up with handfuls of said elephant droppings. Horrified, he wiped the offending hands all over his brand new jacket.

Let's face it. Childless couples don't have to deal with the mounds of elephant and other droppings that parents do. They probably stay reasonably dry on rainy days. I am forever standing in a puddle in the rain fastening seat belts and trying to wrestle the car keys out of the fat little fist of someone who thinks it's funny to see Mommy's hair get plastered to her face. My mother talks about the time my brother, age two, locked her out of the house in her nightgown in a snowstorm. For me it was the torrential rainstorm of 1986. I mean, haven't we all, at one time or another, had our front doors kicked in by the police? It's a tradition in our family. I'll bet Stephen and Judie don't have a locksmith listed in their personal phone directory. I see them come and go at odd hours, sometimes many times a day, and a hazy memory forms of a time when I could be spontaneous without hurrying to put on six shoes instead of two, or worse yet, trying to coax the kids into putting on their own shoes. Or standing over two little tooth brushers like a drill sergeant.

Okay, so Judie and Stephen can go where they want, when they want, and they're not at the mercy of baby-sitters or someone else's bowel movements. For their added enjoyment they have furniture without gouges, a clean house, a gorgeous boat and nice tans. Somewhere in our house are the missing pieces to 347 puzzles. We have a swing set with a lot of miles on it and an Aqua-Slide, slightly chewed by an Australian shepherd. But they don't have anybody to color with either, or play jacks or hopscotch or baseball with, or all the other joys of childhood that we're rediscovering.

There are no little arms over there reaching out, not only to get comfort, but to give it. And nobody lives at their house who believes they know everything. Maybe, just maybe, we have a small person living here who will one day make an important scientific or economic or ecological discovery or who will in some other way make this world a better place. As I tucked him into bed a few nights after our anniversary conversation, my son hugged me extra hard and said, "I'm happy you got married and had kids." Me too!

THE
BABY
PAGES

❧ *Consumer information for the greater Seattle area.*

❧ *Coupons are perforated for ease of use.*

❧ *Don't forget to let merchants know you found them through the Seattle Baby Resource Guide.*

Seattle Baby Pages are separate from the editorial portion of this book. I'm Expecting was not paid for its editorial content of the book by participants in the Baby Pages, nor does I'm Expecting endorse any of the merchants in this section.

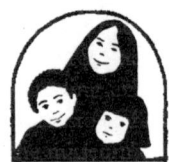
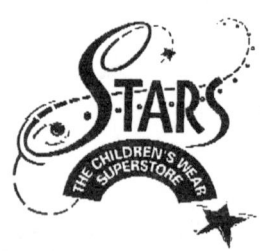
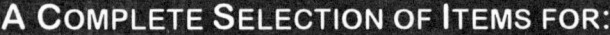

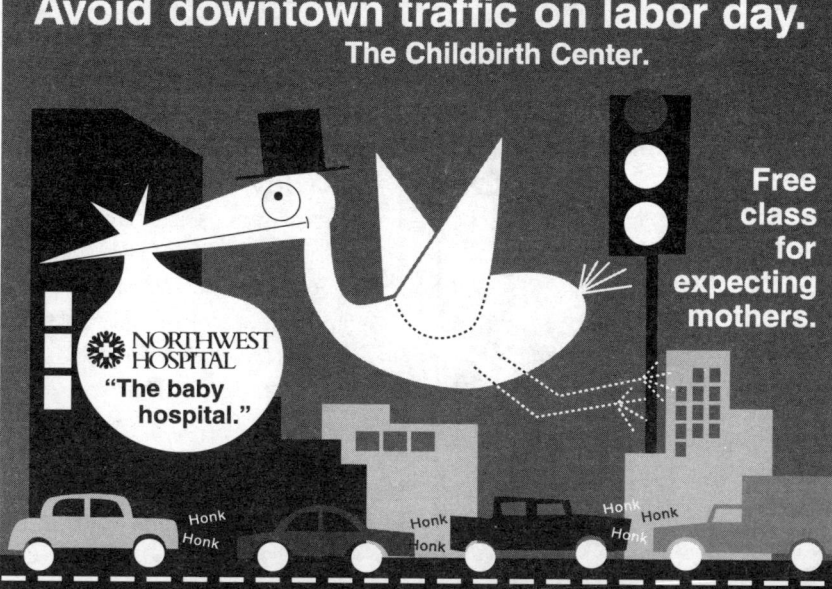

Avoid downtown traffic on labor day.
The Childbirth Center.

Free class for expecting mothers.

NORTHWEST HOSPITAL
"The baby hospital."

Need a physician, nurse midwife or more information? Call 364-BABY- we've got the answers.

Northwest Hospital —"The Baby Hospital"
A leader in the family-centered birth experience.
- wide range of birthing options available
- single-room maternity care
- 24-hour available obstetrical anesthesia care
- comprehensive prenatal & parenting education
- available Jacuzzi and whirlpool baths
- certified lactation consultants
- postpartum follow-up program
- cost-conscious pricing

Call 364-BABY

for information or a physician or midwife referral.

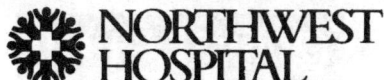

NORTHWEST HOSPITAL

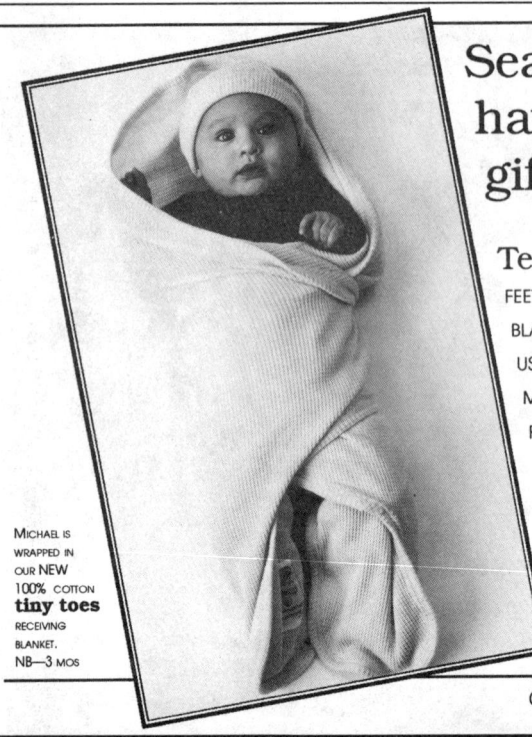

MICHAEL IS WRAPPED IN OUR NEW 100% COTTON **tiny toes** RECEIVING BLANKET. NB—3 MOS

Seattle's "Gotta have it" baby gift!

Teddy Toes—THE BLANKET WITH FEET® FROM SISTERS 3 IS PRACTICAL, BLANKET-WRAP OUTERWEAR. EASY TO USE WITH CAR SEATS, STROLLERS AND MORE, IT SIMPLIFIES BABY CARE AND FITS FROM NEWBORN TO 18 MONTHS.

IN SEATTLE CALL 284-3404 FOR STORE INFORMATION. IF YOU ARE OUT OF THE 206 AREA CALL 1•800•51•TEDDY.

Puget Sound Birth Center

Pregnancy, Birth & Postpartum Care
"A balanced approach between technology & the human touch"

Offering safe, sensitive Midwifery care
where you get the <u>time</u> you deserve

Puget Sound Birth Center, P.S.
13128 Totem Lake Blvd., N.E. #101
Kirkland, WA 98034

(206) 823-1919

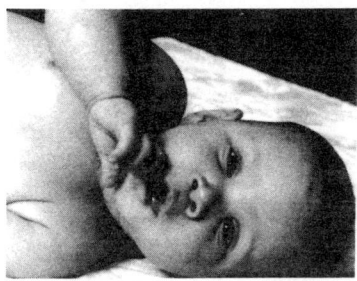
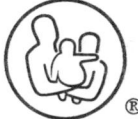

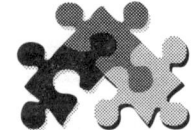
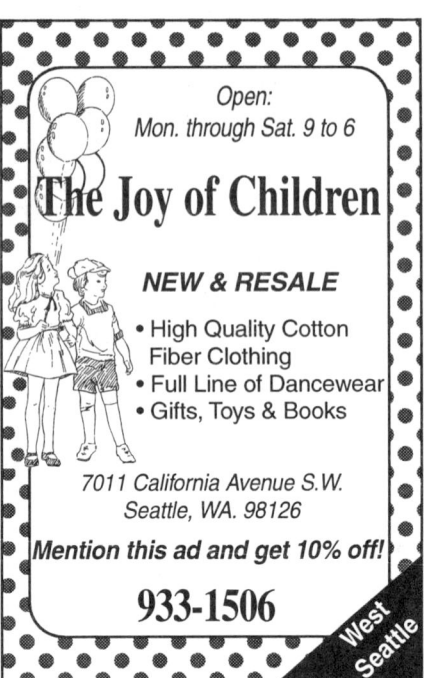
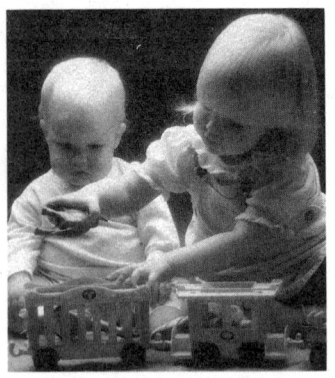
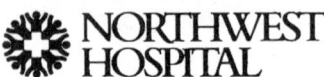

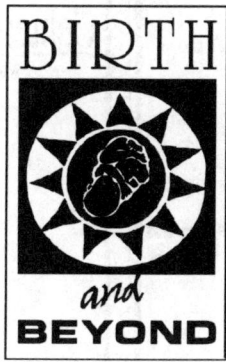
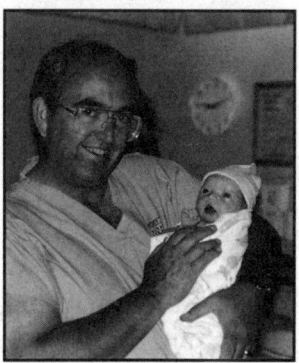
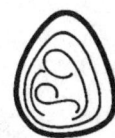

*Clothes as unique
as your child*

K i n d e r   B r i t c h e s

422 Main St.
Edmonds, WA
(206) 778-7600 • Fax (206) 744-0863

✼ Baby Joggers ✼ Flapdoodles
✼ Golden Rainbow
✼ Guess ✼ Esprit
✼ Cow & Lizard ✼ Sweet Potatoes
✼ Wes & Willy
✼ Christening Wear

Centered Method *for* Birthing™
A Step by Step Approach to Maternity through hypnotherapy

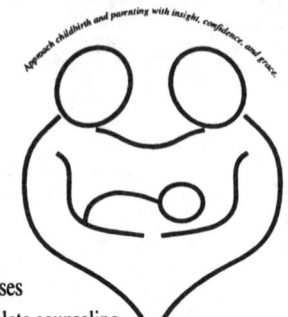

Pre-natal classes
Simple, complete counseling ™
for couples/individuals
Doctor & mid-wife recommended
Call for references in your area.

206-391-8569

Valerie Chantal De Soto, Certified Clinical Hypnotherapist & Doula
Gilman Village, Issaquah, Washington

We're Proud to Deliver
at Northwest Hospital

JAMES A. JOKI, M.D.
Obstetrics and Gynecology
Board Certified

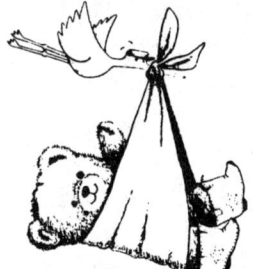

Northwest Hospital Campus
1570 North 115th, Suite 9
Seattle, WA 98133
(206) 362-5654

RALPH M. NEIGHBOR, M.D.
Obstetrics and Gynecology
Board Certified

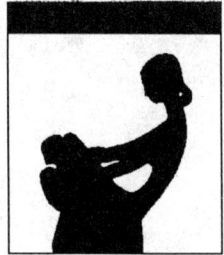

Northwest Hospital Campus
1570 North 115th, Suite 5
Seattle, WA 98133
(206) 367-5699

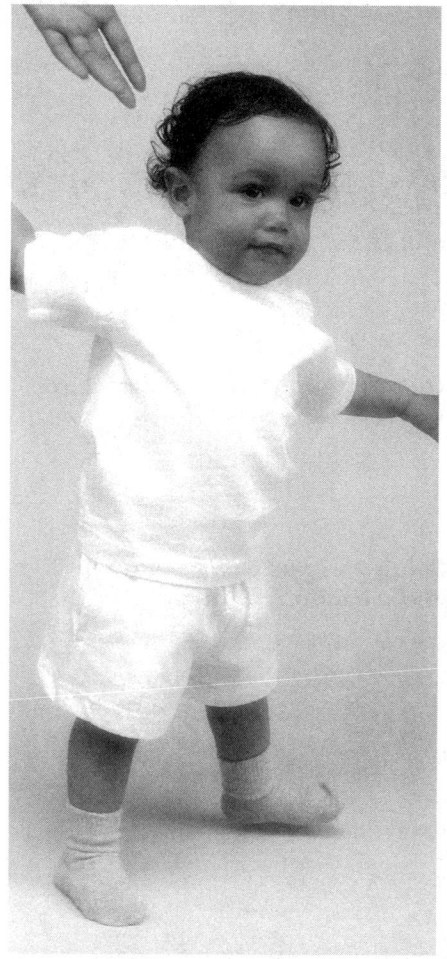

He's not an infant anymore. But if you're thinking of switching your toddler from infant formula to cow's milk, there's a better choice than milk.

After the bottle.

New Next Step® Toddler Formula. Next Step is specially designed for toddlers. A pediatrician approved formula, Next Step is better than milk for your toddler's first year of life. And

Before the milk.

because it's fortified with iron, it has the iron cow's milk lacks for your toddler's second year of life. Next Step Toddler Formula, from the makers of Enfamil®, comes in powder, concentrate,

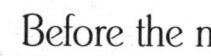

Something new for toddlers.

ready-to-use liquid, and soy powder. So when your toddler reaches that age when he's ready for a switch, Next Step is the right step. For more information, call 1-800-BABY123.

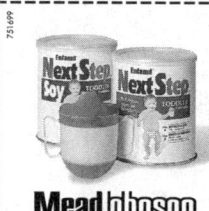
 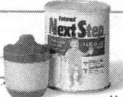

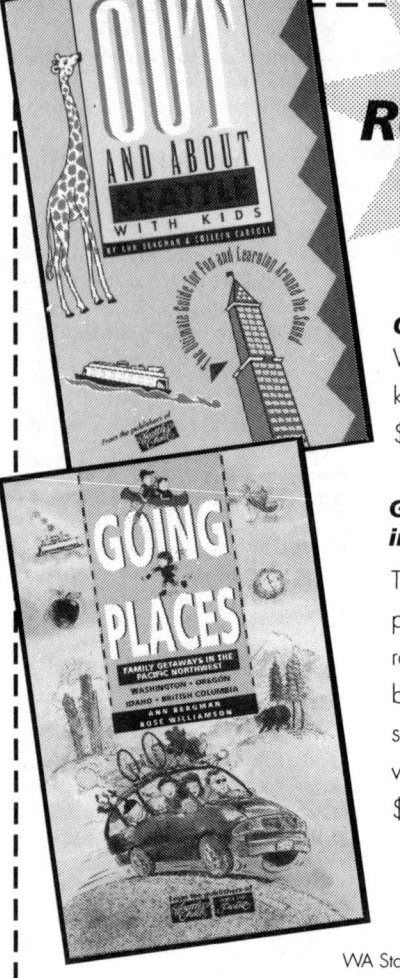

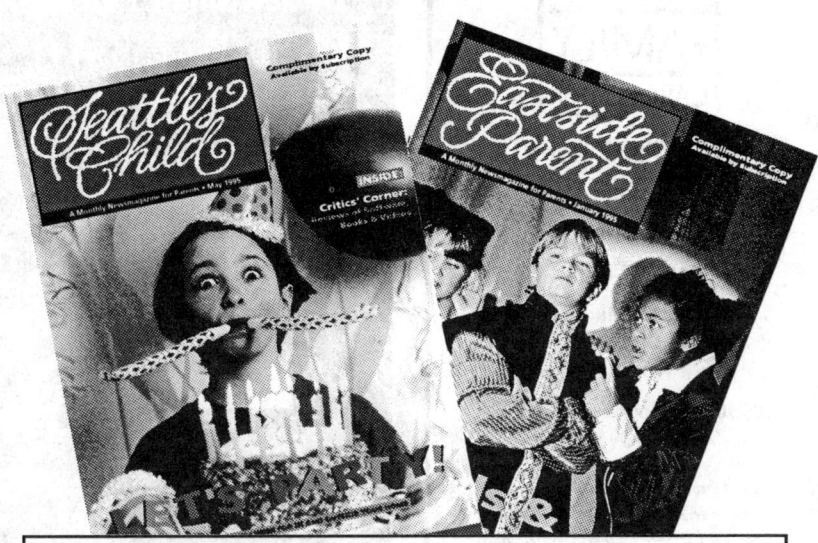

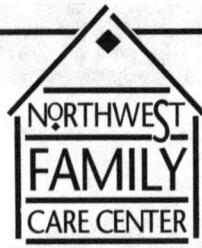
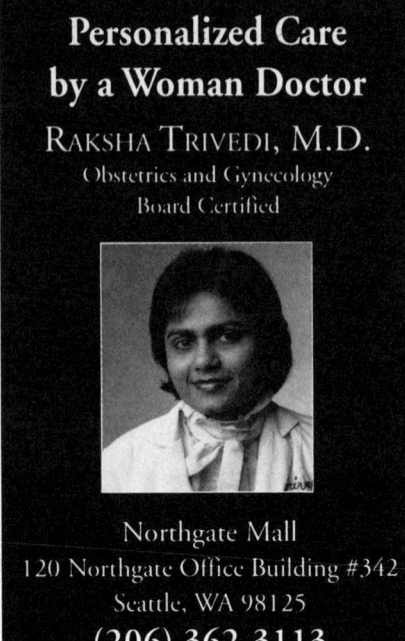

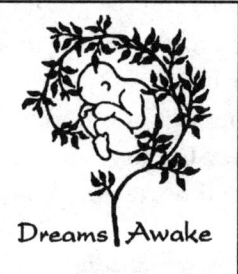
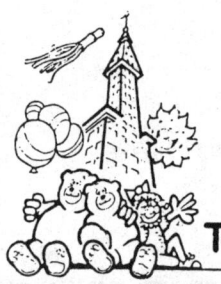
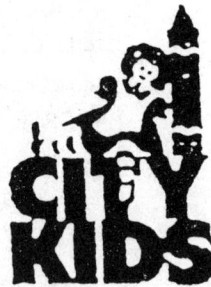

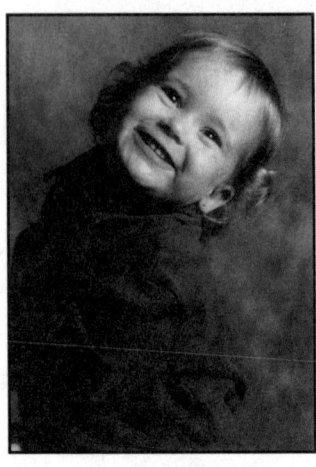
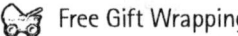

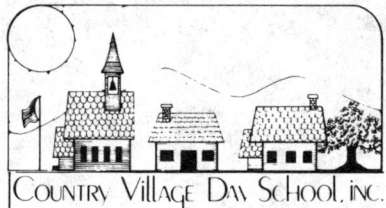
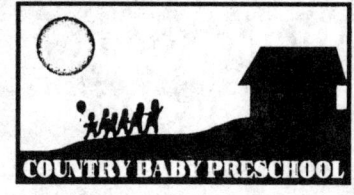
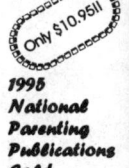
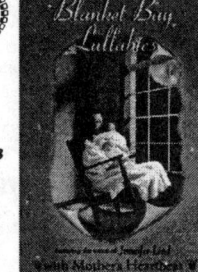

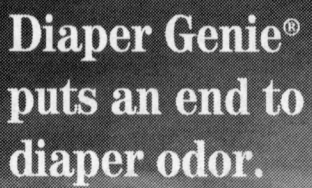

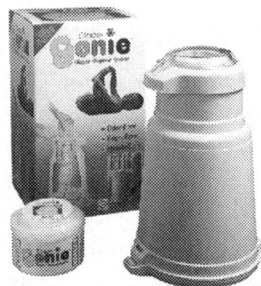

Go To Your Room
528-0711
Roosevelt Square
6411 12th Ave. N.E.
Seattle

453-2990
13000 Bel-Red Rd.
Bellevue

Hours: Mon.-Sat. 10-6
        Sun. 12-5

A complete children's
store!

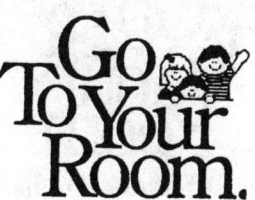

Go To Your Room.

10% Off Total Purchase

Valid at time of purchase only
Only one coupon per customer

SEATTLE BABY PAGES™

Village Maternity
523-5167
University Village

Hours: M-F 10 - 8
        Sat. 10 - 6
        Sun. 11 - 5

Maternity and children's
clothing with that
comfortable Seattle feel.

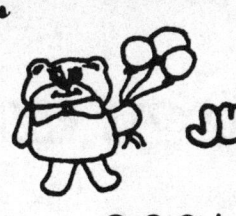

$5.00 OFF

Any $20.00 Purchase
Maternity or Kids Clothing*
*Nursing and sale merchandise not included

SEATTLE BABY PAGES™

Just For You
542-3993
1114 N. 183rd St.
Seattle, WA

A children's consignment
shop filled with toys,
clothing and all sorts of
good stuff for today's
parent!

JUST FOR YOU

20% OFF

Any item in the store!

SEATTLE BABY PAGES™

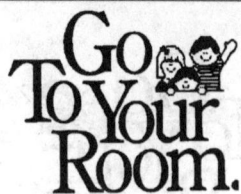
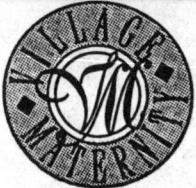
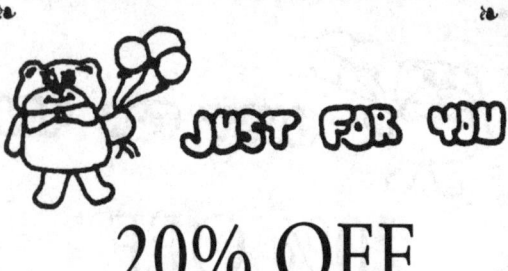

Bellini
451-0126
Located in Park Row
201 Bellevue Way NE
Bellevue, WA 98004

- *Quality, Beautiful Furniture*
- *Personal Service*
- *Unique Items*

Hours:
M-Sat.   10 - 6
Thurs.   10 - 8
Closed Sunday

**Designer Maternity
Factory and Kids Rack**
451-1945
11010 N.E. 8th St.
Bellevue, WA 98004

*Voted Best Maternity Store
by Eastside Parent
Newsmagazine*

Dreams Awake
527-2956
1820 12th Ave.
Seattle, WA 98122

- *Hypnotherapy*
- *HypnoBirthing™ Classes*
- *Prenatal Counseling*
- *Labor Support*

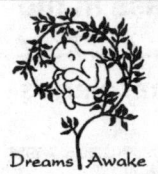

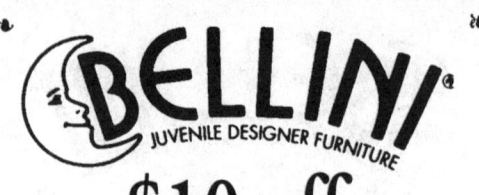

$10 off
Any purchase over $40

Read the store reviews to find out more about Bellini

Bellini
451-0126
Located in Park Row
201 Bellevue Way NE
Bellevue, WA 98004

&a. *Quality, Beautiful Furniture*
&a. *Personal Service*
&a. *Unique Items*

Hours:
M-Sat.   10 - 6
Thurs.   10 - 8
Closed Sunday

&a. **VOTED BEST MATERNITY STORE**
EASTSIDE PARENT NEWSMAGAZINE   &a.

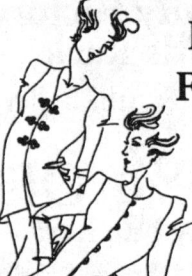

Designer Maternity Factory & Kids Rack

20% off
any one item

Designer Maternity Factory and Kids Rack
451-1945
11010 N.E. 8th St.
Bellevue, WA 98004

See the stores section to learn more about the Designer Maternity Factory and Kids Rack

---

Peace Begins At Birth

25 % Off

any class in the
Body/Mind in Birth™
Seminar Series

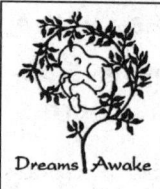

Dreams | Awake   Barbara Kaye, CHt., CHbP. (206) 527-2956

Dreams Awake
527-2956
1820 12th Ave.
Seattle, WA 98122

&a. *Hypnotherapy*
&a. *HypnoBirthing*™ *Classes*
&a. *Prenatal Counseling*
&a. *Labor Support*

Baby Diaper Service
634-2229 Seattle
383-2229 Tacoma
1-800-562-2229
400 N. 36th St.
Seattle, WA 98103

Nothing Less Than the Best...
For Your Baby's Comfort

Quality & Service

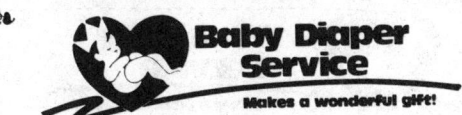
Safety for Toddlers
885-3460
or
800-775-3460
12865 N.E. 85th St.
Suite 296
Kirkland, WA 98033

Safety for Toddlers is
well known in Seattle
for custom installation,
in-home consulations
& safety products.

The Maternity Shop
252-3811
3612 Colby Ave.
Everett, WA 98201

Hours:
M-F   10 - 6
Sat.   10 - 5

A full-service maternity and
nursing store

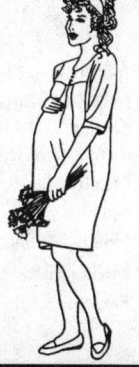

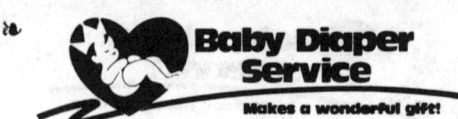
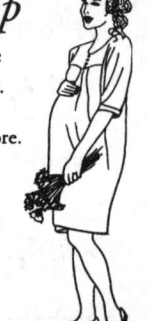

Kids on 45th
633-KIDS
1720 N. 45th St.
Seattle, WA 98103

Hours:
Mon.-Sat. 10-6
Sun.   11-5

*See the stores section to
learn more about
Kids on 45th!*

Andrea Wagner, L.M.P.
464-4828
150 Nickerson St., Ste. 211
Seattle, WA 98109

*Swedish, Deep Tissue and
Pregnancy Massage*

**Breastfeeding Mothers
Resource**
706-0740

*Breastfeeding is the most
natural source of nourishment and security for your
baby, and it's FREE!*

*See the chapter on
breastfeeding to find out
more.*

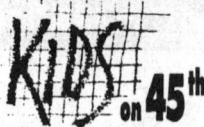
Kids on 45th
633-KIDS
1720 N. 45th St.
Seattle, WA 98103

Hours:
Mon.-Sat. 10-6
Sun. 11-5

Read the stores section to learn more about Kids on 45th.

Andrea Wagner, L.M.P.
464-4828
150 Nickerson St., Ste. 211
Seattle, WA 98109

Treat yourself or someone you know to a Swedish, Deep Tissue or Pregnancy Massage

Breastfeeding Mothers Resource
706-0740

Breastfeeding is the most natural source of nourishment and security for your baby, and it's FREE!

See the chapter on breastfeeding to find out more.

Fifth Avenue Kids
526-5683
8312 5th Ave. N.E.
Seattle, WA 98115

Hours:
Tues.   10-5
Wed.   11-6
Thurs.   12-8
Fri.-Sat.   11-5

Baby Love Maternity

Bellevue Square
2nd Level
454-2122

Southcenter Mall
246-7111

Northgate Mall
362-1021

Alderwood Mall
776-1262

Northwest Parent
Publishing
441-0191
2107 Elliott Ave., Ste. 303
Seattle, WA 98121

Publishers of:
Seattle's Child
Eastside Parent
Puget Sound Parent
Portland Parent

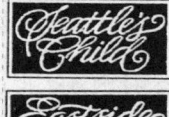
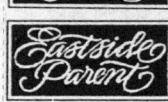

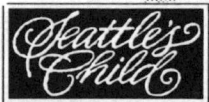 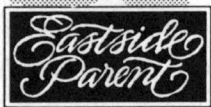

Bootyland
328-0636
1321 East Pine St.
Seattle, WA 98122

Hours: Mon.-Sat. 10 - 6
Closed Sundays

Hey! Recycle that kid stuff!

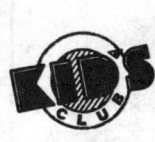
Kid's Club
643-5437
Crossroads Center
15600 N.E. 8th
Bellevue, WA

524-2553
University Village
2676 N.E. University
Village Mall
Seattle, WA

*See the stores review to
learn more about
Kid's Club.*

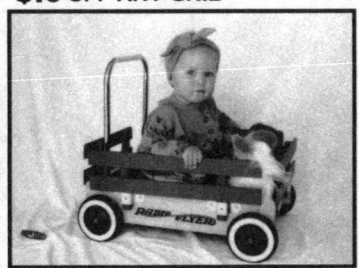
Craig Larsen Studio
885-5553
14630 N.E. 95th St.
Redmond, WA 98052
Fax (206) 881-7915
E-mail:
clarsen_studio@msm.com

*Rediscover the timeless beauty
of black & white portraiture.*

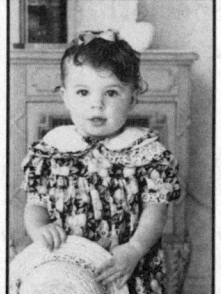

Bootyland
328-0636
1321 East Pine St.
Seattle, WA 98122

*Located on Capitol Hill
at 14th & Pine*

Hours:　Mon.-Sat. 10 - 6
Closed Sundays

*Read the stores section to find
out more about Bootyland!*

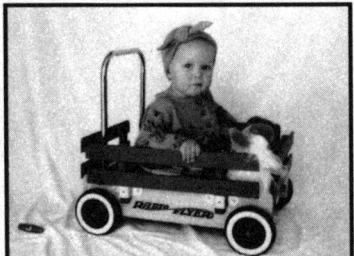
Kid's Club
643-5437
Crossroads Center
15600 N.E. 8th
Bellevue, WA

524-2553
University Village
2676 N.E. University
Village Mall
Seattle, WA 98105

*See the stores review to
learn more about Kid's
Club.*

Craig Larsen Studio
885-5553
14630 N.E. 95th St.
Redmond, WA 98052
Fax (206) 881-7915
E-mail:
clarsen_studio@msm.com

*Rediscover the timeless beauty
of black & white portraiture.*

AirTouch Paging
(800) 678-2370, ext. 4600
or (206) 451-2370
3625 132nd Ave. S.E. #200
Bellevue, WA 98006

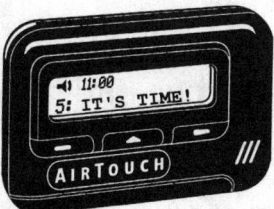
University Bookstore
634-3400
4326 University Way N.E.
Seattle

632-9500
990 102nd Ave. N.E.
Bellevue

❧ *Complete selection of
   parenting and children's
   books*
❧ *Baby shower wishlist*
❧ *Free gift wrapping*

**NW Medical Supply
Breast Pump
Rental Station**
368-11961530 N. 115th
#112
Seattle, WA 98133

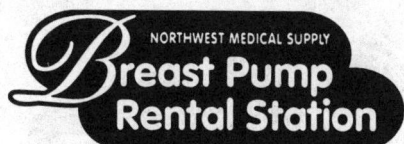

AirTouch Paging
(800) 678-2370, ext. 4600
or (206) 451-2370
3625 132nd Ave. S.E. #200
Bellevue, WA 98006

A pager makes a great baby gift!

University Bookstore

634-3400
4326 University Way N.E.
Seattle

632-9500
990 102nd Ave. N.E.
Bellevue

❧ *Complete selection of parenting and children's books*
❧ *Baby shower wishlist*
❧ *Free gift wrapping*

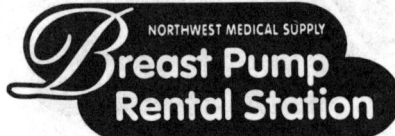
NW Medical Supply
Breast Pump
Rental Station
1530 N. 115th #112
Seattle, WA 98133
368-1196

PCC
Store Locations:
West Seattle • 937-8481
Kirkland • 828-4621
Seward Park • 723-2720
View Ridge • 526-7661
Ravenna • 525-1450
Greenlake • 789-7144
Fremont • 632-6811

*Look in the organic food
section for more about PCC.*

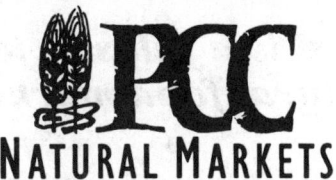
**Tot Stoppers Child
Safety, Inc.**
800-585-1988

✿ *Child Safety Products*
✿ *Professional Installation*
✿ *In-Home Safety Consultations*
✿ *Class Presentations*

*Regional Directors—
International Association of
Child Safety
National Safe Kids Campaign
Baby Proofers International*

Baby Express
337-3739
13416 Bothell-Everett Hwy.
Mill Creek, WA 98012

Hours:
M-Sat. 10:00 a.m.-6:00 p.m.
Sun.   Noon-5:00 p.m.

*A complete baby, maternity
and children's store!
Ask us about our women's
clothing store, SISTERS!*

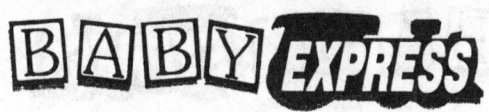

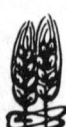
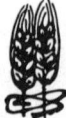

Forget-Me-Not
789-6463
5918 Phinney Ave. N.
Seattle, WA

Hours:
M-Sat. 10 a.m. - 6:00 p.m.
Sun. 12 p.m. - 5:00 p.m.
Call for summer hours

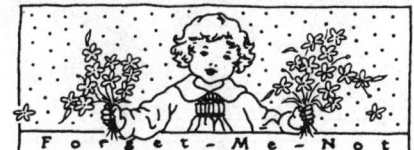
Stork Express
649-5490

Personalized rental signs to deliver the news of your baby to family and friends

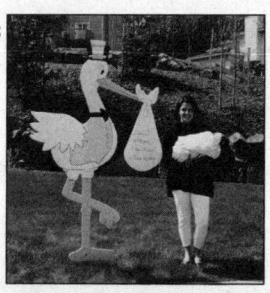
Heaven Sent
Federal Way:
946-BABY or 952-2124
1200 South 324th #5
Federal Way, WA 98003

Lakewood:
581-2526
9514 Gravelly Lk. Dr. S.W.
Tacoma, WA 98499

Children's Quality Resale since 1983

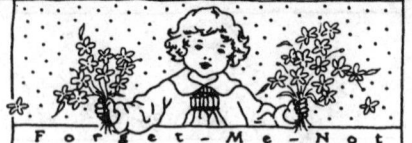

Children's Clothing & Collectibles
new & consignment clothing . toys . equipment . furniture . gifts
NEAR THE ZOO
5918 Phinney Avenue North, Seattle ❧

Children's Clothing & Collectibles

new & consignment clothing . toys . equipment . furniture . gifts

NEAR THE ZOO
5918 Phinney Avenue North, Seattle

Not good with any other offer. One coupon per customer.

Forget-Me-Not
5918 Phinney Ave. N.
Seattle, WA
789-6463

Hours:
M-Sat. 10 a.m. - 6:00 p.m.
Sun.   12 p.m. - 5:00 p.m.
Call for summer hours

STORK EXPRESS

Personalized lawn signs deliver the news
of your baby to family and friends.

$10 off
one week's rental

Not good with any other offer. One coupon per customer.

Stork Express
649-5490

*Personalized rental signs to
deliver the news of your baby
to family and friends*

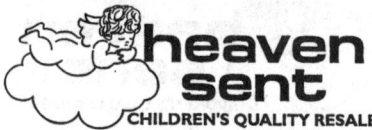

Heaven Sent provides moms and dads with
the necessities their "little angels" need.
Everything from clothing for a special
occasion, a stroller for a walk with Mom, or a
crib for a night filled with dreams.

Not good with any other offer. One coupon per customer.

Heaven Sent
Federal Way:
946-BABY or 952-2124
1200 South 324th #5
Federal Way, WA 98003

Lakewood:
581-2526
9514 Gravelly Lk. Dr. S.W.
Tacoma, WA 98499

*Children's Quality Resale
since 1983*

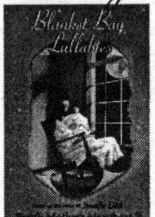
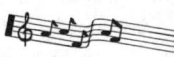

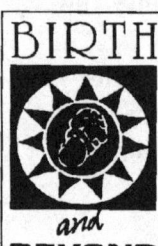

Baby Me

433-1195
Southcenter Mall
The cart near Nordstrom

471-7708
4502 S. Steele #1101
Tacoma, WA

*Read the stores section
to learn more about
Baby Me!*

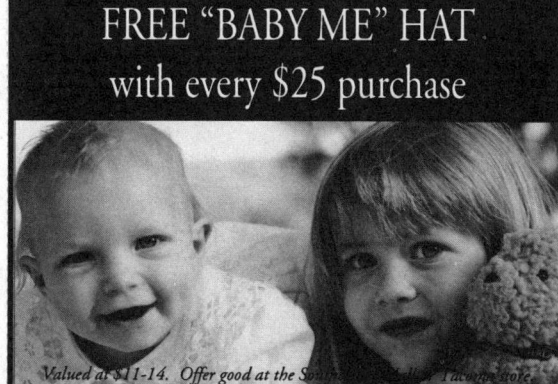
The Take Care Store

Northgate
(206) 527-7878

Seattle
(206) 326-3496

Redmond
(206) 883-5052

Olympia
(360) 923-7678

Mail Order
800-447-2839

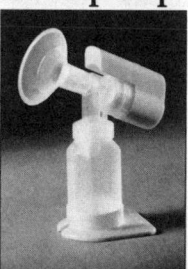
Northwest Hospital

364-BABY
364-(2229)
1550 N. 115th St.
Seattle, WA 98133

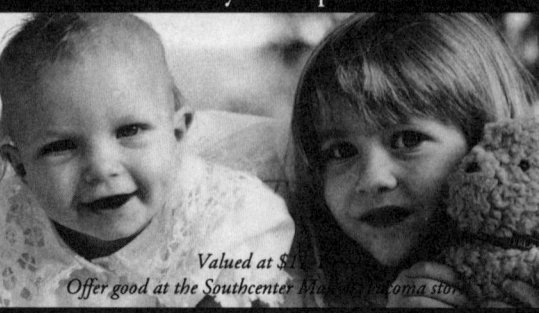
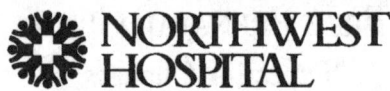